Autism and Child Psychopathology Series

Editor
Johnny L. Matson
Baton Rouge, Louisiana, USA

More information about this series at http://www.springer.com/series/8665

Thompson E. Davis III • Susan W. White
Thomas H. Ollendick

Editors

Handbook of
Autism and Anxiety

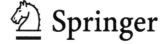 Springer

Editors
Thompson E. Davis III
Department of Psychology
Louisiana State University
Baton Rouge
Louisiana
USA

Susan W. White
Department of Psychology
Child Study Center
Virginia Tech
Blacksburg
Virginia
USA

Thomas H. Ollendick
Department of Psychology
Child Study Center
Virginia Tech
Blacksburg
Virginia
USA

ISSN 2192-922X   ISSN 2192-9238 (electronic)
ISBN 978-3-319-06795-7   ISBN 978-3-319-06796-4 (eBook)
DOI 10.1007/978-3-319-06796-4
Springer Cham Heidelberg New York Dordrecht London

Library of Congress Control Number: 2014939564

Printed on acid-free paper

Springer is part of Springer Science+Business Media (www.springer.com)

To Allison, who is not only my wife but also my best friend. Her constant patience, kindness, encouragement, and love have been the key to my success professionally and personally.

Thompson E. Davis III

To my husband Brad White, who is always my biggest supporter, and my sons Alden and Calvin for providing perspective and unconditional love.

Susan W. White

To Mary, my wife, daughters Laurie and Katie, sons-in-law David and Billy, and grandchildren, Braden, Ethan, Calvin, Addison, Victoria, and William. Without them, life would be much less meaningful and enjoyable.

Thomas H. Ollendick

Foreword

Thompson Davis III, Susan White, and Thomas Ollendick are to be congratulated for having produced an important edited volume which brings together the clinical and research aspects of two conditions: autism and anxiety disorders. These two conditions are given scholarly attention separately and together. Different contributors to this novel collection consider the diagnostic overlap between these two conditions, whether the traditional treatment methods for anxiety disorders apply to autism, and what may account for the considerable comorbidity between autism and anxiety disorders. The issue of anxiety has for 70 years been neglected within autism spectrum conditions (ASC), and in this new book it is brought into central focus.

ASC is also referred to as ASD (autism spectrum disorders) but some authors prefer the more neutral term "condition" to the more value-laden term "disorder." ASC is a neurodevelopmental condition affecting social cognition alongside unusually narrow interest and difficulties in coping with change/a need for sameness. It is commonly accepted clinically that if you put a person with ASC (whether they have classic autism or Asperger Syndrome) into social situations that are unpredictable and unfamiliar, they will experience high levels of social anxiety. And as far as is known, this is true from the earliest age and remains the case across the lifespan.

This may be secondary to the social-cognitive deficits they have, since they report difficulties in "reading" other people's behavior and show impairments on "theory of mind" tests. Such difficulties mean that interpreting and predicting other people's behavior may be challenging for them and lead to confusion, and to social avoidance. Their anxiety may also be secondary to their difficulties in dealing with unpredictability and change more generally, separate to the social world, even if it is the case that most unexpected change comes from the social world.

This book will push clinicians to ask some new questions. If one has a very anxious patient, could this be undiagnosed autism? To answer this would entail an assessment of domains (such as obsessional interests and social skills) that might otherwise be overlooked. Equally, if one has a patient with autism, might their anxiety be treated using methods such as systematic desensitization or cognitive behavioral therapy, or do such approaches need to be modified to be useful to a person with autism? Finally, what is the relationship between autism and anxiety, and do they co-occur because of a common neural substrate, for example, in amygdala dysfunction? This book will be of great value both clinician-scientists in both the autism and anxiety fields, and will do what any valuable book should do, which is to make connections that open up new questions, hopefully lead to new knowledge, and improved clinical practice.

Autism Research Centre   Simon Baron-Cohen
Cambridge University
Cambridge
UK

Preface

It is currently an exciting, but turbulent, time for those studying, assessing, treating, and researching autism spectrum disorder (ASD). It is also a challenging time for individuals with ASD and their families, as they grapple with the upshots of the recent changes in the DSM and what the diagnostic labels mean to them both personally and with respect to service procurement. For the last several decades, estimates of the prevalence of ASD have increasingly indicated the disorder is becoming more and more common, with rates of 1 in 1000 children in 1980, to 1 in 150 children in 2000 to 1 in 88 children as of 2008 (Centers for Disease Control and Prevention [CDC] 2013). As more research has been conducted, it has become clear that ASD is also a disorder that does not occur in isolation. Comorbidity with other psychopathologies has become the rule rather than the exception for those with ASD (Matson and Nebel-Schwalm 2007). Piggybacking the relative explosion in research on ASD has been the subsequent development and ongoing refinement of assessment and treatment methodologies. Amidst all of these changes, a great reorienting of the clinical compass also occurred in May 2013 with the release of the *Diagnostic and Statistical Manual for Mental Disorders—5th edition* (*DSM-5*) and its changes in diagnostic criteria (e.g., collapsing the various Pervasive Developmental Disorders into one disorder) and with pronouncements from the National Institute of Mental Health (NIMH) with its strong endorsement of Research Domain Criteria (RDoC). This latter development has resulted in an increased movement away from research based solely on *DSM-5* diagnostic research.

In addition, ASD was not the only diagnosis to emerge as a changeling from the *DSM-5* work groups: many longstanding diagnoses and diagnostic categories were revised, including a number of anxiety disorders. Importantly, anxiety disorders have been found to be one of the most common comorbid conditions experienced by those with ASD. Beginning with the earliest observations of ASD, there appeared to be a connection between the constellation of social, communicative, and behavioral symptoms and fear and anxiety. Kanner (1943) recorded one mother's description of her son as being "afraid of mechanical things; he runs from them. He used to be afraid of my egg beater, is perfectly petrified of my vacuum cleaner. Elevators are simply a terrifying experience to him. He is afraid of spinning toys" (pp. 222–223). White, Oswald, Ollendick, and Scahill (2009) have noted that the rate of anxiety disorders and symptoms in those with ASD is as high as 84%. Previous guidelines, especially as applied to the assessment and treatment of children and adolescents (e.g., Davis et al.

2011; Silverman and Ollendick 2005) in those with anxiety disorders provided a rough vision for what might work and be modified to help those with ASD (Moree and Davis 2010). Moreover, recent reviews and discussions of ASD, anxiety, and how the two might be intertwined have proven influential (Davis 2012; Kerns and Kendall 2012; Ollendick and White 2012) and pushed the field beyond mere downward and lateral iterations of anxiety in otherwise typically developing individuals to work specifically focused on the intersection of ASD and anxiety (Davis 2012). As a result, decades of research and myriad recent changes to our definitions and understanding of ASD make this an opportune time to evaluate the current state of the literature, elucidate and reinforce best practices, and speculate about the future of these two distinct, but oft intertwined psychopathologies. Seven decades after Kanner's observations, the time seems right to begin to summarize all of these findings in light of new diagnostic and research guidelines.

This volume has emerged largely by standing on the shoulders of those researchers and clinicians who have tirelessly worked to better understand and help those with ASD. We are pleased to have been able to secure contributions from many leaders in the field. Even so, in both editing and writing portions of this book, we have tried to create a volume that would be useful to clinical and academic professionals alike. This book has been organized to be a resource for researchers and educators (e.g., as a training volume) and for practitioners serving clients (e.g., to better understand current issues with anxiety comorbidity). To these ends, we have divided the volume into four broad parts. Part I focuses on laying the groundwork for understanding ASD and anxiety. The volume begins with an historical review of ASD from the past to the present, and then proceeds with chapters devoted to variability in ASD presentation. Anxiety disorders in those with and without ASD and other comorbidities are then introduced and subsequent chapters deal with the increasingly difficult job of disentangling ASD and anxiety—or if they should or even can be disentangled. Part I concludes with a chapter on where we believe the future of ASD and anxiety research lies, in understanding the complex etiologic and transdiagnostic processes involved in the ASD and anxiety interplay. Part II of the volume then introduces specific anxiety diagnoses for consideration alongside ASD symptoms. For example, the common quandaries of whether symptoms are consistent with ASD or obsessive-compulsive disorder, or social anxiety disorder, or phobia are discussed. Part III tackles common issues of ASD and anxiety assessment and treatment, as well as implementation issues within clinics and schools. Finally, we are very pleased to have three diverse perspectives represented in Part IV where we turn to commentaries on the new *DSM-5* criteria and RDoC recommendations. The future of ASD research and practice is highlighted in these final chapters.

Thompson E. Davis III
Susan W. White
Thomas H. Ollendick

References

American Psychiatric Association. (2013). *Diagnostic and Statistical Manual of Mental Disorders* (5th ed.). Arlington: American Psychiatric Publishing.

Centers for Disease Control and Prevention. (June 27, 2013). *Autism spectrum disorders (ASD): Data & statistics.* from http://www.cdc.gov/ncbddd/autism/data.html.

Davis III, T. E. (2012). Where to from here for ASD and anxiety? Lessons learned from child anxiety and the issue of DSM-5. *Clinical Psychology: Science and Practice, 19,* 358–363.

Davis III, T. E., May, A. C., & Whiting, S. E. (2011). Evidence-based treatment of anxiety and phobia in children and adolescents: Current status and effects on the emotional response. *Clinical Psychology Review, 31,* 592–602.

Kanner, L. (1943). Autistic disturbances of affective contact. *Nervous Child, 2,* 217–250.

Kerns, C. M., & Kendall, P. C. (2012). The presentation and classification of anxiety in autism spectrum disorder. *Clinical Psychology: Science & Practice, 19,* 323–347.

Matson, J. L., & Nebel-Schwalm, M. (2007). Comorbid psychopathology with autism spectrum disorder in children: An overview. *Research in Developmental Disabilities, 28,* 341–352.

Moree, B., & Davis III, T. E. (2010). Cognitive-behavioral therapy for anxiety in children diagnosed with Autism Spectrum Disorders: Modification trends. *Research in Autism Spectrum Disorders, 4,* 346–354.

Ollendick, T. H., & White, S. W. (2012). The presentation and classification of anxiety in autism spectrum disorder: Where to from here? *Clinical Psychology: Science and Practice, 19,* 352–355. doi:10.1111/cpsp.12013.

Silverman, W. K., & Ollendick, T. H. (2005). Evidence-based assessment of anxiety and its disorders in children and adolescents. *Journal of Clinical Child and Adolescent Psychology, 34,* 380–411.

White, S. W., Oswald, D., Ollendick, T. H., & Scahill, L. (2009). Anxiety in children and adolescents with autism spectrum disorders. *Clinical Psychology Review, 29,* 216–229.

Acknowledgments

The extensive and remarkable contributions of many others to a project such as this cannot be emphasized or acknowledged enough. First and foremost, this volume was made possible through considerable clinical research and practice from many of our colleagues. Our respect and appreciation also goes out to the many adults, adolescents, children, parents, and families who have generously given of their time and patience to further our understanding of ASD. Their participation in clinical case studies, randomized clinical trials, and basic research allows us to further understand, assess, and treat these disorders. We would also like to extend our special thanks to all our esteemed authors for their time, expertise, and contributions to this volume. This volume would also not be possible without Judy Jones' assistance and all of the staff at Springer—we are very grateful for their support and guidance.

Contents

Contributors

Renae Beaumont School of Psychology, University of Queensland, St. Lucia, QLD, Australia

Audrey Blakeley-Smith Departments of Psychiatry and Pediatrics, School of Medicine, JFK Partners, University of Colorado Anschutz Medical Campus, Aurora, CO, USA

Thompson E. Davis III Department of Psychology, Louisiana State University, Baton Rouge, Louisiana, USA

Geraldine Dawson Duke Center for Autism Diagnosis and Treatment, Duke University, Durham, NC, USA

Andrea Nichole Evans Marcus Autism Center, Atlanta, GA, USA

Ellen Flannery-Schroeder Department of Psychology, University of Rhode Island, Kingston, RI, USA

Katherine Gotham Department of Psychiatry, Vanderbilt University Medical Center, Nashville, TN, USA

Louis Hagopian The Kennedy Krieger Institute and Johns Hopkins University School of Medicine, Baltimore, MD, USA

Susan Hepburn Departments of Psychiatry and Pediatrics, School of Medicine, JFK Partners, University of Colorado Anschutz Medical Campus, Aurora, CO, USA

John D. Herrington Center for Autism Research, The Children's Hospital of Philadelphia, Philadelphia, PA, USA

Heather Jennett Little Leaves Behavioral Services, Silver Spring, MD, USA

Philip C. Kendall Temple University, Philadelphia, PA, USA

Connor Morrow Kerns AJ Drexel Autism Institute, Drexel University, Philadelphia, PA, USA

Nicole L. Kreiser Kennedy Krieger Institute, Department of Neuropsychology, Baltimore, MD, USA

Luc Lecavalier Nisonger Center and Departments of Psychology and Psychiatry, The Ohio State University, Columbus, OH, USA

Christopher Lopata Institute for Autism Research, Canisius College, NY, USA

Catherine Lord Center for Autism and the Developing Brain, Weill Cornell Medical College, New York-Presbyterian Hospital, New York, USA

Carla A. Mazefsky Psychiatry Department, The University of Pittsburgh School of Medicine, Pittsburgh, PA, USA

James C. McPartland Yale Child Study Center, Yale School of Medicine, New Haven, CT, USA

Peter Muris Department of Clinical Psychological Science, Faculty of Psychology and Neuroscience, Maastricht University, Maastricht, MD, The Netherlands

Marie Nebel-Schwalm Department of Psychology, Illinois Wesleyan University, Bloomington, IL, USA

Thomas H. Ollendick Department of Psychology, Child Study Center, Virginia Tech, Blacksburg, Virginia, USA

Judy Reaven Departments of Psychiatry and Pediatrics, School of Medicine, JFK Partners, University of Colorado Anschutz Medical Campus, Aurora, CO, USA

Brian Reichow A.J. Pappanikou Center for Excellence in Developmental Disabilities, University of Connecticut, Storrs, CT, USA

Brittany M. Rudy University of South Florida, St. Petersburg, FL, USA

Lawrence Scahill Marcus Autism Center, Emory University, Atlanta, GA, USA

Amie R. Schry Department of Psychology, Durham Veterans Affairs Medical Center, Blacksburg, VA, USA

Laura D. Seligman Department of Psychology, University of Texas Pan American, Edinburg, TX, USA

Kate Sofronoff School of Psychology, University of Queensland, St. Lucia, QLD, Australia

Eric A. Storch University of South Florida, St. Petersburg, FL, USA

Erin F. Swedish Department of Psychology, University of Toledo, Toledo, OH, USA

Marcus L. Thomeer Institute for Autism Research, Canisius College, NY, USA

Elizabeth Turin Kennedy Krieger Institute, Johns Hopkins University School of Medicine, Baltimore, MD, USA

Fred R. Volkmar Child Study Center, Yale University, New Haven, CT, USA

Jonathan A. Weiss York University, Toronto, ON, Canada

Susan W. White Department of Psychology, Child Study Center, Virginia Tech, Blacksburg, Virginia, USA

Julie Worley Center for Autism Research at the Children's Hospital of Philadelphia, Philadelphia, PA, USA

Monica S. Wu University of South Florida, St. Petersburg, FL, USA

Part I
Introduction and Overview

The History of Autism: From Pillar to Post

Lawrence Scahill, Elizabeth Turin
and Andrea Nichole Evans

Introduction

Historical accounts on autism in modern textbooks almost invariably begin with Leo Kanner's 1943 report of 11 children with a set of symptoms that came to be called autism (Kanner 1943). But earlier descriptions suggestive of autism can be identified. In his classic 1809 book *Observations of Madness and Melancholy,* the notorious Haslam (1809) described a 7-year-old boy with delayed language, impaired socialization, and preoccupations. The boy was brought to the Bethlem Hospital for consultation with Haslam, who was the hospital's apothecary. At age 13, the boy showed improvement in language, but only spoke in short sentences, often inserting his name rather than using the first-person personal pronoun. He had also developed a preoccupation with soldiers and tried to return conversations to that preferred topic. Although the case is of interest, it is difficult to assign a diagnosis to the child. Narrative descriptions of children with conditions reminiscent of what we now call autism spectrum disorder (ASD) were included in other nineteenth-century books as well (Down 1887; Schüle 1886). These authors did not use the word autism, but they provided detailed case descriptions of children with little or no language, limited interaction with others, "living in their own world," and exhibiting stereotypic movements (see Shorter and Wachtel 2013).

The term *autism* was coined by Swiss psychiatrist Eugen Bleuler in 1911. Bleuler (1950) used the term to indicate withdrawal into fantasy and self-centered thinking observed in schizophrenia. The term was subsequently adopted by Emil Kraepelin (1913) to characterize early-onset schizophrenia, which he called *dementia praecox.* He acknowledged Bleuler as the source of the term *autism* and described children with characteristics suggestive of autism. Although he described autistic thinking in children, his observations suggested an unfolding disease process (e.g., retreat to internal world, loss of ability to direct thought) rather than a condition present at birth (Parnas 2011).

Thereafter, the term autism became central to the understanding of childhood schizophrenia (Künkel 1920).Ernst Kretschmer (1921), then professor of psychiatry in Tübingen, Germany, used the term autistic in his description of adults with schizoid personality. The Russian pediatric neurologist G. E. Ssucharewa may be properly credited with coining the term *autism* in the modern sense, i.e., a condition marked by profound social isolation. An associate professor at the Moscow University, and physician at the Moscow Sanatorium–School of the

L. Scahill (✉)
Marcus Autism Center, Emory University, Atlanta, GA 30329 USA
e-mail: lawrence.scahill@emory.edu

E. Turin
Kennedy Krieger Institute, Johns Hopkins University School of Medicine, Baltimore, MD, USA

A. N. Evans
Marcus Autism Center, Atlanta, GA, USA

T. E. Davis III et al. (eds.), *Handbook of Autism and Anxiety,* Autism and Child Psychopathology Series, DOI 10.1007/978-3-319-06796-4_1, © Springer International Publishing Switzerland 2014

Children's Clinic for Psychoneurology, she was keen to apply Kretschmer's ideas about autism and schizoid personalities to the children under her care. In 1926, she described six boys with childhood-onset social isolation, repetitive behavior, phobias, peculiar thoughts, eccentricities, and developmental delays—though some were "highly intelligent" (translated by Wolff 1996). Although none of these boys were described as psychotic, Ssucharewa considered each of these boys to be cases of childhood schizophrenia. She delineated autism, catatonia, and psychosis, but did not attempt to differentiate autism from childhood schizophrenia. Albatz, from the same Moscow clinic in 1934, however, did attempt to distinguish subgroups of childhood schizophrenia. He described one group of children (*schizoid psychopaths*) with normal intelligence and a second group with more developmental disabilities and thought disorder (Grebelskaya-Albatz 1934).

For Kanner, the central features of autism were the preference for aloneness, intolerance of change (sameness), fascination with objects, impairments in the use of language, and restricted interests. Although not a part of the current definition, Kanner noted the tendency of the children in his case series to overreact to loud noises and he speculated that social interaction induced anxiety in children with autism. As noted, the term autism was borrowed from Bleuler, but Kanner drew a clear distinction between autism and schizophrenia. Unlike schizophrenia, Kanner proposed that the "withdrawal" in autism was present from birth. The controversy on whether autism is the childhood equivalent of schizophrenia returned in the 1950s.

Although the case descriptions in Kanner's report are compelling and mark a clear connection to the current definition of ASD, he drew at least two erroneous conclusions from his biased sample. He commented that children in his case series looked intelligent and, therefore, were not intellectually disabled (though he did report specifically about IQ test results). Kanner also noted that the parents of the children in his case series were generally well-educated professionals—though he did not assert that indifferent, professional parents were the cause of autism.

He apparently did not consider the possibility of an ascertainment bias—that well-off professional parents would have the resources to obtain expert consultation. Although there is continued debate about the prevalence of intellectual disability in children with autism, a substantial percentage of children with autism are also intellectually disabled. It is also clear that autism occurs across all socioeconomic strata (Centers for Disease Control and Prevention 2012).

Soon after the publication of Kanner's influential paper was a report by Hans Asperger (1944). In his paper *Die autistischen Psychopathen im Kindesalter* he described four children with what he called "autistic psychopathy." These children had average or above-average intelligence, age-appropriate or even advanced language skills (Asperger noted they spoke like "little professors") but had poor capacity for reciprocal social interaction, impaired motor skills, and narrow interests. His work went largely unnoticed for almost 40 years, until Lorna Wing (1981) referred to the work of Asperger in a clinical report describing similar cases and applied the term "Asperger's syndrome." Asperger's original paper was not translated into English until 1991 (Frith 1991). Over the ensuing decades, there has been considerable debate on whether Asperger's syndrome is separate from autism or a part of the autism spectrum. The preponderance of available evidence supports the view that it is a milder form of autism (Wing 2005). Indeed, the *DSM 5* neurodevelopmental disorders workgroup concluded that, in the absence of convincing evidence, Asperger's disorder should not be considered separate from autism (American Psychiatric Association 2013). As is true for many other debates in autism, this matter is not completely resolved (see Kite et al. 2013; Volkmar et al. 2012).

Post-World War Two Era: Autism, Psychosis, and Psychodynamics

In the 1950s, several authors returned to the distinction between autism and psychosis in children. The highly respected psychoanalyst Margaret Mahler proposed that early infancy is an "autistic phase" of development. In this phase, the infant lives in a symbiotic relationship with the mother. Overtime, the normally developing infant understands that the mother is separate and the infant gradually perceives selfhood. The child who fails to manage this separation-individuation from the mother may retreat to an undifferentiated state that she labeled *symbiotic psychosis.* As this retreat continues, the child becomes less and less responsive to maternal invitation for interaction in a manner resembling Kanner's autism. In Mahler's view, this developmental failure to distinguish self from other and subsequent psychological retreat was due to an inborn vulnerability rather than maternal failure (Mahler 1952).

Continuing on the theme that autism was biological in origin, several other authors proposed that autism was the childhood version of schizophrenia (Bender 1953; Fish et al. 1966).

In their study of the antipsychotic drug trifluoperazine, Fish et al. (1966) described 22 "*autistic schizophrenic*" children between 2 and 6 years of age with profound impairment in social interaction and language delay (14 were nonverbal; 8 had language delay). The investigators specifically noted that the study subjects resembled cases described by Kanner. The severity ratings used to characterize the subjects included levels of language delay, social awareness, and "mood and motility." This last dimension was not well defined but was apparently intended to capture irritability (overreaction to environmental stimuli) or apathy (inactivity and withdrawal). The investigators placed particular attention on the degree of language impairment, which was posited as the most important predictor of long-term outcome.

Rutter (1972) settled the debate about autism and childhood schizophrenia. In a detailed review, he argued that the term "childhood schizophrenia" had been broadened to the degree that it was no longer useful as a diagnostic category. He proceeded to deconstruct the differences between autism and schizophrenia. As Kanner had observed three decades earlier, Rutter noted that the social withdrawal in autism was apparent early in life and was due to a failure of development—rather than regression. By contrast, schizophrenia was marked by social withdrawal and retreat to

fantasy later in life (e.g., end of the second decade of life in most cases). The defining features of delusions and hallucinations of schizophrenia are not often observed in autism. Although both autism and schizophrenia are chronic conditions, schizophrenia is marked by psychotic episodes followed by partial remission. We now know that with treatment, children with autism can show improvement, but the course is not episodic. Autism occurs far more commonly in boys. The prevalence of schizophrenia does not differ by gender. Seizures and intellectual disability are associated with autism but not common in schizophrenia. Rutter echoed Kanner's observation that parents of children with autism were often highly intelligent individuals with professional careers. Unlike the parents of patients with schizophrenia who have a higher likelihood of also having schizophrenia, schizophrenia is uncommon in the parents of children with autism. Indeed, Rutter reiterated the accepted view that autism was more common in highly intelligent and professional parents. Nonetheless, his delineation of autism and schizophrenia was persuasive.

The observation that autism seemed to be associated with highly intelligent and professional parents fit with psychoanalytic theories that exerted great influence on the discourse in the post-war period—particularly in the USA and France. Several authors suggested that the mother's failure to nurture the child in early infancy could cause autism. A strong proponent of this view was Bruno Bettelheim, a psychologist and founder of the Orthogenic School in Chicago. In his book *The Empty Fortress,* Bettelheim (1967) asserted that autism was caused by maternal indifference resulting in a failure to bond with the infant. This failure to bond resulted in the emotional withdrawal by the infant to protect against further emotional pain. At the center of this debate is whether autism is regarded as inborn or the consequence of parental (particularly maternal) failure. Kanner proposed that autism was present at birth—implying a genetic etiology. In this view, the seeming maternal indifference could be a consequence of the infant's inborn affective deficit—rather than the mother's indifference leading to the infant's withdrawal.

This nature versus nurture debate persisted through the 1970s until the publication of a pivotal twin study by Folstein and Rutter (1977). The study included 21 twin pairs (11 monozygotic and 10 dizygotic twins) in which the index twin was diagnosed with autism. Four of the monozygotic co-twins were concordant for autism, but none of the dizygotic co-twins were diagnosed with autism. The authors went on to examine the frequency of cognitive deficits, language delay, and learning difficulties in the twin groups. When this broader phenotype was considered, the difference between monozygotic and dizygotic twin pairs widened (82% of monozygotic co-twins were affected with autism or cognitive delays vs. 10% among dizygotic co-twins). Based on a review of birth records, the authors proposed that interaction between genetic influences and perinatal complications influence the risk of autism or related milder cognitive deficits. This biological argument dismantled the proposed psychogenic origin of autism. In addition, the findings of this study set the stage for the concept of autism spectrum.

The concept of *autism spectrum* was further developed by Wing and Gould (1979). These investigators conducted a ground-breaking study in the borough of Camberwell in London. Using administrative data, Wing and Gould identified 163 children under the age of 15 with intellectual disability, developmental delays, communication delays, and repetitive behavior. In addition to describing the subjects, the sample of 163 children was evaluated with available quantitative measures. The stated goal was to identify cases of autism as well as borderline cases of autism and children with delays but without "autistic features." The children with developmental delays who showed interest in social interaction and responded to requests for social contact from others were classified as *sociable*. Children with social disability were likely to show poor verbal and nonverbal communication, impoverished imagination, and repetitive behavior. Within this group of children with social disability, Wing and Gould described three subgroups: (a) aloof (uninterested in social interaction, associated with behavioral problems), (b) passive (unlikely to initiate social interaction but may be responsive to interactions initiated by others), and (c) active but odd (exhibited unusual and inappropriate approaches and responses to others). According to Wing and Gould (1979), the aloof subgroup was the most impaired. However, subgroup membership was not fixed. Some children with a history suggesting membership in the aloof subgroup could move to less impaired subgroups. Despite improvement with maturity, these children were unlikely to move beyond their social impairment.

Tracking the Official Nomenclature

In their original papers, neither Kanner nor Asperger put forth explicit diagnostic criteria. Subsequently, Eisenberg and Kanner (1956) were the first to propose criteria for autism. Much later in her case series, Wing (1981) enumerated essential characteristics of Asperger's syndrome. The American Psychiatric Association did not officially include autistic disorder as a diagnosis until 1980 with the publication of *DSM-III*. Indeed, *DSM-III* marked a fundamental change in approach to psychiatric diagnosis. First, *DSM-III* moved away from theoretically driven approaches to diagnosis that pervaded earlier versions of the manual. Instead, *DSM-III* enumerated specific symptom criteria to define psychiatric disorders. Table 1.1 presents the essential diagnostic criteria for autism in *DSM-III*. For a diagnosis of autism, *DSM-III* required patients to meet all listed criteria by history and clinical assessment. Although the inclusion of autism in *DSM-III* was an important milestone, this requirement constrained the diagnosis to a narrow phenotype. This narrow definition persisted until 1987 with the release of *DSM-III-R*. The definition was broadened even further with the release of *DSM-IV* in 1994.

DSM-IV followed the trend articulated by Wing, Gould, and others toward the notion of autism spectrum ranging from mild to severe. For the first time, *DSM-IV* also included Asperger's disorder. Retained in *DSM-IV* was the requirement for early age of onset (before 36 months of age). The diagnostic criteria in *DSM-IV* presented three domains of interest: marked impairment

Table 1.1 *DSM-III* Diagnostic criteria for infantile autism

A	Onset before 30 months of age
B	Pervasive lack of responsiveness to other people
C	Gross deficits in language development
D	If speech is present, peculiar speech patterns such as immediate and delayed echolalia, metaphorical language, and pronominal reversal
E	Bizarre responses to various aspects of the environment, e.g., resistance to change, peculiar interest in or attachments to animate or inanimate objects
F	Absence of delusions, hallucinations, loosening of associations, and incoherence as in schizophrenia

Reprinted with permission from the *Diagnostic and Statistical Manual of Mental Disorders,* Third Edition (Copyright 1980). American Psychiatric Association (1980)

in social interaction, delayed and/or deviant language development, and repetitive behavior and/or circumscribed interests (American Psychiatric Association 2000). Social impairment included failure to use and detect nonverbal behaviors in social interaction with others and impaired reciprocal interaction. Restricted interests and repetitive behavior included stereotypic movements, preoccupation with narrow interests, and insistence on routines in everyday activities. The communication domain considered delayed or deviant language, the use of stereotyped phrases, and lack of age-appropriate ability for make-believe play. The diagnosis of autistic disorder in *DSM-IV* required the presence of two symptoms in the social domain and at least one symptom in each of the communication and repetitive behavior domains. Language delay was not required for Asperger's disorder. Although it may be said that *DSM-IV* followed, rather than initiated, the trend toward broadening the diagnosis of *ASD,* the official broadening of the phenotype had a large impact on prevalence (Fombonne 2009).

The prevalence of the more narrowly defined diagnosis of autism in DSM-III ranged from 3 to 15 per 10,000 children. For community prevalence surveys of autism using *DSM-IV* criteria, the estimates ranged from 16 to 40 per 10,000 (Fombonne 2009). Considering the wider definition of ASD described in *DSM-IV* (autistic disorder, Asperger's disorder, and pervasive developmental disorder—not otherwise specified), the current estimate from the Centers for Disease Control and Prevention (2012) is 11.3 per 1000 children. There is little doubt that broadening the diagnostic criteria has played an important role in the dramatic rise in prevalence. However,

several other factors also warrant consideration. First, investigators began to move beyond clinically ascertained samples and to count cases in the community that were not previously identified. Because clinic cases are affected by known and unknown ascertainment biases, clinically referred cases are likely to be an undercount. Second, better assessment methods improved the demarcation of the diagnostic threshold. These improved diagnostic assessments resulted in reclassification of children with intellectual disability and those with normal intelligence with social disability as children with an ASD. Indeed, the largest increase in new cases has occurred in children with average or above-average intellectual ability (Centers for Disease Control and Prevention 2012). The incremental increase in the detected prevalence has also contributed to increased awareness and increased demand for services by parents (Grinker 2007).

With the official nomination of the term *ASD,* it may be said that *DSM 5* reflects the culmination of the trend set in motion early on by Folstein and Rutter (1977). In contrast to *DSM IV, DSM 5* describes two broad domains: (a) deficits in social communication and social interaction and (b) repetitive behavior and restricted interests. The diagnostic criteria in *DSM 5* urge clinicians to consider gradations of severity in these domains rather than simply the presence or absence of a symptom. Thus, in the social domain, the criteria note varying degrees of deficits in reciprocal social interaction, deficits in the use of verbal and nonverbal communication, and deficits in the capacity to negotiate age-appropriate social situations. Similarly, the domain of restrictive and repetitive behavior considers the range of symptoms such as stereotyped motor movements (hand flapping, spinning objects, ordering and arranging objects), repeating stock phrases, rigid insistence on daily routines, circumscribed interests that interfere with daily living). As in *DSM-III* and *DSM-IV, DSM 5* retains the criterion that symptoms must be identifiable early in life. However, *DSM 5* allows for the possibility that the social disability, for example, may not be apparent until the complexity of social relationships exceeds the child's capacity.

Causes, Cures, and Controversies

The finally forsaken view that autism followed infant emotional withdrawal caused by maternal indifference sparked a gradual, inexorable demand by parents for improved recognition and treatment of autism. In the mid-1960s, Bernard Rimland, a psychologist and a father of a son with autism, launched one of the first parent-centered advocacy organizations, Autism Society of America. His book *Infantile autism: The syndrome and its implications for a neural theory of behavior* was among the first of many intended to dismantle the stigma of autism and search for treatments (Rimland 1964). In a pre-Internet era, he created the Autism Research Center, which was a clearing house of information on autism. He also published a newsletter, in which he argued that autism was biological in origin. He called for deeper understanding of autism and for biologically based treatments. In the years that followed his initial pioneering efforts, he championed several treatments—including vitamin B6 with magnesium and, later, secretin. The impact of Rimland's effort is large and difficult to estimate. The mobilization of parents fundamentally changed the discourse on autism. Indeed, subsequent books authored by parents honored his tireless efforts on behalf of children and families with autism (Hamilton 2009).

The array of proposed cures for autism is stunning, ranging from plausible to far-fetched and even dangerous. Applied behavior analysis, facilitated communication, gluten-free and casein-free diets, vitamin B6, fenfluramine, secretin, chelation, hyperbaric oxygen, fluoxetine, oxytocin and the testosterone blocker, and leuprolide are but a few. The writings of Rimland and many others that followed revealed growing tensions between parent groups and the medical establishment (Grinker 2007; Offit 2008). Many parents and advocacy groups such as Defeat Autism Now believed that the improved detection of autism reflected a true rise in incidence (which is defined by a rise in the rate of diagnosis in a given time period). A true rise in prevalence is a daring claim—suggesting that one or more environmental factors are conspiring to increase the number of new cases over a previously stable base rate. This conviction prompted a search for environmental and postnatal exposures (Grinker 2007; McCarthy 2007; Offit 2008). Parental reports of deterioration in language and social engagement after receiving the combined diphtheria-tetanus-pertussis (DPT) vaccine raised a furor that autism could be caused by the mercury-containing preservative thimerosal. Despite the enormous body of evidence to the contrary, many parents continued to believe that vaccines caused their child's rapid regression to autism. As medical investigators debunked the theory, some parents expressed profound indignation that the medical establishment was not listening (McCarthy 2007). For a period of time, even as the expanding weight of evidence was overwhelming, the mass media often presented both sides of the debate—in the name of balanced reporting (Kirby 2006). The thimerosal controversy and its resolution have been chronicled in a carefully researched book entitled *Autism's False Prophets: Bad Science, Risky Medicine, and the Search for a Cure* by Paul Offit (2008). Briefly, thimerosal contains the preservative ethyl mercury, which was used in the USA as a preservative in DPT vaccines until 2001 (Offit 2008). It is also true that exposure to vaccines containing thimerosal gradually increased in the late 1980s and 1990s due to the increase in the number of vaccines routinely given. However, ethyl mercury has a short half-life and does not accumulate in the body (in contrast to methyl mercury that has not been used in vaccines). In addition, the trend toward increased prevalence of autism continued even after thimerosal was removed from vaccines in 2001 (Schechter and Grether 2008). Among the adverse effects of misguided beliefs that mercury in vaccines caused autism was a rise in the number of parents who refused DPT injection and a resultant increase in pertussis—which is not a benign disease (Feikin et al. 2000).

The conviction that the mercury-containing preservative was a cause of autism also led to assertions that chelation could remove mercury from the child's system and improve the deleterious effects of the heavy metal toxicity. Chelation is a standard approach to removing heavy metals such as lead or mercury from the body. There are several methods of chelation: oral, transdermal, and intravenous. If a child does not have heavy metal poisoning, however, chelation is not warranted and may pose certain risks. Although the oral and transdermal methods of chelation are not dangerous, the intravenous injection of the chelating agent can be dangerous for children who do not have mercury toxicity or if the dose is miscalculated. For children who do not have mercury poisoning, chelation may escort other necessary minerals from the body, leading to cardiac arrest (Baxter and Krenzelok 2008).

A parallel vaccine controversy unrelated to thimerosal erupted over the mumps-measles-rubella (MMR) vaccine. This is a live vaccine that has been in use in various forms since 1971 (Centers for Disease Control 2009; Offit 2008). In 1998, a paper by Andrew Wakefield and colleagues (1998) appeared in the *Lancet* describing 12 cases of children who reportedly had normal development until they received the MMR vaccine. The authors proposed that, in vulnerable children, the MMR vaccine causes a gastrointestinal inflammation. This inflammation results in a "leaky gut" allowing chemical toxins to enter systemic circulation and the brain causing autism. This became another banner for some parents and advocacy organizations (Offit 2008). The support for this theory was based on several shaky claims. First, as noted above, proponents were convinced that the prevalence of autism was on the rise. Second, gastrointestinal problems were purported to be more common in children

with autism than typically developing children. This claim was based on case reports from gastroenterology services—raising fundamental questions about ascertainment bias. Indeed, in unselected populations of children with ASD, not drawn from specialty gastroenterology clinics, the rate of gastrointestinal problems in children with ASD does not appear to be elevated (Buie et al. 2010; Nikolov et al. 2009). In a stunning turn of events, Wakefield's paper was retracted—following charges of scientific misconduct (retraction published February 2010; General Medical Council 2010).

In the midst of the furor over the MMR vaccine was the tangled story of secretin. Secretin is a gastrointestinal hormone that plays a role in acid balance in the small intestine. A standard test in a gastroenterology clinic is a secretin challenge to evaluate acid–base balance in the small intestine. Three children with autism reportedly showed spontaneous and dramatic improvement following the routine injection of secretin (Horvath et al. 1998). A mother of one of these children, Victoria Beck, began touting secretin as a possible cure for autism. There was a rush to study secretin and the hubbub continued for several years. One by one, the double-blind, placebo-controlled trials showed that secretin was no better than placebo. Ironically, secretin is among the most studied treatments in autism—despite the long list of negative results. The small pharmaceutical company Repligen yoked its future on the hope that secretin would be an effective treatment for autism and went bankrupt when its pivotal trial showed no benefit (Repligen 2004).

Separate from these highly charged controversies, several voluntary organizations founded by parents have made extraordinary contributions. Groups such as Cure Autism Now, Simons Foundation, Autism Society of America, Organization of Autism Research, National Alliance for Autism Research, Doug Flutie Foundation, and Autism Speaks have raised awareness, raised money, and sponsored research. Autism Speaks manages a large genetic repository. The efforts of parents in these organizations have had a positive influence on public policy and mobilized federal funding to research the causes and treatments of ASD. For example, the federally funded Research Units on Pediatric Psychopharmacology Autism Network has completed several multisite trials since it was launched in 1997 (Scahill et al. 2013). The Autism Centers of Excellence are currently engaged in important genetic studies and treatment trials. The setting of priorities for research in ASD is articulated in an annual report by the Interagency Autism Coordinating Committee (2012). This deliberative body includes representatives from voluntary organizations, the National Institutes of Health, and investigators.

Conclusions

Leo Kanner is recognized for his description of autism as a rare, congenital, chronic condition of early childhood onset. Independently and soon thereafter, Hans Asperger described a case series of children that we now consider a variant of autism. Historical accounts, however, suggest that autism is not a mid-twentieth phenomenon. In the years following Kanner's description (while Asperger's report resided in relative obscurity), there were active debates on whether autism was present at birth, whether it was the result of indifferent and uncaring mothers, or the childhood equivalent of schizophrenia. Gradually, these debates waned as evidence and argument mounted to show a genetic etiology and a natural history that was inconsistent with schizophrenia. Most importantly, the notion that autism was caused by indifferent and uncaring mothers toppled under the weight of evidence. The introduction of *DSM-III* in 1980 and release of the *DSM-IV* in 1994 were important milestones in the modern history of autism. *DSM-III* provided clear, but narrow, diagnostic criteria for autism that were consistent with the notion that autism was relatively a rare and severe disorder. In the 1980s, there was a growing opinion favoring the notion that autism should be viewed as a spectrum. Much of this important work was carried out by investigators in Britain and later in the USA (Frith 2004; Lord and Schopler 1989; Schopler 1965; Volkmar et al. 1994; Wing and Gould 1979). Thus, *DSM-IV* offered broader diagnostic criteria along with

qualitative breaks in the autism spectrum (autistic disorder, Asperger's disorder, and pervasive developmental disorder—not otherwise specified).

Meanwhile, there have been several ground swells among parents of children with ASD. Parent advocacy groups emerged in several regions of the USA and other countries as well. Indignant parents rejected old notions of refrigerator mothers and demanded action. Fanned by the flames of questionable science and high profile (through spurious findings), some parent groups decried the seeming indifference of the medical establishment and rallied around a series of causes and cures. Concerns and convictions about the toxicity of thimerosal in vaccines and MMR-induced inflammatory bowel conditions produced a wedge between established medicine and some advocacy groups (Offit 2008). Parents turned to unconfirmed treatments such as megavitamins, secretin, gluten-free diets, hyperbaric oxygen, and more dangerous interventions such as chelation (Grinker 2007). Ironically, the more established medicine questioned or denounced these unconfirmed treatments, the stronger some parents embraced these treatments.

Contention between advocacy groups and medical investigators, however, has not been the whole story. Several voluntary organizations have joined with governmental organizations and the scientific community to mobilize resources for early detection, and psychosocial and pharmacological treatments (Interagency Autism Coordinating Committee 2012). *DSM 5* reflects a new synthesis. The qualitative diagnostic breaks in *DSM-IV* have been resolved to a single category called *ASD*. As noted in this chapter, the notion of autism spectrum is not new having been articulated by Folstein and Rutter (1977) and Wing and Gould (1979). Findings from more recent genetic studies also support the *autism spectrum* concept (State and Sestan 2012).

Many questions remain for the autism field as we go forward. First, there is general conviction that early detection and early intervention are paramount. Recent findings provide tantalizing evidence that an earlier detection may be possible (Jones and Klin 2013). Against the backdrop of the *autism spectrum,* ranging from mild to severe, it is difficult to be certain about the types and intensity of early intervention that are appropriate. Children with intellectual disability and significant language delay will require more intensive intervention than children with milder forms of autism. A related issue reflects the evolving methods of early detection and the problem of false-positive and false-negative cases. False positives may generate alarm in families faced with this information and prematurely label a child as a case of ASD. False negatives may have the unfortunate result of withholding early intervention.

Systematic delivery of educational and behavioral techniques has been the backbone of early intervention in autism (National Research Council 2001). Drug treatment has also emerged as an important component of comprehensive treatment planning in children with ASD. Currently, two medications (risperidone and aripiprazole) are approved by the US Food and Drug Administration for the treatment of irritability in children with *DSM-IV*-defined autistic disorder. In clinical practice, however, a wide range of medications are used in the treatment of children with ASD (Oswald and Sonenklar 2007). Although a handful of commonly used medications have empirical support in this population, many do not (Scahill et al. 2014). Recent and future findings from preclinical studies and genetics may provide exciting leads for drug treatment focused on the core features of ASD (e.g., social disability and repetitive behavior) as well as highly relevant coexisting problems such as anxiety and depression (State and Sestan 2012; Oberman 2012; Scahill et al. 2014; Lecavalier et al. 2013). Thus, drug development is an obligation and a challenge. Drug development from the ground up entails multiple steps including studies on the proof of mechanism as well as studies of tolerability and efficacy. This next generation of studies will almost certainly involve compounds that are not currently on the market. Although the commercial interest on the part of pharmaceutical companies may not be immediately compelling, promising compounds that are not on the market are not available without collaboration with pharmaceutical companies. Thus, successful drug development will require collaboration between the pharmaceutical industry, government, and academia.

References

American Psychiatric Association. (1980). *Diagnostic and statistical manual of mental disorders* (3rd ed.). Washington, DC: American Psychiatric Association.

American Psychiatric Association. (2000). *Diagnostic and statistical manual of mental disorders* (4th ed., text rev.). Washington, DC: American Psychiatric Association.

American Psychiatric Association. (2013). *Diagnostic and statistical manual of mental disorders* (5th ed.). Arlington: American Psychiatric Publishing.

Asperger, H. (1944). Die "autistischen psychopathen" im Kindersalter. *Archives fur Psychiatrie und Nervenkrankheiten, 117,* 76–136.

Baxter, A. J., & Krenzelok, E. P. (2008). Pediatric fatality secondary to EDTA chelation. *Clinical toxicology, 46*(10), 1083–1084.

Bender, L. (1953). Childhood schizophrenia. *Psychiatric Quarterly, 27*(1), 663–681.

Bettelheim, B. (1967). *Empty fortress.* New York: Simon and Schuster.

Bleuler, E. (1950). *Dementia Praecox, or the group of schizophrenias* (trans: J. Zinkin). New York: International Universities Press. (Original work published in 1911).

Buie, T., Campbell, D. B., Fuchs, G. J., Furuta, G. T., Levy, J., VandeWater, J., Winter, H., et al. (2010). Evaluation, diagnosis, and treatment of gastrointestinal disorders in individuals with ASD: A consensus report. *Pediatrics, 125*(Suppl. 1), S1–S18.

Centers for Disease Control and Prevention. (2009). Measles vaccination: Who needs it? Retrieved From: http://www.cdc.gov/VACCINES/VPD-VAC/measles/default.htm. Accessed 21 November 2013.

Centers for Disease Control and Prevention. (2012). Prevalence of autism spectrum disorders: Autism and developmental disabilities monitoring network, 14 sites, United States, 2008. Morbidity and Mortality Weekly Report. Surveillance Summaries. Vol. 61, No. 3. Retrieved from http://www.cdc.gov/mmwr/pdf/ss/ss6103.pdf. Accessed 21 November 2013.

Down, J. L. (1887). *On some of the mental affections of childhood and youth.* London: J. & A. Churchill.

Eisenberg, L., & Kanner, L. (1956). Childhood schizophrenia symposium, 1955. 6. Early infantile autism, 1943–55. *American Journal of Orthopsychiatry, 26*(3), 556–566.

Feikin, D. R., Lezotte, D. C., Hamman, R. F., Salmon, D. A., Chen, R. T., & Hoffman, R. E. (2000). Individual and community risks of measles and pertussis associated with personal exemptions to immunization.

JAMA: the Journal of the American Medical Association, 284(24), 3145–3150.

Fish, B., Shapiro, T., & Campbell, M. (1966). Long-term prognosis and the response of schizophrenic children to drug therapy: A controlled study of trifluoperazine. *American Journal of Psychiatry, 123,* 32–39.

Folstein, S., & Rutter, M. (1977). Infantile autism: A genetic study of 21 twin pairs. *Journal of Child Psychology and Psychiatry, 18*(4), 297–321.

Fombonne, E. (2009). Epidemiology of pervasive developmental disorders. *Pediatric Research, 65*(6), 591–598.

Frith, U. (1991). Translation and annotation of "autistic psychopathy" in childhood, by H. Asperger (pp. 37–92). (U. Frith, *Autism and Asperger syndrome*).

Frith, U. (2004). Emanuel Miller lecture: Confusions and controversies about Asperger syndrome. *Journal of child psychology and psychiatry, 45*(4), 672–686.

General Medical Council. (2010). Andrew Wakefield: Determination of serious professional misconduct 24 May 2010. www.gmc-uk.org/Wakefield_SPM_and_SANCTION.pdf_32595267.pdf.

Grebelskaya-Albatz, E. (1934). Zur Klinik der Schizophrenien des frühen Kindesalters. *Schweizer Archiv für Neurochirurgie und Psychiatrie, 34*(244), 35.

Grinker, R. R. (2007). *Unstrange minds: Remapping the world of autism*. New York: Basic Books.

Hamilton, L. M. (2009). *Facing autism: Giving parents reasons for hope and guidance for help*. New York: Random House, Digital, Inc.

Haslam, J. (1809). *Observations on madness and melancholy: Including practical remarks on those diseases; Together with cases: and an account of the morbid appearances on dissection*. London: Printed for J. Callow, by G. Hayden. Retrieved from www.gutenburg.org/ebooks/37144. Accessed 07 November 2013.

Horvath, K., Stefanatos, G., Sokolski, K. N., Wachtel, R., Nabors, L., & Tildon, J. T. (1998). Improved social and language skills after secretin administration in patients with autistic spectrum disorders. *Journal of the Association for Academic Minority Physicians: the official publication of the Association for Academic Minority Physicians, 9*(1), 9–15.

Interagency Autism Coordinating Committee. (2012). US Department of Health & Human Services. IACC/OARC autism spectrum disorder publications analysis: the global landscape of autism research, July 2012.

Jones, W., & Klin, A. (2013). Attention to eyes is present but in decline in 2-6-month-old infants later diagnosed with autism. *Nature.* doi:10.1038/nature12715.

Kanner, L. (1943). Autistic disturbances of affective contact. *Nervous Child, 2*(3), 217–250.

Kirby, D. (2006). *Evidence of harm: Mercury in vaccines and the autism epidemic: A medical controversy*. New York: Macmillan.

Kite, D. M., Gullifer, J., & Tyson, G. A. (2013). Views on the diagnostic labels of autism and Asperger's disorder and the proposed changes in the DSM. *Journal of Autism and Developmental Disorders, 43*(7), 1692–1700.

Kretschmer, E. (1921). *Physique and character: An investigation of the nature of constitution and the theory of temperament*. New York: Harcourt Brace.

Kraepelin, E. (1913). *Psychiatrie; ein Lehrbuch für Studierende und Ärzte* (Vol. 3). Leipzig: Barth.

Künkel, F. W. (1920). The childhood development of schizophrenic patients. *Monatsschrift für Psychiatrie, 48,* 254–272.

Lecavalier, L., Wood, J. J., Halladay, A. K., Jones, N. E., Aman, M. G., Cook, E. H., Handen, B. L., King, B. H., Pearson, D. A., Hallett, V., Sullivan, K. S., Grondhuis, S., Bishop, S. L., Horrigan, J. P., Dawson, G., & Scahill, L. (2013). Measuring anxiety as a treatment endpoint in youth with autism spectrum disorder. *Journal of Autism and Developmental Disorders, 44*(5), 1128–1143.

Lord, C., & Schopler, E. (1989). Stability of assessment results of autistic and non-autistic language-impaired children from preschool years to early school age. *Journal of Child Psychology and Psychiatry, 30*(4), 575–590.

Mahler, M. S. (1952). On child psychosis and schizophrenia: Autistic and symbiotic infantile psychoses. *The Psychoanalytic Study of the Child, 7,* 286–305.

McCarthy, J. (2007). *Louder than words: A mother's journey in healing autism*. New York: Penguin.

National Research Council (US). Committee on Educational Interventions for Children with Autism. (2001). *Educating children with autism*. Washington, DC: National Academies.

Nikolov, R. N., Bearss, K. E., Lettinga, J., Erickson, C., Rodowski, M., Aman, M. G., McCracken, J. T., McDougle, C. J., Tierney, E., Vitiello, B., Arnold, L. E., Shah, B., Posey, D. J., Ritz, L., & Scahill, L. (2009). Gastrointestinal symptoms in a sample of children with pervasive developmental disorders. *Journal of Autism and Developmental Disorders, 39*(3), 405–413.

Oberman, L. M. (2012). mGluR antagonists and GABA agonists as novel pharmacological agents for the treatment of autism spectrum disorders. *Expert Opinion on Investigational Drugs, 21*(12), 1819–1825.

Offit, P. (2008). *Autism's false prophets: Bad science, risky medicine, and the search for a cure*. New York: Columbia University Press.

Oswald, D. P., & Sonenklar, N. A. (2007). Medication use among children with autism spectrum disorders. *Journal of Child and Adolescent Psychopharmacology, 17*(3), 348–355.

Parnas, J. (2011). A disappearing heritage: The clinical core of schizophrenia. *Schizophrenia Bulletin, 37*(6), 1121–1130.

Repligen. (2004). Phase 3 study of secretin for autism fails to meet dual primary endpoints development of secretin for schizophrenia to continue [Press release]. Accessed 15 March 2004.

Rimland, B. (1964). *Infantile Autism: The Syndrome and its Implications for a neural theory of Behaviour*. New York: Appleton-Century-Crofts.

Rutter, M. (1972). Childhood schizophrenia reconsidered. *Journal of Autism and Developmental Disorders, 2*(3), 315–337.

Scahill, L., Hallett, V., Aman, M., McDougle, C. J., Arnold, L. E., McCracken, J. T., Tierney, E., Dziura, J., Deng, Y., & Vitiello, B. (2013). Brief report: Social disability in autism spectrum disorder: Results from research units on pediatric psychopharmacology (RUPP) autism network trials. *Journal of Autism and Developmental Disorders, 43*(3), 739–746.

Scahill, L., Tillburg, C. S., & Martin, A. (2014). Pychopharmacology. In F. Volkmar (Ed.) *Handbook of Autism and Pervasive Developmental Disorders* (4th ed.). Hoboken, New Jersey: John Wiley and Sons.

Schechter, R., & Grether, J. K. (2008). Continuing increases in autism reported to California's developmental services system: Mercury in retrograde. *Archives of General Psychiatry, 65*(1), 19–24.

Schopler, E. (1965). Early infantile autism and receptor processes. *Archives of General Psychiatry, 13*(4), 327–333.

Schüle, H. (1886). Klinische psychiatrie. *DMW-Deutsche Medizinische Wochenschrift, 13*(01), 15–15.

Shorter, E., & Wachtel, L. E. (2013). Childhood catatonia, autism and psychosis past and present: Is there an 'iron triangle'? *Acta Psychiatrica Scandinavica, 128*(1), 21–33.

State, N. W., & Sestan, N. (2012). Neuroscience. The emerging biology of autism spectrum disorders. *Science, 337*(6100), 1301–1303.

Volkmar, F. R., Klin, A., Siegel, B., Szatmari, P., Lord, C., Campbell, M., Freeman, B. J., Cicchetti, D. V., Rutter, M., Kline, W., Buitelaar, J., Hattab, Y., Fombonne, E., Fuentes, J., Werry, J., Stone, W., Kerbeshian, J., Hoshino, Y., Bregman, J., Loveland, K., Szymanski, L., Towbin, K., (1994). Field trial for autistic disorder in DSM-IV. *The American Journal of Psychiatry, 151*(9), 1361–1367.

Volkmar, F. R., Reichow, B., & McPartland, J. (2012). Classification of autism and related conditions: Progress, challenges, and opportunities. *Dialogues in clinical neuroscience, 14*(3), 229–237.

Wakefield, A. J., Murch, S. H., Anthony, A., Linnell, J., Casson, D. M., Malik, M., Berelowitz, M., Dhillon, A. P., Thomson, M. A., Harvey, P., Valentine, A., Davies, S. E., & Walker-Smith, J. A. (1998). Ileal-lymphoid-nodular hyperplasia, non-specific colitis, and pervasive developmental disorder in children. *The Lancet, 351*(9103), 637–641. (Retraction published February 2010 *The Lancet*, 375(9713), p. 445).

Wing, L. (1981). Language, social and cognitive impairments in autism and severe mental retardation. *Journal of Autism and Developmental Disorders, 10*, 31–44.

Wing, L. (2005). Reflections on opening Pandora's box. *Journal of Autism and Developmental Disorders, 35*(2), 197–203.

Wing, L., & Gould, J. (1979). Severe impairments of social interaction and associated abnormalities in children: Epidemiology and classification. *Journal of Autism and Developmental Disorders, 9*(1), 11–29.

Wing, L., Gould, J., & Gillberg, C. (2011). Autism spectrum disorders in the DSM-V: Better or worse than the DSM-IV? *Research in Developmental Disabilities, 32*(2), 768–773.

Wolff, S. (1996). The first account of the syndrome Asperger described. Translation of a paper entitled 'Die schizoiden Psychopathien im Kindesalter.' *European Child and Adolescent Psychiatry, 5*, 119–132.

Phenotypic Variability in Autism Spectrum Disorder: Clinical Considerations

Luc Lecavalier

Introduction

The qualitative impairments in social-communicative behaviors and repetitive and restrictive behaviors and interests that define autism spectrum disorder (ASD) are known to be highly variable. This heterogeneity leads to important challenges for diagnosis and classification, epidemiology, treatment, and the understanding of pathogenesis. Major diagnostic systems attempt to allow for the variability, but it has proven challenging to find a systematic way of doing so. After all, it is a formidable task to find a set of criteria that reliably distinguishes a group of people who have different developmental levels. Rarely do two children with ASD present with identical symptoms, and factors such as developmental level, language ability, and intelligence quotient (IQ) further complicate the presentation of symptoms. Perhaps the most parsimonious way we currently have to decrease heterogeneity of the ASD phenotype is with level of intellectual functioning. This is certainly not a panacea and there are other ways this could be done, but IQ does help to decrease and/or explain phenotypic variability in ASD.

In this section, high- and low-functioning ASD are contrasted and discussed in terms of prevalence, etiology, diagnosis, clinical presentation, and outcome. It is important to note that high- and low-functioning ASD could be defined in several ways. Here, they are broadly defined as ASD with or without intellectual disability (ID), which is defined as an IQ below 70 in most writings. ID is a state of functioning characterized by intellectual and adaptive deficits with an onset in the developmental period. It is objectively defined, but the cutoffs used are arbitrary (AAIDD 2010; APA 2013). Even this artificial dichotomy might not be ideal as there are increased neurobiological abnormalities in people with IQs below 50 (Jacobson et al. 2007; van Bokhoven 2011). Furthermore, other proxies for cognitive ability such as adaptive behavior or language are sometimes used to define high and low functioning when discussing important clinical domains in people with ASD. Finally, sometimes the terms are only used to refer to a median split of the sample under study.

Prevalence

The topic of high- and low-functioning ASD is quite germane to the rise in prevalence observed in the past 40 years. Surveys have clearly shown that prevalence figures published after 2000 have yielded higher rates of case identification (Fombonne 2009). The change in our conceptualization of ASD to include children from all levels

L. Lecavalier (✉)
Nisonger Center and Departments of Psychology and Psychiatry, The Ohio State University, 371-D McCampbell Hall, 1581 Dodd Drive, Columbus, OH 43210, USA
e-mail: lecavalier.1@osu.edu

T. E. Davis III et al. (eds.), *Handbook of Autism and Anxiety,* Autism and Child Psychopathology Series, DOI 10.1007/978-3-319-06796-4_2, © Springer International Publishing Switzerland 2014

of functioning and those with other neuropsychiatric and medical disorders is one factor that has contributed to this increase. Recent surveys have suggested much higher rates of about 60–70/10,000 (Fombonne 2009). It is now believed that most children on the autism spectrum do not function in the range of ID. Indeed, approximately 40–50% fall in the ID range, although rates were higher for *Diagnostic and Statistical Manual of Mental Disorder, Fourth Edition's* (*DSM-IV*; APA 2000) autistic disorder, which by definition consisted of more symptoms than Asperger syndrome and pervasive developmental disorder-not otherwise specified (PDD-NOS). In autistic disorder, rates of ID have been reported to hover around 70%. They also clearly vary according to the level of intellectual deficits, with approximately 30% having mild-to-moderate impairments and 40% having severe-to-profound impairments (Fombonne 2009).

In addition to changes in our conceptualization and measurement of ASD, a number of policy changes have contributed to increased prevalence. The introduction of the 1990 Individuals with Disabilities Educational Act in the USA was followed by diagnostic practice changes, whereby children previously diagnosed with ID were being diagnosed with ASD, either with (accretion) or without (substitution) a co-occurring diagnosis of ID. There is evidence of simultaneous decreases in the population prevalence of ID along with increases in ASD (Shattuck 2006). In other words, some children who in the past would have received a diagnosis of ID have received an ASD diagnosis in more recent times when presenting with similar behaviors. Exactly how much of the increase is due to "diagnostic substitution" is not known. King and Bearman (2009) analyzed data from the California Department of Developmental Services database and found that children previously classified with "mental retardation" accounted for one-quarter of the measured increase in autism prevalence between 1992 and 2005. These definitional issues are reminiscent of the diagnostic substitutions between learning disability and mental retardation seen in the 1990s (*see* MacMillan and Speece 1999*)*.

In addition to policy changes, the epidemiology of ASD has been impacted by a number of social factors. For instance, Palmer et al. (2005) reported that the proportion of economically disadvantaged children per school district was inversely associated with the proportion of autism cases in the Texas Education Agency database. The prevalence estimate of autism for school districts in the top decile in terms of revenue was six times higher than for school districts in the bottom decile of revenue. In other words, children were more likely to be educationally classified as having autism if they were in a school district with more financial resources. The exact reasons for this are likely multiple, but the ability to navigate convoluted bureaucracies to be deemed eligible for services can impact identification rates and advantage families of higher socioeconomic status.

In summary, multiple factors have impacted the rise in ASD prevalence. Definitional changes and inconsistencies as well as changes in social policy have clearly impacted prevalence rates. These variables have impacted high- and low-functioning ASD differently, but the result is that more people are being diagnosed with ASD today than 20–30 years ago, and many of them are considered high-functioning individuals.

Etiology

The past 15 years have brought remarkable progress in the understanding of the etiology of ASD (e.g., Amaral et al. 2008; Ameis and Szatmari 2012; Dodds et al. 2011; Geschwind 2011; Grafodatskaya et al. 2010). One thing is clear: The etiology of ASD is multifactorial and complex. There are multiple genes and environmental factors that contribute to ASD susceptibility. Several lines of evidence suggest that epigenetics also plays an important role in the causes of ASD by integrating genetic and environmental influences to dysregulate neurodevelopmental processes. It is clear that ASD arises from many different etiologies and represents the final outcome of multiple pathological processes.

There is a complex relationship between ASD and ID. The strength and origin of the association remain unclear, but it is hoped that a better understanding of this relationship will lead to a better understanding of the etiology of ASD. On the one hand, the overlap between ASD and ID suggests genetic similarities. Indeed, genetic disorders that are characterized in part by ID, such as fragile X, tuberous sclerosis, or Smith–Lemli–Opitz syndrome, occur at substantially higher rates in individuals with ASD compared to the general population (e.g., Grafodatskaya et al. 2010; Geschwind 2011). We also know that copy number variations explain up to 10% of idiopathic ASD and are also implicated in ID. Such an overlap between ASD and ID argues for a search of common genes influencing both conditions. On the other hand, studies have also reported limited associations between ASD traits and IQ, suggesting separate genetic influences on specific traits. For instance, Hoekstra et al. (2009) reported on the association between autistic traits and ID in a population-based sample of twins between 7 and 9 years old. Only modest correlations were found between IQ and autistic traits (correlations between −.01 and −.40). The association was driven by communication problems characteristic of ASD and suggested that autistic traits are substantially genetically independent of ID. It could be that the genetic risks for ASD and ID are distinctly different, and it is the combination of these conditions that leads to a recognizable ASD. Skuse (2007) proposed that individuals who are genetically susceptible to ASD who also have adequate cognitive skills can compensate for the social-cognitive deficits that are associated with the genetic vulnerability toward ASD. Individuals with the same genetic risk for ASD who function at a lower level are more likely to develop an ASD due to the absence of protective cognitive skills and the increased likelihood of clinical identification.

One of the most well-established findings in the genetic epidemiology of ASD is the fourfold male predominance (Fombonne 2009). In addition, several studies have shown that when females are affected by ASD, they exhibit a more severe form of the disorder, at least when severity is defined in terms of lower IQ or adaptive functioning deficits. This has been clearly demonstrated in epidemiological studies which show that the gender ratio approaches equality at the level of severe ID, but has many more boys than girls in the normal IQ range. The reasons behind this relationship remain a mystery. It has been proposed that females at risk are protected in some way, so that only those with the greatest genetic liability are affected. The relationship between gender and IQ is likely muddled by other variables. For instance, Banach et al. (2009) compared 194 simplex and 154 multiplex families on measures of severity, including nonverbal IQ. Among simplex families (only one child with autism in the family), girls had lower nonverbal IQs than boys, but no such differences were seen among multiplex families (more than one child with autism in the family). Similarly, the affected brothers of girls with autism were no different from affected brothers of male probands. These data suggest that both simplex and multiplex families differ with respect to the relationship between gender and level of functioning.

A final word on etiology and its relationship to level of functioning: It is well-documented that people with ASD have higher rates of neurological problems such as cerebral palsy, microcephaly, and sleep disturbances. One of the more commonly reported co-occurring medical problems is epilepsy (Caniato 2007). Whereas the prevalence of epilepsy in the general population is between 0.5 and 1%, the prevalence in ASD is substantially higher with figures ranging from 5 to 40% (Caniato 2007). ID has been identified as one factor that may account for the variability in prevalence rates. Amiet et al. (2008) synthesized the literature on epilepsy and intellectual functioning in people with ASD in a meta-analysis. They found that the prevalence of epilepsy was higher in individuals with ASD and ID as compared to those without ID. Pooled prevalence rates indicated a rate of 21.4% for individuals with ASD and ID versus 8% in individuals with ASD without ID. Additionally, it was reported that within the sample of individuals with comorbid ID, the prevalence of epilepsy increases with the severity of ID.

Diagnostic and Clinical Features

Level of functioning is associated with a host of clinical features. Related to this are a few general diagnostic issues that warrant consideration. First, level of functioning is associated with age of identification. For instance, Shattuck et al. (2009) analyzed data from 13 sites participating in the Centers for Disease Control and Prevention's 2002 multisite ongoing autism surveillance program. They used data from health and education records to examine factors that influence the timing of community-based identification and diagnosis. Several factors were associated with a younger age of identification, including being male and having an IQ of 70 or lower.

A second point is that level of functioning impacts the psychometric properties of the different instruments used to identify and diagnose people with ASD (e.g., Gotham et al. 2009; Hus et al. 2013; Norris and Lecavalier 2010). Generally speaking, diagnostic accuracy is better in school-age children with mild-to-moderate ID. Diagnostic criteria and rating instruments are not as accurate in toddlers, preschoolers, adolescents, or in individuals with more severe ID or no ID. The take-home message here is that level of functioning impacts who is identified, when in life they are identified, and diagnostic complexity/certainty.

Finally, level of functioning impacts the classification of ASD. For a diagnostic system to be meaningful, individuals in one category should be similar to one another on key variables such as clinical features, psychological profiles, history, and course, but different from people in other categories (Cantwell 1996; Robins and Guze 1970). In other words, a good classification scheme minimizes within-group variability and maximizes between-group variability. Diagnostic groups cannot be valid if they are not reliable. Taken as a whole, the literature on *DSM-IV*-defined ASD subtypes suggested blurry lines between categories. In fact, one could argue that the reliability problems were largely related to level of functioning. In their review of 22 studies comparing ASD subtypes, Witwer and Lecavalier (2008) concluded that the differences observed across ASD subtypes might be better explained by IQ than diagnostic subtypes. For example, many of the differences across ASD subtypes in terms of core diagnostic features, executive functioning, motor functioning, or behavior problems were equally explained by IQ differences (i.e., differences across groups disappeared when analyses controlled for IQ). The model of ASD in the *DSM-IV* did not provide enough diagnostic clarity on how to distinguish ASD subtypes, especially for higher-functioning children. The subsequent study by Lord et al. (2012) further elaborated on this phenomenon. They examined 2102 children with ASD across 12 university-based autism centers. Although the distribution of children's behaviors on standardized measures was similar across sites, the distributions of clinical best-estimate diagnoses were dramatically different. In other words, even when using the same diagnostic instruments and standardized procedures across sites, there was regional variability in which ASD subtype was given to a child. Clinicians used non-ASD specific behavioral characteristics such as hyperactivity, age, and IQ to assign ASD subtypes. For example, some sites gave children with higher IQs a diagnosis of Asperger's syndrome, while other sites used PDD-NOS.

The inability to establish the reliability and validity of ASD subtypes in *DSM-IV* was an impetus for a new definition of ASD. In contrast to *DSM-IV, DSM-5* identifies a smaller number of more general symptoms in social communication. These symptoms are expected to be present in *all* individuals with ASD regardless of age and developmental level, but symptoms can be manifested in many different ways. Clinicians will now specify the presence of ID, making it an explicit consideration in the ASD diagnosis. The new edition of the *DSM* shows promise, but its validity, particularly its incremental validity over predecessors, will only be determined with time.

Core Diagnostic Features

Correlational and cross-sectional analyses of IQ and ASD symptoms have found evidence for negative correlations between level of functioning and a number of ASD symptoms. Lower verbal IQ and lower nonverbal IQ have been associated with more ASD symptoms (Gotham et al. 2009; Spiker et al. 2002). In fact, Spiker et al. (2002) found that ASD symptoms and nonverbal IQ represented parallel dimensions of severity such that children with lower nonverbal IQ also tended to have the most severe ASD symptoms, particularly in the social-communicative domain. Another example is the study by Ben Itzchak et al. (2008), which grouped 44 preschoolers with autism by cognitive level to form three groups: Normal (IQ>90), Borderline (70<IQ<89), and Impaired (50<IQ<69). They compared the groups' scores on the *Autism Diagnostic Observation Schedule* (Lord et al. 2000). Compared to the two other groups, the Impaired group had significantly higher scores in the reciprocal social interaction domain. The Impaired group also had higher scores than the Borderline group in the stereotyped behavior domain. Differences were not found between the Borderline and Normal groups.

In recent years, more attention has been paid to the relationship between IQ and restrictive repetitive behaviors and interests (RRBI). Several studies have proposed two main groups of RRBI (Bishop et al. 2013; Bishop et al. 2006; Cuccaro et al. 2003; Szatmari et al. 2006). One group consists of repetitive sensory and motor behaviors (RSMB) such as hand/finger mannerisms, unusual sensory interests, repetitive use of objects/parts of objects, and rocking. The other group of RRBI, often referred to as "insistence on sameness" (IS), consists of behaviors related to rigidity or resistance to change which include difficulties with changes in routine, resistance to trivial changes in environment, and compulsions/rituals.

The two broad groups of RRBI seem to have different relationships with level of functioning. Whereas RSMB have been found to be negatively related to age and IQ in some people, IS behaviors have shown either no relationship or positive relationships with level of functioning. Most of the studies examining the relationship between level of functioning and different types of RRBI have been conducted with some combination of the 12 items found on the *Autism Diagnostic Interview—Revised* (ADI-R; Rutter et al. 2003). Of course, this fairly small pool of items limits the associations that can be found. For instance, in most studies, self-injurious behaviors (SIB) and circumscribed interests (CI) were not included. In one of these studies, in a sample of 830 children who ranged from 15 months to 11 years of age, Bishop et al. (2006) found a significant interaction between nonverbal IQ and chronological age, such that nonverbal IQ was more strongly related to the prevalence of several RRBI in older children. The prevalence of a number of repetitive behaviors (e.g. repetitive use of objects, hand and finger mannerisms) was negatively associated with nonverbal IQ. However, the prevalence of certain behaviors (e.g. circumscribed interests) was positively associated with nonverbal IQ. In a sample of 339 individuals with ASD, Szatmari et al. (2006) reported RSMB to be negatively correlated with adaptive skills, while IS was positively correlated with autistic symptoms in the communication and language domain. In addition, analyses suggested moderate familial aggregation among affected sibling pairs within the IS but not the RSMB factor, suggesting that IS may be under familial/genetic control, while RSMB appears to simply reflect variation in developmental level. Lam et al. (2008) reported three factors in their sample of 316 people with autism: RSMB, IS, and CI. They also reported that RSMB were associated with a variety of subject characteristics such as IQ, age, social/communication impairments, and the presence of regression or skill loss. IS was associated with social and communication impairments, whereas CI appeared to be independent of subject characteristics. Based on sib-pair correlations, they also reported that IS and CI (but not RSMB) appear to be familial. Finally, one recent study replicated these findings using both the ADI-R and the *Repetitive Behavior Scale—Revised* (Bodfish et al. 2000) in a large independent sample (Bishop et al. 2013) recruited from the Simons Simplex Collection, a North American multisite university-based research study that includes families with only one child with an ASD.

Adaptive Behavior

A number of large-scale studies on adaptive behavior have been published in the past 10 years or so. Evidence suggests that as children with ASD become older, their adaptive skills are more impaired relative to age-matched peers (Kanne et al. 2011; Szatmari et al. 2003). This implies that individuals are failing to acquire skills commensurate with their chronological and cognitive growth. The "typical autism profile" is described as one marked by the most substantial delays in socialization, lesser delays in adaptive communication, and relative strengths in daily living skills (Bolte and Poustka 2002). Even this "typical" adaptive behavior profile is impacted by the level of cognitive ability. The profile has been documented in higher-functioning ASD samples (e.g., Klin et al. 2007; Perry et al. 2009; Saulnier and Klin 2007). Yet, in lower-functioning individuals, adaptive behavior has been found to be commensurate or higher than mental age in some cases (e.g., Fenton et al. 2003; Perry et al. 2009). In other words, the "autism profile" is less likely to manifest as the gap increases between chronological and mental age. Kanne et al. (2011) reported on this relationship using the *Vineland Adaptive Behavior Scales-II* (Sparrow et al. 2005) in a large sample of verbal youth with ASD. Specifically, children with an IQ < 70 (n = 223; average IQ = 54) had an average adaptive behavior composite score of 66, whereas the children with an IQ > 70 (n = 855; average IQ = 98) had an average adaptive behavior composite score of 79.

Behavior and Psychiatric Problems

As used here, the term "behavior problems" describes those challenging and impairing behaviors often seen in people with ASD such as self injury, tantrums, aggression, and property destruction. Behavior problems are contrasted with the psychiatric disorders defined in the DSM. The relationship between behavior and psychiatric problems is not well understood. There is little doubt that they co-occur but there is no evidence to suggest a systematic relationship between the two. Rather, the evidence seems to suggest that behavior problems are nonspecific indicators of distress and dysfunction (Witwer and Lecavalier 2010).

It is well-documented that children with ASD present with high rates of behavior problems (Brereton et al. 2006; Lecavalier 2006). As previously discussed, ID has been commonly associated with more severe ASD (Fombonne 2009). In addition, behaviors challenging to caregivers such as aggression have also been associated with ASD severity (Jang et al. 2010). A few studies have specifically reported on the relationship between level of functioning and behavior problems. In a sample of 487 young people with ASD between the ages of 3 and 21 years, Lecavalier (2006) reported that children with more impaired adaptive skills had significantly more problems on most of the prosocial and problem behavior subscales of the *Nisonger Child Behavior Rating Form* (Aman et al. 1996). Estes et al. (2007) reported on the relation between level of functioning and behavior problems in a sample of 74 6–9-year-olds. Participants were classified as lower and higher functioning using nonverbal IQ, verbal IQ, and communication scores on the *Vineland Adaptive Behavior Scales* at age 6 years. Likewise, problem behaviors were assessed with a variety of rating scales. Results suggested that higher-functioning children at age 6 years displayed increased internalizing symptoms by age 9 years, whereas lower-functioning children displayed higher hyperactivity, attention problems, and irritability by the age of 9 years. These data suggest that level of intellectual functioning may be a risk factor for different patterns of associated symptoms by later childhood. The trend of greater behavior problems in lower-functioning individuals is also true for adolescents and adults with ASD. In their longitudinal study, Shattuck et al. (2007) found that individuals with comorbid ID had more behavior problems than those without ID. Furthermore, behavior problems in individuals with comorbid ID improved less over a period of 4.5 years as compared to those without ID.

SIB and aggression are two of the most vexing behavior problems. There are actually few large-scale studies examining the relationship between level of functioning and these two behavior problems in ASD. This is rather surprising given their clinical importance and the amount of resources allocated to them. One exception is the recent study by Duerden et al. (2012) who investigated the relationship between SIB and intellectual functioning in a sample of 250 children with an average chronological age of 88 months. Children with lower IQ were more likely to engage in SIB. IQ explained a small portion of the variance in the SIB data, but not as much as IS (i.e., IS was more predictive of SIB than IQ). This association between low cognitive functioning and high rates of SIB in children with autism is consistent with some prior findings but at odds with studies suggesting that IS is either not correlated or positively correlated with IQ (e.g., Bishop et al. 2006; Szatmari et al. 2006). The exact reason for higher rates of SIB in lower-functioning individuals is a mystery although several explanations have been proposed, including impaired memory systems that lead to an inability to learn about pain. From research among individuals with ID without ASD, we have known for decades that SIB tends to increase with severity of functional handicap (Schroeder et al. 2001).

Dominick et al. (2007) conducted one of the few studies examining factors associated with aggression in 67 children with ASD. They found that the presence of aggression was associated with lower IQ, poorer expressive and receptive language, and RRBI. In a much larger sample, Kanne and Mazurek (2011) did not find an association between aggression and level of intellectual or adaptive functioning, language ability, or ASD severity. This was a large (n = 1380) and well-characterized sample taken from the Simons Simplex Collection. Of note, however, is the fact that only four items from the ADI-R (current and ever ratings of *aggression towards caregivers or family members* and *aggression towards non-*

caregivers or nonfamily members) were used to measure aggression.

Similar to behavior problems, high rates have also been reported for psychiatric problems (Gadow et al. 2005; Simonoff et al. 2008). Commonly reported psychiatric symptoms include attention-deficit/hyperactivity disorder (ADHD), disruptive behavior disorders, and anxiety and fears. Conceptualization of these syndromes in ASD is a matter of debate. On the one hand, it is possible that psychiatric disorders are independent of ASD and reflect co-occurring conditions. On the other hand, it is possible that they are inherently associated with core features of ASD and are distributed from low to high in children with ASD, similar to language and intellectual skills. It could also be that psychiatric symptoms and ASD are separate but not independent, in that the presence of one amplifies the other because of certain genetic and environmental influences. There are currently not enough data to declare a winner in the debate, but there are some studies that lend support to the *DSM-IV* as a valid conceptualization of psychiatric disorders in children with ASD. For instance, Lecavalier et al. (2009) submitted parent and teacher ratings of *DSM*-based symptoms to confirmatory factor analysis. The sample in this study consisted of 498 children aged between 6 and 12 years. The authors found support for ADHD, oppositional defiant disorder (ODD), conduct disorder, generalized anxiety disorder (GAD), and mood/dysthymic disorder as diagnostic categories in ASD. In fact, they reported similar indices of fit for children with ASD and a comparison group of typically developing children. If the DSM was not a valid conceptualization for these children, symptoms would not correlate with one another in this organized fashion. Interestingly, fit indices improved when analyses were only conducted on children with an IQ > 70, which could suggest that the DSM conceptualization becomes less valid as IQ declines. Along the same lines, Gadow and colleagues provided additional support for the validity of psychiatric disorders in ASD by examining patterns of comorbidity and genetic and psychosocial risk factors (Gadow et al. 2008a, 2008b, 2008c; Gadow et al. 2006; Gadow et al. 2012).

The differential patterns of comorbidity and risk factors observed in ASD were similar to those observed in typically developing children. One thing is clear, whether these problems are part of ASD or independent from them, they are impairing, fairly common, and appropriate targets for psychosocial or pharmacological treatment (Kaat et al. 2013).

A few studies have examined the relationship between level of functioning and psychiatric problems using structured psychiatric interviews. Witwer and Lecavalier (2010) used the parent version of the *Children's Interview for Psychiatric Symptoms* (P-ChIPS), a structured interview based on the *DSM-IV,* to compare psychiatric symptom endorsement rates of children with ASD. They found that children with an IQ<70 had fewer reported symptoms than those with an IQ≥70. Lower-functioning individuals were more likely to be subsyndromal (defined as having symptoms for a disorder and related impairments, but falling short of full diagnostic criteria by one or two symptoms) for GAD and nonverbal individuals were more likely to be subsyndromal for ODD. Symptom endorsement also varied based on language levels. Contrasting results were reported in the only epidemiological sample examining risk factors for psychiatric disorders in children with ASD (Simonoff et al. 2008). In this sample of 112 10–14-year-olds, neither IQ nor adaptive behavior scores were associated with increased rates of psychiatric disorders. The authors explained the lack of association between IQ and psychiatric disorders as possibly indicating that ASD trumps other risk factors, whereby the influence of IQ is diminished in this population due to the more potent risk factor of ASD itself.

Anxiety in ASD has been the object of several recent published reports (Hallett et al. 2013; van Steensel et al. 2011; White et al. 2009). Unlike externalized behavior problems, it may be difficult to infer which behaviors are driven by anxiety and which are due to ASD in the absence of direct verbal expression from the individual. In addition to expressive verbal ability, the problem of attribution is likely to be influenced by IQ. Gotham et al. (2013) reported on the relationship between anxiety and IS in a sample of 1429 individuals, also recruited from the Simons Simplex Collection. These constructs were minimally associated with each other and with chronological age and verbal IQ. Neither anxiety nor IS was associated with other core autism diagnostic scores. Anxiety was associated with a variety of other psychiatric and behavioral symptoms, including irritability, attention problems, and aggression, while IS was not. These data showed that anxiety and IS appear to function as distinct constructs, each with a wide range of expression in children with ASD across age and IQ levels.

Hallett et al. (2013) examined parent-reported anxiety symptoms in a sample of 415 children with ASD who participated in one of four multisite psychopharmacological trials. They used 20 items measuring anxiety from the *Child and Adolescent Symptom Inventory* (CASI-Anxiety; Gadow and Sprafkin 1997, 2002; Sukhodolsky et al. 2008). Items measuring panic, post-traumatic stress symptoms, and obsessions are not included on the CASI-Anxiety. They observed that high scores on the CASI-Anxiety were associated with being verbal, having an IQ of 70 or above, and showing higher levels of inappropriate speech, irritability, and hyperactivity. They also observed that children in the upper quartile on the CASI-Anxiety had higher Vineland scores, which is consistent with previous findings showing positive associations between IQ and anxiety in ASD (Weisbrot et al. 2005; Witwer and Lecavalier 2010). Interestingly, considering the individual items of the CASI-Anxiety, the most- and least-endorsed statements were the same in the high- and low-functioning groups. Items such as "*acts restless or edgy,*" "*has difficulty falling asleep,*" and "*is extremely tense and unable to relax*" are directly observable and were most commonly endorsed by parents. The high language requirements for items starting with "worries" or "complains" apparently limited the rate of endorsement in the lower IQ group, which in turn contributed to the lower CASI-Anxiety mean score. Nonetheless, youth with IQ of 70 or greater had significantly higher mean scores than the ID group on the 10 scale items with low verbal demand. This suggests that, even when considering the more observable aspects of anxiety, higher-functioning children exhibited more anxiety than children with lower IQ.

In contrast to these findings, the meta-analysis by van Steensel et al. (2011) found higher rates of anxiety disorders in children with lower levels of intellectual functioning (defined by the cross-study median split IQ of 87), suggesting that children with lower IQ do experience anxiety and exhibit anxiety-driven behaviors even if the anxiety is not expressed verbally. In the Hallett et al. (2013) study, children with the highest levels of anxiety also had more behavior problems than those who were less anxious. This could reflect the overall behavioral disturbance of the children in this sample, albeit this relationship has been reported elsewhere (Gotham et al. 2013). These associations could also suggest that anxiety may amplify other behavioral problems or that a combination of higher IQ coupled with more severe behavior problems poses a greater risk for anxiety difficulties. This is particularly interesting as irritability and hyperactivity have been associated with lower IQ (e.g., Estes et al. 2007). Clearly, more research on the correlates of anxiety is needed.

Outcome

Level of functioning has been shown to impact the natural course of ASD and response to treatment. The long-term course of ASD is generally understood to involve lifelong impairments with a modest trend toward improvement (Seltzer et al. 2004). However, individual characteristics such as severity of cognitive deficits influence the trajectory of the disorder and its eventual outcome. The most frequently cited characteristics that influence the course of ASD are ID and overall language ability. The absence of ID and the presence of better language skills in early childhood have been consistently associated with a greater likelihood of improvement over time in children and better adult outcomes (Baghdadli et al. 2007; Howlin et al. 2004; Shattuck et al. 2007; Szatmari et al. 2003).

In their seminal follow-up study of 68 adults who met criteria for ASD as children and had a nonverbal IQ above 50, Howlin et al. (2004) found that individuals with a childhood nonverbal IQ of 70 or higher had a significantly better outcome in adulthood. Outcome was quite variable and, on an individual level, neither verbal nor nonverbal IQ proved to be consistent prognostic indicators. Howlin and colleagues found that social and adaptive outcomes were more highly correlated with verbal IQ than with nonverbal IQ. They concluded that having an IQ over 70 is necessary but not sufficient for an optimal outcome. In their sample of 241 adolescents and adults with ASD, Shattuck et al. (2007) examined change in autism symptoms over a 4.5-year period. Although the majority of the sample showed improvement, those individuals with comorbid ID improved less over time. In fact, the absence of ID was the most robust predictor of change in symptoms.

The term "optimal outcome" has been used to describe children who once met criteria for ASD but now present without significant symptoms of ASD and function in the average range of intelligence (Fein et al. 2013). Helt et al. (2008) reviewed long-term outcome studies and concluded that between 3 and 25 % of individuals with ASD eventually lost their diagnosis, although very few of the studies reporting these outcomes explicitly addressed the question of whether their social and communication abilities were fully typical. They also concluded that early predictors of better outcomes included higher IQ, receptive language, imitation, motor skills, earlier diagnosis and treatment, and a diagnosis of PDD-NOS rather than autistic disorder. A recent study by Fein et al. (2013) confirmed that optimal outcome is more likely in individuals with higher cognitive functioning and somewhat milder initial symptoms.

Studies of early interventions in children with ASD have also found IQ, age at treatment initiation, and early language skills to be among the strongest predictors of response to treatment. These findings have been reported among a variety of intervention types (e.g., Ozonoff and Cathcart 1998), but mainly for early intensive behavioral intervention (Howlin et al. 2009). In spite of the convergence across studies in terms of identified predictors of successful response to treatment, it is important to note that there is great variability at the individual level and there have been few sufficiently powered studies to allow adequate testing of moderators of treatment response. Nonetheless, studies with different research designs have reached similar conclusions. For instance, Sallows and Graupner (2005) examined the predictors of best response to a 4-year applied behavioral analysis-based treatment for 24 children with ASD. Treatment outcome was best predicted by pretreatment imitation, language, and social responsiveness. Children with higher pretreatment IQs were more likely eventually to have IQs in the average range (75 % of children with IQs between 55 and 64 vs. 17 % of children with IQs between 35 and 44). Similarly, a study of 44 preschool children who received 2 years of early intensive behavioral intervention indicated that the best outcomes were achieved by those who had higher IQs and adaptive skills at baseline (Remington et al. 2007). Finally, Ben Itzchak and Zachor (2007) examined predictors of outcome of early behavioral intervention in preschool children with autism who underwent 1 year of intensive behavioral interventions at 35 h per week. Children with ID demonstrated slower acquisition of receptive and expressive language skills, play skills, and nonverbal communication skills after 1 year of treatment. In this study, progress in the receptive language domain was highly related to pretreatment cognitive and social abilities. Children with higher pretreatment cognitive ability or with better social reciprocal abilities made more gains in their receptive language.

Unfortunately, there are few long-term follow-up studies of children with ASD who attended intensive intervention programs in their preschool years. Magiati et al. (2011) reported on 36 children with ASD (mean age of 3.4 years) enrolled in relatively intense, specialist preschool programs (minimum of 15 h of intervention per week for 2 years). They assessed the children 2 years (mean age 5.5 years) and 7 years (mean age 10.3 years) posttreatment on cognitive skills,

language, adaptive behavior, and severity of ASD symptoms. Baseline IQ and language and adaptive behavior skills were predictive of outcome 7 years posttreatment. This study highlighted that while overall group improvements may be evident, the rate and nature of these improvements is highly variable across individual children. Further investigation of the specific child characteristics that affect treatment effectiveness is required as level of functioning alone does not explain the variability in response rates.

Current evidence on the role of IQ for positive outcomes in early intervention might be the most compelling we have. One reason for this is that many of the recent psychosocial treatment studies such as social skills training or cognitive behavior therapy for anxiety have focused on high-functioning individuals (Kaat and Lecavalier 2014; Lang et al. 2010). The story is quite different when it comes to the use of psychotropic medicines, which may very well be the most commonly used type of treatment for people with ASD (Lecavalier and Gadow 2008). Overall, multiple surveys show that approximately half of people with ASD take psychotropic medicines and that older age and lower level of functioning are associated with increased patterns of use (Rosenberg et al. 2010; Witwer and Lecavalier 2005). Of course, factors external to clinical presentation likely affect odds of psychotropic medication use. For instance, in the Rosenberg et al. (2010) study, people residing in a poorer county or in the south or midwest regions of the USA had increased rates of psychotropic medication use. Beyond the actual use of medicines, the key question is whether or not children with high- and low-functioning ASD respond differently to the same agents. Much like the early intervention studies, there are few sufficiently powered controlled trials that allow the study of moderation (Siegel and Beaulieu 2012). Some of the largest studies that have been conducted in the field to date have not found an effect of level of functioning on clinical response (Arnold et al. 2010; Research Units on Pediatric Psychopharmacology (RUPP) Autism Network 2005; King et al. 2009). On some levels this is surprising as there is evidence that IQ impacts response rates for some medicines in non-ASD populations. For instance, Aman et al. (2003) reported that children with low IQ and ADHD clearly respond to methylphenidate, but their rate of beneficial response appears to be well under that of average-IQ children and more varied.

Conclusions

ASD represents a heterogeneous group of neurodevelopmental disorders that overlap with ID. Differences in intellectual ability help to explain some of the vast heterogeneity associated with ASD. The past decade has taught us that the etiology of ASD is complex, but there is a relationship with level of functioning. High- and low-functioning individuals with ASD have different profiles in terms of core and associated clinical features. Lower-functioning individuals tend to have more social-communicative deficits and RSMB. There is great diversity across individuals, but the natural course of ASD and response to treatment seems to be impacted by level of functioning. Several studies have shown higher levels of functioning to be significantly associated with better clinical outcomes. Ultimately, it is hoped that identifying more phenotypically homogenous subgroups will facilitate efforts to understand the causes and treatment of ASD.

References

Aman, M. G., Tassé, M. J., Rojahn, J., & Hammer, D. (1996). The Nisonger CBRF: A child behavior rating form for children with developmental disabilities. *Research in Developmental Disabilities, 17,* 41–57. doi:10.1016/0891-4222(95)00039-9.

Aman, M. G., Buican, B., & Arnold, L. E. (2003). Methylphenidate treatment in children with borderline IQ and mental retardation: Analysis of three aggregate studies. *Journal of Child and Adolescent Psychopharmacology, 13,* 29–40. doi:10.1089/104454603321666171.

Amaral, D. G., Schumann, C. M., & Nordahl, C. W. (2008). Neuroanatomy of autism. *Trends in Neurosciences, 31,* 137–145. doi:10.1016/j.tins.2007.12.005.

AAIDD. (2010). *Intellectual disability: Definition, classification, and systems of supports* (11th ed.). Washington, DC: American Association on Intellectual and Developmental Disabilities.

APA. (2000). *Diagnostic and statistical manual of mental disorders* (4th ed. text revised). Washington, DC: American Psychiatric Association. doi:10.1176/appi.books.9780890423349.

APA. (2013). *Diagnostic and statistical manual of mental disorders* (5th ed.). Arlington: American Psychiatric Association.

Ameis, S. H., & Szatmari, P. (2012). Imaging-genetics in autism spectrum disorder: Advances, translational impact, and future directions. *Frontiers in Psychiatry, 3,* 46. doi:10.3389/fpsyt.2012.00046.

Amiet, C., Gourfinkel-An, I., Bouzamondo, A., Tordjman, S., Baulac, M., Lechat, P., et al. (2008). Epilepsy in autism is associated with intellectual disability and gender: Evidence from a meta-analysis. *Biological Psychiatry, 64,* 577–582. doi:10.1016/j.biopsych.2008.04.030.

Arnold, L. E., Farmer, C., Kraemer, H. C., Davies, M., Witwer, A. N., Chang, S., et al. (2010). Moderators, mediators, and other predictors of risperidone response in children with autistic disorder and irritability. *Journal of Child and Adolescent Psychopharmacology, 20,* 83–93. doi:10.1089/cap.2009.0022.

Baghdadli, A., Picot, M. C., Michelon, C., Bodet, J., Pernon, E., Burstezjn, C., et al. (2007). What happens to children with PDD when they grow up? Prospective follow-up of 219 children from preschool age to mid-childhood. *Acta Psychiatrica Scandinavica, 115,* 403–412. doi:10.1111/j.1600-0447.2006.00898.x.

Banach, R., Thompson, A., Szatmari, P., Goldberg, J., Tuff, L., Zwaigenbaum, L., & Mahoney, W. (2009). Brief report: Relationship between non-verbal IQ and gender in autism. *Journal of Autism and Developmental Disorders, 39,* 188–193. doi:10.1007/s10803-008-0612-4.

Ben Itzchak, E., & Zachor, A. D. (2007). The effects of intellectual functioning and autism severity on outcome of early behavioral intervention for children with autism. *Research in Developmental Disabilities, 28,* 287–303. doi:10.1016/j.ridd.2006.03.002.

Ben Itzchak, E., Lahat, E., Burgin, R., & Zachor, A. D. (2008). Cognitive, behavior, and intervention outcome in young children with autism. *Research in Developmental Disabilities, 29,* 447–458. doi:10.1016/j.ridd.2007.08.003.

Bishop, S. L., Richler, J., & Lord, C. (2006). Association between restricted and repetitive behaviors and nonverbal IQ in children with autism spectrum disorders. *Clinical Neuropsychology, 12,* 247–267. doi:10.1080/09297040600630288.

Bishop, S. L., Hus, V., Duncan, A., Huerta, M., Gotham, K., Pickles, A., et al. (2013). Subcategories of restricted and repetitive behaviors in children with autism spectrum disorders. *Journal of Autism and Developmental Disorders, 43,* 1287–1297. doi:10.1007/s10803-012-1671-0.

Bodfish, J. W., Symons, F. J., Parker, D. E., & Lewis, M. H. (2000). Varieties of repetitive behavior in autism: Comparisons to mental retardation. *Journal of Autism and Developmental Disorders, 30*, 237–243. doi:10.1023/A:1005596502855.

Bolte, S., & Poustka, F. (2002). The relation between general cognitive level and adaptive behavior domains in individuals with autism with and without co-morbid mental retardation. *Child Psychiatry and Human Development, 33*, 165–172. doi:10.1023/A:1020734325815.

Brereton, A. V., Tonge, B. J., & Einfeld, S. L. (2006). Psychopathology in children and adolescents with autism compared to young people with intellectual disability. *Journal of Autism and Developmental Disorders, 36*, 863–870. doi:10.1007/s10803-006-0125-y.

Caniato, R. (2007). Epilepsy in autism spectrum disorders. *European Child and Adolescent Psychiatry, 16*, 61–66. doi:10.1007/s00787-006-0563-2.

Cantwell, D. P. (1996). Classification of child and adolescent psychopathology. *Journal of Child Psychology and Psychiatry, 37*, 3–12. doi:10.1111/j.1469-7610.1996.tb01377.x.

Cuccaro, M. L., Shao, Y., Grubber, J., Slifer, M., Wolpert, C. M., Donnelly, S. L., et al. (2003). Factor analysis of restricted and repetitive behaviors in autism using the Autism Diagnostic Interview-Revised. *Child Psychiatry and Human Development, 34*, 3–17. doi:10.1023/A:1025321707947.

Dodds, L., Fell, D. B., Shea, S., Armson, B. A., Allen, A. C., & Bryson, S. (2011). The role of prenatal, obstetric and neonatal factors in the development of autism. *Journal of Autism and Developmental Disorders, 41*, 891–902. doi:10.1007/s10803-010-1114-8.

Dominick, K. C., Davis, N. O., Lainhart, J., Tager-Flusberg, H., & Folstein, S. (2007). Atypical behaviors in children with autism and children with a history of language impairment. *Research in Developmental Disabilities, 28*, 145–162. doi:10.1016/j.ridd.2006.02.003.

Duerden, E. G., Oatley, H. K., Mak-Fan, M. K., McGrath, P. A., Taylor, M. J., Szatmari, P., & Roberts, S. W. (2012). Risk factors associated with self-injurious behaviors in children and adolescents with autism spectrum disorders. *Journal of Autism and Developmental Disorders, 42*, 2460–2470. doi:10.1007/s10803-012-1497-9.

Estes, A. M., Dawson, G., Sterling, L., & Munson, J. (2007). Level of intellectual functioning predicts patterns of associated symptoms in school-age children with autism spectrum disorder. *American Journal on Mental Retardation, 112*, 439–449.

Fein, D., Barton, M., Eigsti, I.-M., Kelly, E., Naigles, L., Schultz, R., et al. (2013). Optimal outcome in individuals with a history of autism. *Journal of Child Psychology and Psychiatry, 54*, 195–205. doi:10.1111/jcpp.12037.

Fenton, G., D'Ardia, C., Valente, D., Vecchio, I. D. V., Fabrizi, A., & Bernabei, P. (2003). Vineland adaptive behavior profiles in children with autism and moderate to severe developmental delay. *Autism: The International Journal of Research and Practice, 7*, 269–287. doi:10.1177/1362361303007003004.

Fombonne, E. (2009). The epidemiology of pervasive developmental disorders. *Pediatric Research, 65*, 591–598. doi:10.1203/PDR.0b013e31819e7203.

Gadow, K. D., & Sprafkin, J. (1997). *Adolescent symptom inventory-4 screening manual*. Stony Brook: Checkmate Plus.

Gadow, K. D., & Sprafkin, J. (2002). *Child symptom inventory-4 screening and norms manual*. Stony Brook: Checkmate Plus.

Gadow, K. D., DeVincent, C. J., Pomeroy, J., & Azizian, A. (2005). Comparison of DSM-IV symptoms in elementary school-age children with PDD versus clinic and community. *Autism: The International Journal of Research and Practice, 9*, 392–415. doi:10.1177/1362361305056079.

Gadow, K. D., DeVincent, C. J., & Pomeroy, J. (2006). ADHD symptom subtypes in children with pervasive developmental disorder. *Journal of Autism and Developmental Disorders, 36*, 271–283. doi:10.1007/s10803-005-0060-3.

Gadow, K. D., DeVincent, C. J., & Drabick, D. A. G. (2008a). Oppositional defiant disorder as a clinical phenotype in children with autism spectrum disorder. *Journal of Autism and Developmental Disorders, 38*, 1302–1310. doi:10.1007/s10803-007-0516-8.

Gadow, K. D., DeVincent, C., & Schneider, J. (2008b). Predictors of psychiatric symptoms in children with an autism spectrum disorder. *Journal of Autism and Developmental Disorders, 38*, 1710–1720. doi:10.1007/s10803-008-0556-8.

Gadow, K. D., Roohi, J., DeVincent, C. J., & Hatchwell, E. (2008c). Association of ADHD, tics, and anxiey with dopamine transporter (DAT1) genotype in autism spectrum disorder. *Journal of Child Psychology and Psychiatry, 49*, 1331–1338. doi:10.1111/j.1469-7610.2008.01952.x.

Gadow, K. D., Guttmann-Steinmetz, S., Rieffe, C., & DeVincent, C. J. (2012). Depression symptoms in boys with autism spectrum disorder and comparison samples. *Journal of Autism and Developmental Disorders, 42*, 1353–1363. doi:10.1007/s10803-011-1367-x.

Geschwind, D. H. (2011). Genetics of autism spectrum disorders. *Trends in Cognitive Sciences, 15*, 409–416. doi:10.1016/j.tics.2011.07.003.

Gotham, K., Pickles, A., & Lord, C. (2009). Standardizing ADOS scores for a measure of severity in autism spectrum disorders. *Journal of Autism and Developmental Disorders, 39*, 693–705. doi:10.1007/s10803-008-0674-3.

Gotham, K., Bishop, S. L., Hus, V., Huerta, M., Lund, S., Buja, A., Krieger, A., & Lord, C. (2013). Exploring the relationship between anxiety and insistence on sameness in autism spectrum disorders. *Autism Research, 6*, 33–41. doi:10.1002/aur.1263.

Grafodatskaya, D., Chung, B., Szatmari, P., & Weksberg, P. (2010). Autism spectrum disorders and epigenetics. *Journal of the American Academy of Child and Adolescent Psychiatry, 49*, 794–809. doi:10.1016/j.jaac.2010.05.005.

Hallett, V., Lecavalier, L., Sukhodolsky, D. G., Cipriano, N., McCracken, J. T., et al. (2013). Exploring anxiety in children with pervasive developmental disorders across a broad range of functioning. *Journal of Autism and Developmental Disorders, 43*(10), 2341–2352. doi:10.1007/s10803-013-1775-1.

Helt, M., Kelley, E., Kinsbourne, M., Pandey, J., Boorstein, H., Herbert, M., & Fein, D. (2008). Can children with autism recover? If so, how? *Neuropsychology Review, 18,* 339–366. doi:10.1007/s11065-008-9075-9.

Hoekstra, R. A., Happé, F., Baron-Cohen, S., & Ronald, A. (2009). Association between extreme autistic traits and intellectual disability. *British Journal of Psychiatry, 195,* 531–536. doi:10.1192/bjp.bp.108.060889.

Howlin, P., Goode, S., Hutton, J., & Rutter, M. (2004). Adult outcome for children with autism. *Journal of Child Psychology and Psychiatry, 45,* 212–229. doi:10.1111/j.1469-7610.2004.00215.x.

Howlin, P., Magiati, I., & Charman, T. (2009). Systematic review of early intensive behavioral interventions for children with autism. *American Journal on Intellectual and Developmental Disabilities, 114,* 23–41. doi:10.1352/2009.114:23;nd41.

Hus, V., Bishop, S., Gotham, K., & Huerta, M., & Lord, C. (2013). Factors influencing scores on the social responsiveness scale. *Journal of Child Psychiatry and Psychology, 54,* 216–224. doi:10.1111/j.1469-7610.2012.02589.x.

Jacobson, J. W., Mulick, J. A., & Rojahn, J. (Eds.). (2007). *Handbook of intellectual and developmental disabilities.* New York: Springer. doi:10.1007/0-387-32931-5.

Jang, J., Dixon, D. R., Tarbox, J., & Granpeesheh, D. (2010). Symptom severity and challenging behavior in children with ASD. *Research in Autism Spectrum Disorders, 5,* 1028–1032. doi:10.1016/j.rasd.2010.11.008.

Kaat, A. J., & Lecavalier, L. (2014). Group-based social skills treatment: A methodological review. *Research in Autism Spectrum Disorders, 8,* 15–24.

Kaat, A. J., Gadow, K. D., & Lecavalier, L. (2013). Psychiatric symptom impairment in children with autism spectrum disorders. *Journal of Abnormal Child Psychology, 41,* 959–969. doi:10.1007/s10802-013-9739-7.

Kanne, S., & Mazurek, M. (2011). Aggression in children and adolescents with ASD: Prevalence and risk factors. *Journal of Autism and Developmental Disorders, 41,* 926–937. doi:10.1007/s10803-010-1118-4.

Kanne, S. M., Gerber, A. J., Quirmbach, L. M., Sparrow, S. S., Cicchetti, D. V., & Saulnier, C. A. (2011). The role of adaptive behavior in autism spectrum disorders: Implications for functional outcome. *Journal of Autism and Developmental Disorders, 41,* 1007–1018. doi:10.1007/s10803-010-1126-4.

King, B. H., Hollander, E., Sikich, L., McCracken, J. T., Scahill, L., Bregman, J. D., et al. (2009). Lack of efficacy of cilaopram in children with autism spectrum disorders and high levels of repetitive behavior. *Archives of General Psychiatry, 66,* 583–590. doi:10.1001/archgenpsychiatry.2009.30.

King, M., & Bearman, P. (2009). Diagnostic change and the increased prevalence of autism. *International Journal of Epidemiology, 38,* 1224–1234. doi:10.1093/ije/dyp261.

Klin, A., Saulnier, C. A., Sparrow, S. S., Cicchetti, D. V., Volkmar, F. R., & Lord, C. (2007). Communication abilities and disabilities in higher functioning individuals with autism spectrum disorders: The Vineland and ADOS. *Journal of Autism and Developmental Disorders, 37,* 748–759. doi:10.1007/s10803-006-0229-4.

Lam, K. S. L., Bodfish, J. W., & Piven, J. (2008). Evidence for three subtypes of repetitive behavior in autism that differ in familiality and association with other symptoms. *Journal of Child Psychology and Psychiatry, 49,* 1193–2000. doi:10.1111/j.1469-7610.2008.01944.x.

Lang, R., Regester, A., Lauderdale, S., Ashbaugh, K., & Haring, A. (2010). Treatment of anxiety in autism spectrum disorders using cognitive behavior therapy: A systematic review. *Developmental Neurorehabilitation, 13,* 53–63. doi:10.3109/17518420903236288.

Lecavalier, L. (2006). Behavior and emotional problems in young people with pervasive developmental disorders: Relative prevalence, effects of subject characteristics, and empirical classification. *Journal of Autism and Developmental Disorders, 36,* 1101–1114. doi:10.1007/s10803-006-0147-5.

Lecavalier, L., & Gadow, K. D. (2008). Pharmacology effects and side effects. In J. L. Matson (Ed.), *Clinical assessment and intervention for autism spectrum disorders* (pp. 221–263). New York: Elsevier.

Lecavalier, L., Gadow, K., DeVincent, C. J., & Edwards, M. C. (2009). Validation of DSM-IV model of psychiatric syndromes in children with autism spectrum disorders. *Journal of Autism and Developmental Disorders, 39,* 278–289. doi:10.1007/s10803-008-0622-2.

Lord, C., Risi, S., Lambrecht, L., Cook, E. H., Leventhal, B. L., DiLavore, P. C., Pickles, A., & Rutter, M. (2000). The autism diagnostic observation schedule-generic: A standard measure of social and communication deficits associated with the spectrum of autism. *Journal of Autism and Developmental Disorders, 30,* 205–223. doi:10.1023/A:1005592401947.

Lord, C., Petkova, E., Hus, V., Gan, W., Lu, F., Martin, D. M., et al. (2012). A multisite study of the clinical diagnosis of different autism spectrum disorders. *Archives of General Psychiatry, 69,* 306–313. doi:10.1001/archgenpsychiatry.2011.148.

MacMillan, D. L., & Speece, D. L. (1999). Utility of current diagnostic categories for research and practice. In R. Gallimore, L. P. Bernheimer, D. L. MacMillan, D. L. Speece & S. Vaughn (Eds.), *Developmental perspectives on children with high-incidence disabilities* (pp. 111–113). Mahwah: Erlbaum.

Magiati, I., Moss, J., Charman, T., & Howlin, P. (2011). Patterns of change in children with autism spectrum disorders who received community based comprehensive interventions in their pre-school years: A seven year follow-up study. *Research in Autism Spectrum Disorders, 5,* 1016–1027. doi:10.1016/j.rasd.2010.11.007.

Norris, M., & Lecavalier, L. (2010). Screening accuracy of Level 2 autism spectrum disorder rating scales: A review of selected instruments. *Autism: The International Journal of Research and Practice, 14,* 263–284. doi:10.1177/1362361309348071.

Ozonoff, S., & Cathcart, K. (1998). Effectiveness of a home program intervention for young children with autism. *Journal of Autism and Developmental Disorders, 28,* 25–32. doi:10.1023/A:1026006818310.

Palmer, R. F., Blanchard, S., Jean, C. R., & Mandell, D. S. (2005). School district resources and identification of children with autistic disorder. *American Journal of Public Health, 95,* 125–130. doi:10.2105/AJPH.2003.023077.

Perry, A., Flanagan, H. E., Geier, J. D., & Freeman, N. L. (2009). Brief report: The Vineland Adaptive Behavior Scales in young children with autism spectrum disorders at different cognitive levels. *Journal of Autism and Developmental Disorders, 39,* 1066–1078. doi:10.1007/s10803-009-0704-9.

Remington, B., Hastings, R. P., Kovshoff, H., degli Espinosa, F., Jahr, E., Brown, T., et al. (2007). Early intensive behavioral intervention: Outcomes for children with autism and their parents after two years. *American Journal on Mental Retardation, 112,* 418–438.

Research Units on Pediatric Psychopharmacology (RUPP) Autism Network (2005). Randomized, controlled, crossover trial of methylphenidate in pervasive developmental disorders with hyperactivity. *Archives of General Psychiatry, 62,* 1266–1274. doi:10.1001/archpsyc.62.11.1266.

Robins, E., & Guze, S. B. (1970). Establishment of diagnostic validity in psychiatric illness: Its application to schizophrenia. *American Journal of Psychiatry, 126,* 983–987.

Rosenberg, R. E., Mandell, D. S., Farmer, J. E., Law, J. K., Marvin, A. R., & Law, P. A. (2010). Psychotropic medication use among children with autism spectrum disorders enrolled in a national registry, 2007-2008. *Journal of Autism and Developmental Disorders, 40,* 342–351. doi:10.1007/s10803-009-0878-1.

Rutter, M., Le Couteur, A., & Lord, C. (2003). *Autism diagnostic interview—Revised.* Los Angeles: Western Psychological Services.

Sallows, G. O., & Graupner, T. D. (2005). Intensive behavioral treatment for children with autism: Four-year outcome and predictors. *American Journal on Mental Retardation, 110,* 417–438.

Schroeder, S. R., Oster-Granite, M. L., Berkson, G., Bodfish, J. W., Breese, G. R., Cataldo, M. F., et al. (2001). Self-injurious behavior: Gene-brain-behavior relationships. *Mental Retardation and Developmental Disabilities, 7,* 3–12.

Seltzer, M. M., Shattuck, P., Abbeduto, L., & Greenberg, J. S. (2004). Trajectory of development in adolescents and adults with autism. *Mental Retardation and Developmental Disabilities Research Reviews, 10,* 234–247. doi:10.1002/mrdd.20038.

Shattuck, P. T. (2006). The contribution of diagnostic substitution to the growing administrative prevalence of autism in US special education. *Pediatrics, 117,* 1028–1037. doi:10.1442/peds.2005-1516.

Shattuck, P. T., Seltzer, M. M., Greenberg, J. S., Orsmond, G. I., Bolt, D., Kring, S., Lounds, J., & Lord, C. (2007). Change in autism symptoms and maladaptive behaviors in adolescents and adults with an autism spectrum disorder. *Journal of Autism and Developmental Disorders, 37,* 1735–1747. doi:10.1007/s10803-006-0307-7.

Shattuck, P. T., Durkin, M., Maenner, M., Newschaffer, C., Mandell, D. S., Wiggins, L., et al. (2009). Timing of identification among children with an autism spectrum disorder: Findings from a population-based surveillance study. *Journal of the American Academy of Child and Adolescent Psychiatry, 48,* 474–483. doi:10.1097/CHI.0b013e31819b3848.

Siegel, M., & Beaulieu, A. A. (2012). Psychotropic medications in children with autism spectrum disorders: A systematic review and synthesis for evidence-based practice. *Journal of Autism and Developmental Disorders, 42,* 1592–1605. doi:10.1007/s10803-011-1399-2.

Simonoff, E., Pickles, A., Charman, T., Chandler, S., Loucas, T., & Baird, G. (2008). Psychiatric disorders in children with autism spectrum disorders: Prevalence, comorbidity, and associated factors in a population-derived sample. *Journal of the American Academy of Child and Adoelscent Psychiatry, 47,* 921–929. doi:10.1097/CHI.0b013e318179964f.

Skuse, D. H. (2007). Rethinking the nature of genetic vulnerability to autistic spectrum disorders. *Trends in Genetics, 8,* 387–395. doi:10.1016/j.tig.2007.06.003.

Sparrow, S. S., Cicchetti, D., & Balla, D. A. (2005). *Vineland adaptive behavior scales (2nd ed. manual).* Minneapolis: NCS Pearson.

Spiker, D., Lotspeich, L. J., Dimiceli, S., Myers, R. M., & Risch, N. (2002). Behavioral phenotypic variation in autism multiplex families: Evidence for a continuous severity gradient. *American Journal of Medical Genetics (Neuropsychiatric Genetics), 114,* 129–136. doi:10.1002/ajmg.10188.

Sukhodolsky, D. G., Scahill, L., Gadow, K. D., Arnold, E., Aman, M. G., McDougle, C. J., et al. (2008). Parent-rated anxiety symptoms in children with pervasive developmental disorders: Frequency, distribution, and association with the core autism symptoms and cognitive functioning. *Journal of Abnormal Child Psychology, 36,* 117–128. doi:10.1007/s10802-007-9165-9.

Szatmari, P., Bryson, S. E., Boyle, M. H., Streiner, D. L., & Duku, E. (2003). Predictors of outcome among high functioning children with autism and Asperger syndrome. *Journal of Child Psychology and Psychiatry, 44,* 520–528. doi:10.1111/1469-7610.00141.

Szatmari, P., Georgiades, S., Bryson, S., Zwaigenbaum, L., Roberts, W., Mahoney, W., Goldberg, J., & Tuff, L. (2006). Investigating the structure of the restricted, repetitive behaviors and interests domain of autism. *Journal of Child Psychology and Psychiatry, 47,* 582–590. doi:10.1111/j.1469-7610.2005.01537.x.

van Bokhoven, H. (2011). Genetic and epigenetic networks in intellectual disabilities. *Annual Review of Genetics, 45,* 81–104. doi:10.1146/annurev-genet-110410-132512.

van Steensel, F. J., Bogels, S. M., & Perrin, S. (2011). Anxiety disorders in children and adolescents with autistic spectrum disorders: A meta-analysis. *Clinical Child and Family Psychology Review, 14,* 302–317. doi:10.1007/s10567-011-0097-0.

Weisbrot, D. M., Gadow, K. D., DeVincent, C. J., & Pomeroy, J. (2005). The presentation of anxiety in children with pervasive developmental disorders. *Journal of Child and Adolescent Psychopharmacology, 15,* 477–496. doi:10.1089/cap.2005.15.477.

White, S. W., Oswald, D., Ollendick, T., & Scahill, L. (2009). Anxiety in children and adolescents with autism spectrum disorders. *Clinical Psychology Review, 29,* 216–229. doi:10.1016/j.cpr.2009.01.003.

Witwer, A., & Lecavalier, L. (2005). Treatment incidence and patterns in children and adolescents with autism spectrum disorders. *Journal of Child and Adolescent Psychopharmacology, 15,* 671–681. doi:10.1089/cap.2005.15.671.

Witwer, A. N., & Lecavalier, L. (2008). Examining the validity of autism spectrum disorder subtypes. *Journal of Autism and Developmental Disorders, 38,* 1611–1624. doi:10.1007/s10803-008-0541-2.

Witwer, A. N., & Lecavalier, L. (2010). Validity of comorbid psychiatric disorders in children with autism spectrum disorders. *Journal of Developmental and Physical Disabilities, 22,* 367–380. doi:10.1007/s10882-010-9194-0.

Anxiety Disorders

3

Peter Muris

Introduction

Fear and anxiety are normal phenomena that occur throughout childhood. Most children and adolescents show these emotional reactions every now and then, but normally symptoms are mild and of short duration. Many of these fears and anxieties are closely related to the specific challenges that young people face during their development towards adulthood. For example, toddlers may display clear signs of separation anxiety when they enter school for the first time, latency-aged children may worry about performance at school when they take their first tests, and adolescents invest in personal relations and thus may show fear of being rejected by their peers. In some youths, fear and anxiety symptoms are so frequent, severe, and persistent that they interfere with daily functioning. In these cases, the diagnosis of an anxiety disorder may be appropriate. This chapter will focus on anxiety disorders in children and adolescents, inasmuch as most research on the intersection of anxiety and autism has been conducted in young persons. Normal and abnormal affective experiences of fear and anxiety, and their expressions, in children and adolescents will be discussed. Special attention will be devoted to the classification of anxiety disorders as well as to their epidemiology, course, and comorbidity in youths. Next, a variety of factors will be described that have been shown to be involved in the etiology of this type of psychopathology. Finally, evidence-based treatment options for anxiety disorders will be briefly discussed.

Phenomenology

Normal Fear and Anxiety

Fear and anxiety are interchangeably used terms that refer to an innate basic emotion that, at its core, is adaptive in nature. This emotion typically involves the activation of a threat circuitry in the brain which produces a characteristic set of cognitive (anxious thoughts) and physical (increased heart rate, sweating, etc.) symptoms that lead to a defensive behavioral response (i.e., fight, flight, or freeze) that serves to protect the organism against danger and to increase the chances of survival. Sometimes, fear and anxiety are out of proportion to the actual threat posed by the stimulus or situation. This regularly occurs in young people who are still unfamiliar with a wide range of specific objects and events, and have not yet acquired adequate coping skills. Indeed, various studies have documented that children and adolescents without clinical diagnoses report a fairly large number of fears and anxieties pertaining to the themes of "danger and death" (e.g., being hit by a car), "the unknown" (e.g., the dark), "animals"

P. Muris (✉)
Department of Clinical Psychological Science, Faculty of Psychology and Neuroscience, Maastricht University, P.O. Box 616, 6200 MD, Maastricht, The Netherlands
e-mail: peter.muris@maastrichtuniversity.nl

T. E. Davis III et al. (eds.), *Handbook of Autism and Anxiety,* Autism and Child Psychopathology Series, DOI 10.1007/978-3-319-06796-4_3, © Springer International Publishing Switzerland 2014

(e.g., snakes), and "failure and criticism" (e.g., being teased; see Ollendick et al. 1989).

Research has also shown that normal fear and anxiety follow a predictable course during childhood (Marks 1987). This probably has to do with the developmental challenges posed to children and adolescents as well as the progression of cognitive abilities, which strongly guides youths' conceptualization of threat (Vasey 1993). Thus, at a very young age, fear and anxiety are primarily directed at concrete threats (e.g., loud noises, loss of physical support). As cognitive abilities develop, fear and anxiety become more sophisticated. For example, around 9 months, children learn to differentiate between familiar and unfamiliar faces and, consequently, separation anxiety and fear of strangers become manifest. Following this, fears of imaginary creatures occur and these are thought to be closely linked to the magical thinking of toddlers (e.g., Bauer 1976). Fears of animals also develop during this phase. These fears are believed to be functionally related to the increased mobility of the child and its exploration of the external world. From age 7 onwards, children are increasingly able to infer physical cause–effect relationships and to anticipate potential negative consequences. These cognitive changes broaden the range of fear-provoking stimuli and enhance the more cognitive features of anxiety (e.g., worry). Further cognitive maturation, at the beginning of adolescence, enables youths to develop fear or anxiety of more abstract, psychological threats and to misinterpret physical symptoms in a threatening way (Muris 2007).

Taken together, fear and anxiety in children and adolescents are quite prevalent and often developmentally sequenced. Although occasionally producing considerable distress, they usually dissipate within a short period of time. However, in some youths, fear and anxiety persist and become so intense that they start to interfere with daily life and functioning. These emotional symptoms then hinder the young person in his/her interactions with other people and undermine performance at school and in other domains. In these cases, fear and anxiety can no longer be consid-ered as "normal," and the diagnosis of an anxiety disorder may be warranted.

Anxiety Disorders

The latest edition of the *Diagnostic and Statistical Manual of Mental Disorders* (i.e., DSM-5; American Psychiatric Association (APA) 2013) describes various anxiety disorders which can be diagnosed in children and adolescents as well as adults. DSM-5 adopts a developmental life span perspective, which means that (a) the anxiety disorders are chronologically ordered according to their age of onset, beginning with separation anxiety disorder and concluding with panic disorder, and (b) the anxiety disorders of children and adolescents are comparable to those of adults, although the specific criteria may be slightly different (i.e., different requirements for duration, symptom expression, or symptoms count). Table 3.1 provides an overview of the main characteristics of the anxiety disorders that are listed in DSM-5, with special attention for the adjustments in the criteria made for children and adolescents. The table also indicates differences from the previous edition of the DSM (i.e., DSM-IV-TR; APA 2000).

For reasons of completeness, it should be mentioned that DSM-5 also includes substance/medication-induced anxiety disorder, anxiety disorder due to a medical condition, other specified anxiety disorders, and unspecified anxiety disorder in the anxiety disorders section. These classifications mainly "borrow" symptoms of the other anxiety disorders, have a fairly low prevalence in youths, and therefore will not be discussed further in this chapter.

It is important to note that DSM-5 no longer considers obsessive-compulsive disorder (OCD) and posttraumatic or acute stress disorder as anxiety disorders. OCD is characterized by the presence of obsessions (i.e., recurrent and persistent thoughts, urges, or images that are experienced as intrusive and unwanted) and compulsions (i.e., repetitive behaviors or mental acts that an individual feels driven to perform in response to an obsession or according to rules that must be

Table 3.1 Anxiety disorders that, according to DSM-5, can occur in children and adolescents

Anxiety disorder	Essential feature(s) in DSM-5	Difference(s) with DSM-IV-TR	Specific criteria for youths
Separation anxiety disorder	Developmentally inappropriate and excessive fear or anxiety concerning separation from those to whom the individual is attached	In DSM-IV-TR, this anxiety disorder was limited to childhood/adolescence, but according to DSM-5, this diagnosis can be made in all age groups	The disturbance must last for a period of at least 4 weeks in children and adolescents (in adults, duration is typically 6 months or longer)
Selective mutism	Consistent failure to speak in specific social situations in which there is an expectation for speaking (e.g., at school) despite speaking in other situations	In DSM-IV-TR, selective mutism was not listed as an anxiety disorder but belonged to the category of "Disorders first diagnosed in infancy, childhood, or adolescence"	–
Specific phobia	Marked fear or anxiety about a specific object or situation (e.g., flying, heights, animals, receiving an injection, seeing blood)	The DSM-IV-TR criterion "The person recognizes that the fear is excessive and unreasonable" has been changed to "The fear or anxiety is out of proportion to the actual danger posed by the specific object or situation and to the specific sociocultural context"	The fear or anxiety may be expressed by crying, tantrums, freezing, or clinging
Social anxiety disorder	Marked fear or anxiety of social situations in which the individual may be scrutinized by others in social interaction, observation, or performance situations. The individual fears that he or she will be negatively evaluated	DSM-5 covers the essential features in two separate criteria, whereas DSM-IV-TR combined these in one. Further, the "excessive and unreasonable" criterion adopts an "out of proportion to the actual threat" formulation	The anxiety must occur in peer settings and not just during interactions with adults. Further, in children, fear or anxiety may be expressed by crying, tantrums, freezing, clinging, shrinking, or failing to speak in social situations
Panic disorder	Recurrent unexpected panic attacks, which can be defined as abrupt surges of intense fear or discomfort that reach a peak within minutes, and during which physical (e.g., palpitations) and cognitive (e.g., fear of losing control or "going crazy") symptoms occur	DSM-IV-TR made a distinction between panic disorder with and panic disorder without agoraphobia. DSM-5 unlinks panic disorder and agoraphobia, which is now listed as a separate disorder	–
Agoraphobia	Marked fear and anxiety about certain situations (e.g., using public transport, being in open spaces, being in enclosed places) because of the thought that escape might be difficult or help might not be available in the event of developing panic-like symptoms or other incapacitating or embarrassing symptoms	In DSM-IV-TR agoraphobia was not codable as a separate disorder	–

Table 3.1 (continued)

Anxiety disorder	Essential feature(s) in DSM-5	Difference(s) with DSM-IV-TR	Specific criteria for youths
Generalized anxiety disorder	Excessive anxiety and uncontrollable worry (apprehensive expectation) about a number of events or activities	–	In adults, generalized anxiety disorder is accompanied by at least three symptoms (e.g., restlessness, fatigue, irritability); in children, only one of these symptoms is required

Main differences with criteria as described in the previous edition of the DSM (i.e., DSM-IV-TR; APA 2000) and specific criteria for children and adolescents are also shown
DSM Diagnostic and Statistical Manual of Mental Disorders

applied rigidly), while posttraumatic and acute stress disorders refer to a specific set of symptoms (i.e., trauma-related intrusions, avoidance of trauma-related stimuli, negative cognition and mood, and increased arousal and reactivity) that occur following exposure to one or more traumatic events, differentiated from each other on the basis of duration since trauma. Although fear and anxiety are part of the clinical picture of these disorders, they clearly share features with other mental health problems, thereby justifying their inclusion in other diagnostic categories (i.e., OCD and related disorders and trauma- and stressor-related disorders; see APA 2013).

Prevalence

Epidemiological research has shown that the prevalence of anxiety disorders in children and adolescents varies between 2 and 27 % (see Costello et al. 2004). The variation in these figures is quite large, and this is due to how prevalence is defined in the various studies. That is, the 3-month prevalence of anxiety disorders ranges between 2.2 and 8.6 %, the 6-month prevalence between 5.5 and 17.7 %, the 12-month prevalence between 8.6 and 20.9 %, and the lifetime prevalence varies between 8.3 and 27.0 %. Other variables that account for differences in the prevalence rates across studies involve the types of anxiety disorder investigated, the diagnostic instrument that was used, as well as characteristics of the population under study (e.g., age of participants; clinical vs. community sample).

A comparison of these prevalence figures with those of other psychological disorders reveals that anxiety disorders are among the most prevalent types of psychopathology among children and adolescents. For example, in a large community sample of British youths between 5 and 15 years of age, a 3-month prevalence of 3.7 % was found, indicating that anxiety disorders belonged to the top three of psychological problems in this population. Only disruptive behavior disorders (including oppositional defiant disorder, conduct disorder, and attention-deficit/hyperactivity disorder) were more prevalent. Similar results were obtained in a prospective epidemiological research carried out in the Great Smoky Mountains in the USA (Costello et al. 2003). Moreover, this study indicated that by the age of 16 the cumulative prevalence of anxiety disorders was 9.9 %, indicating that 1 out of 10 children had fulfilled the diagnostic criteria for an anxiety problem at some point during their childhood.

Estimated prevalence of the anxiety disorders in children and adolescents shows that specific phobia, social anxiety disorder, generalized anxiety disorder, and separation anxiety disorder are most common, with mean percentages varying between 2.2 and 3.6 % each. Other anxiety disorders such as agoraphobia, panic disorder, and selective mutism are less frequent among youths (< 2 %; Bergman et al. 2002; Costello et al. 2004).

Research in adults has demonstrated that there is a clear gender difference in the prevalence of anxiety disorders: Most of these problems occur more often in women than in men (APA 2013).

This gender difference is also present in children and adolescents. In the aforementioned study by Costello et al. (2003), for instance, it was found that, before the age of 16, 12.2 % of the girls had fulfilled the diagnostic criteria of any anxiety disorder, whereas this percentage was 7.7 % in boys. Other research has confirmed that the girls to boys ratio in the prevalence of anxiety disorders is about 2:1, and that this difference already emerges at a fairly young age: Around 6 years of age, these problems are already far more prevalent in girls than among boys (Lewinsohn et al. 1998).

Course, Severity, and Comorbidity

Anxiety disorders in youths typically show fairly low stability or persistence over time (Beesdo et al. 2009). For example, in a study of 1,035 German adolescents from the general population, Essau et al. (2002) found that only 22.6 % of the youths still suffered from the same type of anxiety problem at 1-year follow-up (i.e., homotypic continuity). About one third (35.5 %) had developed a new anxiety disorder or another psychological problem (i.e., heterotypic continuity; somatoform disorder, depressive disorder), while the remaining 41.9 % no longer fulfilled diagnostic criteria for a psychological disorder. However, the researchers also noted that many of the adolescents in the latter categories still had symptoms of their initial anxiety disorder. These findings seem to indicate that anxiety disorders in children and adolescents remit spontaneously although symptoms often remain in a subclinical form, and thus the disorder or a related problem may reappear at a later point during development. This notion is also supported by retrospective research of adult patients with anxiety disorders who indicate that their problem on an average had started around the age of 11 (Kessler et al. 2005), which obviously suggests that when looking over longer time periods, anxiety disorders of children and adolescents may have a chronic course.

Although anxiety disorders in youths by definition are associated with significant impairment in daily functioning (APA 2013), there is a tendency among clinicians to consider fear and anxiety problems as fairly mild (Carr 2002). Research, however, shows that this is not the case. For example, Newman et al. (1996) who followed an epidemiological sample of youths from age 11 onwards noted that, by age 21, a substantial proportion of those who had developed an anxiety disorder had sought professional help for their problem (29.5 %), used medication (9.9 %), were admitted to a psychiatric hospital (4.2 %), or had attempted to commit suicide (7.2 %). In addition, a study by Van Ameringen et al. (2003) demonstrated that anxiety disorders have a negative impact on young people's performance in school. Adult anxiety patients were interviewed about their functioning in secondary school. Almost half of the patients (49 %) reported that they had dropped out of school, and a considerable proportion of them (24 %) indicated that anxiety was the main reason for this event (Van Ameringen et al. 2003).

Comorbidity is a common phenomenon in children and adolescents with anxiety disorders. First of all, youths frequently suffer from multiple anxiety disorders. In community samples, about one in five children with an anxiety disorder are also diagnosed with a second anxiety disorder (Essau et al. 2000). In clinically referred youths, this comorbidity is even higher: in about half of these children, the primary anxiety disorder is accompanied by one or more other anxiety disorders (Kendall et al. 2001). In particular, generalized anxiety disorder, separation anxiety disorder, social anxiety disorder, and specific phobia often co-occur in children and adolescents.

Second, anxiety disorders in youths also show high comorbidity with other psychological disorders. Most notable in this regard is the co-occurrence of anxiety disorders and depression. Costello et al. (2003) found an odds ratio of 8.2, indicating that the chance for a child with an anxiety disorder to suffer from a depressive disorder is 8.2 times greater than the risk faced by a child without an anxiety disorder. This high comorbidity of anxiety disorders and depression may in part be explained by commonalities in etiology, but there is also some evidence for a temporal link between both disorders, with most of the research showing that depression arises as a secondary problem because the anxiety disorder hinders the child so much in his/her daily functioning (Seligman and Ollendick 1998).

Other comorbid problems of anxiety disorders are oppositional defiant disorder and attention-deficit/hyperactivity disorder, for which odds ratios of 3.1 and 3.0, respectively, have been found (Costello et al. 2003). Various studies have demonstrated that there is also an association between anxiety disorders and substance use disorders in adolescents, although it is also true that this relation disappears when controlling for concurrent psychological problems (Armstrong and Costello 2002). Finally, anxiety disorders frequently occur in youths with autism spectrum disorders, and this will be discussed in more detail in Chapters 7–12 of this handbook.

Etiology

Contemporary models of the etiology of anxiety disorders assume that normal and abnormal fear and anxiety are part of the same dimension (Craske 2003; Muris 2007). Accordingly, an anxiety disorder should be seen as a radicalized normal fear or anxiety, and so the critical issue is: why do fear and anxiety for most young people stay within the normative range, whereas for some children and adolescents these emotional reactions are so frequent and intense that they start to interfere with daily functioning? Research has made clear that the origins of anxiety disorders in children and adolescents cannot be attributed to a single variable. As with other types of childhood psychopathology, the principle of equifinality applies, which means that the origins of anxiety disorders in youths should be ascribed to multiple factors. The DSM-5 refers to three categories of etiological factors: temperamental, environmental, and genetic/physiological. In the following sections, examples of relevant factors for each of these categories will be examined.

Temperamental Vulnerability

Neuroticism (in the literature also known as negative affectivity or emotionality) is a basic temperamental trait that is characterized by a proneness to experience negative emotions, and is generally considered as a predisposing factor for various types of psychopathology, including the anxiety disorders (Eysenck and Eysenck 1985). The latter has been explained by the fact that neuroticism is associated with a hypersensitivity of subcortical brain areas in which the threat detection system is located (Pine 2007). Extraversion is a second temperamental factor that is relevant for the etiology of anxiety disorders. When extraversion is low, the person is more likely to display a tendency towards avoidance behavior (Eysenck and Eysenck 1985), which according to learning theorists makes an important contribution to the development and continuation of anxiety problems. A combination of neuroticism and low extraversion would constitute a temperamental vulnerability factor for developing pathological anxiety (Muris and Ollendick 2005; Nigg 2006). Interestingly, some children show this temperamental constellation at a very young age. For instance, Kagan (1994) described the typology of behavioral inhibition, which can be defined as the habitual tendency to exhibit fearfulness, restraint, and withdrawal in the face of novel events or situations, including unfamiliar rooms, toys, peers, and adults.

Research has provided support for the idea that behavioral inhibition is indeed a mixture of neuroticism and low extraversion (Muris et al. 2009) and even more importantly that youths with this temperament characteristic are at increased risk for developing anxiety disorders. In a longitudinal study, Biederman et al. (1990, 1993) followed a group of inhibited and noninhibited 3-year-old children for a period of 3 years. At the baseline assessment, inhibited children already displayed clearly more anxiety disorders than the noninhibited children, and this difference became even more prominent at the follow-up assessment. Various other studies have replicated these findings and converge on the notion that behavioral inhibition should be regarded as a temperamental vulnerability factor for the development of anxiety in problems in children and adolescents (Fox et al. 2005).

While neuroticism and (low) extraversion (and their combination, known as behavioral inhibition) increase youths' vulnerability to a broad range of anxiety problems, there are also more specific temperamental factors at work. A case in point is disgust sensitivity, which can be defined as the predisposition to experience feelings of revulsion for stimuli that convey a risk of contamination with disease, and is thought to be involved in the etiology of certain types of childhood phobias (especially animal and blood-injection-injury phobias; Muris and Merckelbach 2001). Another example is anxiety sensitivity, which refers to the fear of sensations experienced in anxiety-eliciting situations, and appears to be of particular importance for the development of panic disorder and agoraphobia during adolescence (e.g., Hayward et al. 2000).

Environmental Risk

It is widely assumed that family factors play a role in the etiology of anxiety disorders in children and adolescents (Bögels and Brechman-Toussaint 2006). A variable that seems to be relevant in this context is the bonding between parent and child. Research has shown that an early attachment relationship is predictive of anxiety problems in later childhood. For example, in their prospective study, Warren et al. (1997) examined whether insecurely attached infants run a greater risk for developing anxiety disorders than infants who are securely attached. At 12 months of age, infants were classified as either securely or insecurely attached using the "strange situation" observation procedure (Ainsworth et al. 1978). When children reached 17.5 years of age, current and past anxiety disorders were assessed by means of a structured diagnostic interview. Results indicated that insecurely attached children more frequently displayed anxiety disorders than children who were securely attached.

Other studies have examined the contribution of specific parental rearing behaviors in the development of anxiety disorders in youths. For example, there is increasing evidence that over-protective parenting plays an important role in this regard (e.g., Hudson and Rapee 2001). Parents with this parenting style are often anxious themselves, and hence try to shield their child from potential danger and distress by intrusively providing unnecessary help and restricting exposure to a broad range of situations. The net effect is that children's fears and worries are enhanced because parents increase the awareness of danger, reduce the level of perceived control, and promote avoidance behavior in their offspring.

Negative learning experiences also seem to be involved in the etiology of childhood anxiety disorders. For example, conditioning events may be important in the formation of the anxiety problem in youths. Systematic research examining the role of this environmental variable is sparse, although there is of course the widely known Little Albert case (Watson and Rayner 1920) which demonstrated that it was possible to elicit pervasive fear in an 11-month-old boy by repeatedly pairing a neutral stimulus (a white rat) with an aversive stimulus (a loud noise produced by striking a steel bar behind the boy's head). Considerably more studies have since been conducted examining the contributions of learning via modeling (Askew and Field 2007) and negative information transmission (Muris and Field 2010) in the acquisition of fear and anxiety, which may also typically occur within families (e.g., Muris et al. 1996, 2010).

Finally, stressful life events may also exacerbate fear and anxiety in children. Clinical support for this idea comes from youths who develop an adjustment disorder with symptoms of nervousness, worry, jitteriness, and/or separation anxiety after being exposed to an identifiable stressor (APA 2013). Empirical studies reveal a clear link between negative life events and fear and anxiety problems in youths. For instance, Tiet et al. (2001) demonstrated that events such as death of a family member, arguing parents, being bullied by peers, changing school, learning difficulties, and psychiatric problems of parents increase the risk for young people to develop an anxiety disorder considerably, and this appeared especially true for generalized anxiety disorder and separation anxiety disorder.

Genetic and Physiological Vulnerability

Behavioral-genetic studies have examined the genetic contribution to childhood fear and anxiety and related disorders. For example, in a recent study by Trzaskowski et al. (2012), parents of more than 3,500 twin pairs completed a questionnaire rating of their children's fear and anxiety symptoms twice, at 7 and 9 years of age. The results indicated that the influence of heritability was moderate (with an average of 54%). Further, it was found that fear and anxiety were fairly stable from 7 to 9 years and that the genetic factor explained most of the homotypic continuity of these symptoms (68%), which of course provides additional support for the notion that heritability plays a significant role. Similar results have been obtained when studying clinical anxiety symptoms in youths. Noteworthy in this regard is a study by Feigon et al. (2001) who asked the mothers of 2,043 3- to 18-year-old twin pairs to rate DSM-defined symptoms of separation anxiety disorder. Results revealed significant effects of genetics (47%). Interestingly, these effects were significantly moderated by gender and age. More precisely, the genetic influence was larger for girls and also appeared to increase as children became older. Admittedly, not all studies have obtained comparable findings, but a qualitative overview of the literature by Eley and Gregory (2004) concluded that the genetic influence on fear and anxiety problems in youths was moderate but nonetheless significant and accounted for roughly 30% of the variance.

It has been proposed that anxiety-prone children and adolescents have hyperexcitable subcortical brain circuits that promote fear and anxiety (Blackford and Pine 2012). In particular, the amygdala is considered highly important in this regard. This medial temporal brain structure is thought to be involved in the detection of threat and the initial formation of a fear/anxiety response. Evidence for the link between anxiety vulnerability and heightened amygdala sensitivity comes from a study by Grillon et al. (1997) who elicited startle responses in behaviorally inhibited and noninhibited children. Briefly, the startle reflex is thought to be an amygdala-mediated defensive response to a sudden and unexpected stimulus. Grillon et al. (1997) demonstrated greater startle responsivity in behaviorally inhibited children as compared to control children. The greater responsivity of the at risk children was not only observed for the first startle but also for the full series of startles, suggesting that these children displayed greater reactivity of the amygdala system as well as less habituation over time.

Some youths may also have a biological predisposition to react with panic and anxiety to respiratory irregularities (Klein 1993). Support for this idea comes from studies showing that children with panic and other anxiety problems more frequently display respiratory abnormalities and respond more intensely to a CO_2 challenge than control children (Pine et al. 2000). Further, there is also research showing that anxiety disorders are more prevalent among children with asthma (Katon et al. 2004).

Maintaining Variables: Avoidance and Cognitive Biases

Once children and adolescents have developed an anxiety disorder, this condition is likely to be maintained, or even intensified, by a variety of influences. The two-stage model proposed by Mowrer (1960) suggests that avoidance behavior is largely responsible for the maintenance of anxiety problems. More precisely, avoidance would minimize direct and prolonged contact with the fear-provoking stimulus or situation, and, hence, the anxious child would not have the opportunity to learn that the stimulus or situation is in fact harmless or safe. While the role of avoidance behavior in the maintenance of anxiety disorders seems self-evident (Ollendick et al. 2001), it is not the only maintenance mechanism. A number of cognitive distortions also promote prolongation of these psychopathological problems. Cognitive distortions refer to cognitive processes that are biased and erroneous, and therefore yield dysfunctional and maladaptive thoughts and behaviors. Typically, in anxiety disorders, such distortions reflect the chronic overactivity of schemas organized around themes of danger and threat (Muris and Field 2008).

One typical cognitive distortion that is involved in the anxiety disorders is attentional bias. Fearful or anxious individuals display increased attention towards (potentially) threatening stimuli (e.g., Bar-Haim et al. 2007). Attentional bias can be demonstrated by means of an experimental procedure known as the dot probe task (Vasey and MacLeod 2001). During this task, two competing stimuli (words or pictures) are briefly presented on a computer screen: one stimulus is threat-relevant, whereas the other is emotionally neutral. Following the disappearance of the stimuli, a small probe appears on the location previously occupied by one of the stimuli. The latency to identify this probe provides an index of the extent to which a child's attention was directed towards the stimulus that just disappeared. Thus, faster latencies to detect a probe following threatening stimuli relative to neutral stimuli would indicate an attention bias towards threat, whereas the opposite pattern would reflect a tendency to direct attention away from the threat. An illustrative study in children and adolescents has been conducted by Roy et al. (2008) who administered a dot probe task involving pictures of faces with threat and positive and neutral expressions to 101 young participants with generalized anxiety disorder, social anxiety disorder, and/or separation anxiety disorder and 51 nonclinical controls (all aged between 9 and 18 years). Compared to nonclinical youths, the children and adolescents with anxiety disorders displayed a greater attentional bias towards threat faces.

Another cognitive distortion that plays a role in anxiety problems is interpretation bias, which refers to the tendency to disproportionally impose threat upon ambiguous situations. An ambiguous vignette paradigm has been successfully used to demonstrate this type of bias in youths. For instance, in an early investigation by Barrett et al. (1996), children with anxiety disorders, children with oppositional defiant disorder, and nonclinical control children (aged between 7 and 14 years) were presented with brief stories of ambiguous situations and asked what would happen in each situation. Then, youths were given two possible neutral outcomes and two possible negative (threatening) outcomes and asked which outcome was most likely to occur. Results indicated that both anxious and oppositional children more frequently interpreted the ambiguous situations as threatening than normal controls. Interestingly, anxious youths more often chose avoidant negative outcomes, whereas oppositional youths more frequently chose aggressive negative outcomes.

Multifactorial Model

During the past decades, knowledge of the factors that are involved in the etiology of anxiety disorders in children and adolescents has steadily increased. This chapter has mainly focused on a number of important variables that seem to be involved. It is important to note that these etiological factors do not operate in isolation. Rather, we should consider multifactorial models in which genetic/physiological, environmental, and temperamental variables as well as resilience and protective influences (e.g., emotion regulation capacity, supportive friends and family) interact with each other to produce an adaptive or a maladaptive outcome (Vasey and Dadds 2001). An example of such a model has been provided by Muris (2007) who assumes that anxiety disorders in children and adolescents are essentially normal fears and anxieties that have radicalized due to an accumulation of risk and vulnerability which exceeds levels of resilience and protection (Fig. 3.1; see also Beesdo-Baum and Knappe 2012).

Treatment

Cognitive-Behavioral Therapy

In the case of anxiety problems, psychotherapy generally implies that youths are taught more effective ways of coping with anxious emotion and acquire more effective strategies for dealing with perceived threat. It is beyond any doubt that cognitive-behavioral therapy (CBT) is the most appropriate psychological intervention for children and adolescents with anxiety problems (March 2009; Seligman and Ollendick 2011). The main principle of CBT is exposure, which involves helping the child to gradually confront with the

Fig. 3.1 Multifactorial
model for the etiology
of anxiety disorders in
children and adoles-
cents. (Based on Muris
2007)

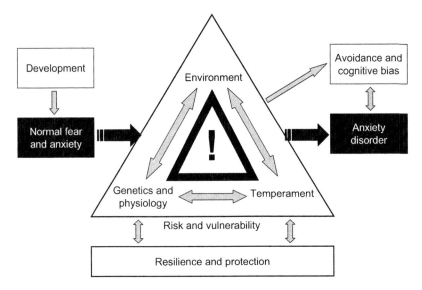

feared situations through completion of a fear
hierarchy, so that extinction of fear takes place
and avoidance or escape behavior is no longer
the dominant response (Marks 1987). Exposure
is often combined with cognitive restructuring,
which pertains to the identification and modification of dysfunctional, anxiety-promoting
thinking patterns (Beck and Emery 1985), and
various other active treatment components such
as psychoeducation, relaxation, problem-solving,
self-evaluation, and reinforcement (Albano and
Kendall 2002).

Since the pioneering work by Kendall (1994)
and Kendall et al. (1997), a host of randomized
controlled outcome studies has appeared in the
literature, all indicating that CBT is effective in
treating anxiety disorders in children and adolescents (see Rapee et al. 2009). A meta-analysis of
this research has yielded a mean Cohen's d of 0.86
for the pre- to posttreatment decrease in anxiety,
which indicates that the effect size as achieved by
this intervention can be qualified as "large" (In-
Albon and Schneider 2007). In general, about
two-thirds of the youth who complete this type
of psychotherapy no longer meet the criteria for
their principal anxiety disorder. Importantly, various studies have demonstrated that the effects
produced by CBT remain clearly visible after long
time periods of up to 10 years after treatment
(Barrett et al. 2001; Kendall et al. 2004).

The exposure and cognitive restructuring
components of CBT are appropriate for all childhood anxiety disorders, but it is important to note
that special protocols have been developed that
employ specific treatment strategies for tackling
characteristic features of the various anxiety disorders. For instance, the cognitive restructuring
component is less prominent in the treatment of
specific phobias, where the emphasis of the intervention should be on gradual real-life exposure
to the feared stimulus or situation, as is done in a
one-session therapy (Ollendick et al. 2009). CBT
can be delivered to children in an individual or a
group format, which in general have been shown
to be equally effective (e.g., Flannery-Schroeder
and Kendall 2000). Various considerations may
guide a clinician in choosing the appropriate
CBT format. In case a number of children apply
for this type of treatment, a group format could
be appropriate simply because it may be more efficient in terms of costs and time. However, an
individual treatment may still be indicated for
some children. For instance, severely trauma-
tized youth may find it difficult to discuss their
experiences, fears, and anxieties in front of other
children.

Based on the notion that family factors play
a role in the etiology of childhood anxiety problems, it is important to involve parents in the
treatment. As for controlled treatment outcome
research conducted in this domain, studies have

mainly focused on CBT-based family interventions, which primarily focus on guiding parents to help their children to handle fear- and anxiety-provoking situations in a more optimal way. Some studies have demonstrated that including parents in the intervention yields better results than a child-focused CBT and that this is especially true when parents suffer from anxiety problems themselves (e.g., Cobham et al. 1998). However, there is also research showing that the addition of a parent component does not always improve the efficacy of a CBT intervention (Nauta et al. 2003; Bodden et al. 2008). Thus, at present, there is still debate on the benefits of the inclusion of parents in CBT for anxiety-disordered youth.

Pharmacotherapy

In the past two decades, there is accumulating evidence indicating that pharmacotherapy, and in particular treatment with selective serotonin reuptake inhibitors (SSRIs), should be considered as an effective intervention for children and adolescents with anxiety disorders (March and Ollendick 2004). In a placebo-controlled trial by the RUPP Anxiety Study Group (2001), 128 children and adolescents (aged between 6 and 17 years) with separation anxiety disorder, generalized anxiety disorder, and/or social anxiety disorder were randomly allocated to a treatment with fluvoxamine or placebo for 8 weeks. Outcome was evaluated using clinician ratings of anxiety symptoms and global improvement. Results indicated that the decline in anxiety symptoms was more than three times larger in the fluvoxamine treatment group as compared to the placebo group. The majority (76%) of the children in the fluvoxamine group responded favorably to the intervention as compared to only 29% in the placebo group. Comparable findings have been obtained with other SSRIs such as sertraline (Rynn et al. 2001), paroxetine (Wagner et al. 2004), and fluoxetine (Birmaher et al. 2003).

A disadvantage of pharmacological treatment alone is that the anxiety problems tend to return once the medication is stopped (e.g., Clark et al.

2005), and therefore it is preferred to combine the pharmacotherapy with a psychological (CBT) intervention. Interestingly, an investigation by Walkup et al. (2008) even indicated that such a combined treatment may yield the most optimal results. In this large-scale multicenter study, the efficacy of sertraline, CBT, a combination of sertraline and CBT, and placebo was compared in 488 youths aged 7–17 years who had a primary diagnosis of separation anxiety disorder, generalized anxiety disorder, or social anxiety disorder. Sertraline proved to be equally effective as CBT, and both produced better treatment effects than the placebo intervention. That is, improvement rates were 54.9% for sertraline and 59.7% for CBT versus only 23.7% in the placebo condition. However, the combination of CBT and sertraline was superior to both monotherapies and by far produced the best effect with an improvement rate of 81%. Highly similar results were documented with a standardized clinician rating scale of anxiety symptoms. At the 12-week assessment, children and adolescents treated with a combination of sertraline and CBT displayed lower anxiety levels than those treated with sertraline or CBT alone, who in turn exhibited lower anxiety levels than those who had received the placebo medication.

Figure 3.2 provides a treatment algorithm for anxiety disorders in children and adolescents. It is clear that CBT has a central position in the clinical management of these disorders. In the case of specific phobias, an exposure-based intervention seems to be the initial choice because a direct correction of fear network by means of real-life experiences with the phobic stimulus is often necessary to produce the therapeutic effect (King et al. 2005). In all other childhood anxiety disorders, exposure certainly needs to be an important part of the intervention, but there is also a clear place for the cognitive restructuring component of CBT. The CBT intervention can be delivered individually or in a group, and as a child-focused or family-based program. There are no clear-cut criteria to guide clinicians in their decision of choosing the appropriate CBT format for a specific child although there is some support for the idea that children will profit more

Fig. 3.2 Treatment algorithm for children and adolescents with anxiety disorders. (Reprinted from Muris 2012). *CBT* cognitive-behavioral therapy, *SSRI* selective serotonin reuptake inhibitor

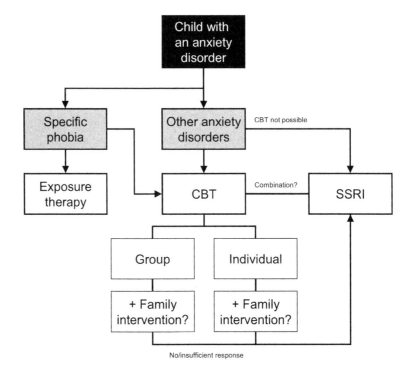

from a family-based intervention if the parents are highly anxious themselves (Cobham et al. 1998). Here, the professional view of the clinician is important, but preferences of the child and his/her parents also need to be taken into account. There are three considerations for employing pharmacotherapy, and more specifically an SSRI, in the intervention of children and adolescents with anxiety disorders: (1) when the delivery of CBT is not possible (e.g., because a cognitive-behavioral therapist is not available), (2) in case of an insufficient response to the CBT intervention, and (3) as a combination treatment with CBT for youth with severe anxiety problems and/or comorbid disorders. Obviously, the two latter considerations seem certainly relevant when treating anxious youths with autism spectrum disorders (Kolevzon et al. 2006).

Conclusions

Anxiety disorders are among the most prevalent forms of psychopathology seen in children and adolescents. Although they often change form during the course of development, fear and anxiety problems tend to run a chronic course and tend to persist into adulthood when left untreated. Moreover, anxiety disorders are associated with an increased risk for developing comorbid disorders, notably depression. With regard to etiology, there is increasing consensus on the notion that anxiety disorders have a multifactorial origin, in which temperamental, environmental and genetic/physiological risk, vulnerability, and protective variables are involved. Once an anxiety disorder exists, it is maintained by operant (avoidance) and cognitive (information processing biases) mechanisms. Anxiety disorders can be effectively treated, preferably by means of CBT, while pharmacotherapy with SSRIs should be seen as a viable alternative or additional intervention.

As noted at the beginning of this chapter, development strongly guides youths' fears and anxieties, and hence is also relevant for the study of their abnormal variations as seen in phobias and anxiety disorders. It is clear that youths with autism spectrum disorders typically show pervasive aberrations in their cognitive, emotional, and social development, and therefore the co-occurrence of anxiety problems should not come as a surprise. In upcoming chapters of this handbook, the phenomenology, etiology, and treatment of anxiety problems in youths with autism and related disorders will be highlighted.

References

Ainsworth, M., Blehar, M. C., Waters, E., & Wall, S. (1978). *Patterns of attachment: A psychological study of the strange situation.* Hillsdale: Erlbaum.

Albano, A. M., & Kendall, P. C. (2002). Cognitive behavioral therapy for children and adolescents with anxiety disorders: Clinical research advances. *International Review of Psychiatry, 14,* 129–134.

American Psychiatric Association. (2000). *Diagnostic and statistical manual of mental disorders, fourth edition-text revision.* Washington, DC: American Psychiatric Association.

American Psychiatric Association. (2013). *Diagnostic and statistical manual of mental disorders, fifth edition.* Arlington: American Psychiatric Association.

Armstrong, T. D., & Costello, E. J. (2002). Community studies on adolescent substance use, abuse, or dependence and psychiatric comorbidity. *Journal of Consulting and Clinical Psychology, 71,* 1224–1239.

Askew, C., & Field, A. P. (2007). Vicarious learning and the development of fears in childhood. *Behaviour Research and Therapy, 45,* 2616–2627.

Bar-Haim, Y., Lamy, D., Pergamin, L., Bakermans-Kranenburg, M. J., & Van IJzendoorn, M. H. (2007). Threat-related attentional bias in anxious and nonanxious individuals: A meta-analytic study. *Psychological Bulletin, 133,* 1–24.

Barrett, P. M., Rapee, R. M., Dadds, M. R., & Ryan, S. M. (1996). Family enhancement of cognitive style in anxious and aggressive children. *Journal of Abnormal Child Psychology, 24,* 187–203.

Barrett, P. M., Duffy, A. L., Dadds, M. R., & Rapee, R. M. (2001). Cognitive-behavioral treatment of anxiety disorders in children: Long-term (6-year) follow-up. *Journal of Consulting and Clinical Psychology, 69,* 135–141.

Bauer, D. H. (1976). An exploratory study of developmental changes in children's fears. *Journal of Child Psychology and Psychiatry, 17,* 69–74.

Beck, A. T., & Emery, G. (1985). *Anxiety disorders and phobias: A cognitive perspective.* New York: Basic Books.

Beesdo-Baum, K., & Knappe, S. (2012). Developmental epidemiology of anxiety disorders. *Child and Adolescent Psychiatric Clinics of North America, 21,* 457–478.

Beesdo, K., Knappe, S., & Pine, D. S. (2009). Anxiety and anxiety disorders in children and adolescents: Developmental issues and implications for DSM-V. *Psychiatric Clinics of North America, 32,* 483–524.

Bergman, R. L., Piacentini, J., & McCracken, J. (2002). Prevalence and description of selective mutism in a school-based sample. *Journal of the American Academy of Child and Adolescent Psychiatry, 41,* 938–946.

Biederman, J., Rosenbaum, J. F., Hirshfeld, D. R., Faraone, S. V., Bolduc, E. A., Gersten, M., & Reznick, J. S. (1990). Psychiatric correlates of behavioral inhibition in young children of parents with and without psychiatric disorders. *Archives of General Psychiatry, 47,* 21–26.

Biederman, J., Rosenbaum, J. F., Bolduc-Murphy, E. A., Faraone, S. V., Chaloff, J., Hirshfeld, D. R., & Kagan, J. (1993). A 3-year follow-up of children with and without behavioral inhibition. *Journal of the American Academy of Child and Adolescent Psychiatry, 32,* 814–821.

Birmaher, B., Axelson, D. A., Monk, K., Kalas, C., Clark, D. B., Ehmann, M., & Brent, D. A. (2003). Fluoxetine for the treatment of childhood anxiety disorders. *Journal of the American Academy of Child and Adolescent Psychiatry, 42,* 415–423.

Blackford, J. U., & Pine, D. S. (2012). Neural substrates of childhood anxiety disorders: A review of neuroimaging findings. *Child and Adolescent Psychiatric Clinics of North America, 21,* 501–525.

Bodden, D., Bögels, S. M., Nauta, M. H., De Haan, E., Ringrose, J., Appelboom, C., & Appelboom-Geerts, K. (2008). Child versus family cognitive-behavioral therapy in clinically anxious youth: An efficacy and partial effectiveness study. *Journal of the American Academy of Child and Adolescent Psychiatry, 47,* 1384–1394.

Bögels, S. M., & Brechman-Toussaint, M. L. (2006). Family issues in child anxiety: Attachment, family functioning, parental rearing and beliefs. *Clinical Psychology Review, 26,* 834–856.

Carr, A. (2002). *The handbook of child and adolescent clinical psychology.* New York: Brunner-Routledge.

Clark, D. B., Birmaher, B., Axelson, D., Monk, K., Kalas, C., Ehmann, M., & Brent, D. (2005). Fluoxetine for the treatment of childhood anxiety disorders: Open-label, long-term extension to a controlled trial. *Journal of the American Academy of Child and Adolescent Psychiatry, 44,* 1263–1270.

Cobham, V. E., Dadds, M. R., & Spence, S. H. (1998). The role of parental anxiety in the treatment of childhood anxiety. *Journal of Consulting and Clinical Psychology, 66,* 893–905.

Costello, E. J., Mustillo, S., Erkanli, A., Keeler, G., & Angold, A. (2003). Prevalence and development of psychiatric disorders in childhood and adolescence. *Archives of General Psychiatry, 60,* 837–844.

Costello, E. J., Egger, H. L., & Angold, A. (2004). Developmental epidemiology of anxiety disorers. In T. H. Ollendick & J. S. March (Eds.), *Phobic and anxiety disorders in children and adolescents. A clinician's guide to effective psychosocial and pharmacological interventions* (pp. 61–910). New York: Oxford University Press.

Craske, M. G. (2003). *Origins of phobias and anxiety disorders. Why more women than men?* Oxford: Elsevier.

Eley, T. C., & Gregory, A. M. (2004). Behavioral genetics. In T. L. Morris & J. S. March (Eds.), *Anxiety disorders in children and adolescents* (pp. 71–97). New York: Guilford.

Essau, C. A., Conradt, J., & Petermann, F. (2000). Frequency, comorbidity, and psychosocial impairment of anxiety disorders in German adolescents. *Journal of Anxiety Disorders, 14,* 263–279.

Essau, C. A., Conradt, J., & Petermann, F. (2002). Course and outcome of anxiety disorders in adolescents. *Journal of Anxiety Disorders, 16,* 67–81.

Eysenck, H. J., & Eysenck, M. W. (1985). *Personality and individual differences: A natural science approach.* New York: Plenum.

Feigon, S. A., Waldman, I. D., Levy, F., & Hay, D. A. (2001). Genetic and environmental influences on separation anxiety disorder symptoms and their moderation by age and sex. *Behavior Genetics, 31,* 403–411.

Flannery-Schroeder, E. C., & Kendall, P. C. (2000). Group and individual cognitive-behavioral treatment for youth with anxiety disorders: A randomized clinical trial. *Cognitive Therapy and Research, 24,* 251–278.

Fox, N. A., Henderson, H. A., Marshall, P. J., Nichols, K. E., & Ghera, M. M. (2005). Behavioral inhibition: Linking biology and behaviour within a developmental framework. *Annual Review of Psychology, 56,* 235–262.

Grillon, C., Dierker, L., & Merikangas, K. R. (1997). Startle modulation in children at risk for anxiety disorders and/or alcoholism. *Journal of the American Academy of Child and Adolescent Psychiatry, 36,* 925–932.

Hayward, C., Killen, J. D., Kraemer, H. C., & Taylor, C. B. (2000). Predictors of panic attacks in adolescents. *Journal of the American Academy of Child and Adolescent Psychiatry, 39,* 207–214.

Hudson, J. L., & Rapee, R. M. (2001). Parent–child interactions and anxiety disorders: An observational study. *Behaviour Research and Therapy, 39,* 1411–1427.

In-Albon, T., & Schneider, S. (2007). Psychotherapy of childhood anxiety disorders: A meta-analysis. *Psychotherapy and Psychosomatics, 76,* 15–24.

Kagan, J. (1994). *Galen's prophecy. Temperament in human nature.* New York: Basic Books.

Katon, W. J., Richardson, L., Lozano, P., & McCauley, E. (2004). The relationship of asthma and anxiety disorders. *Psychosomatic Medicine, 66,* 349–355.

Kendall, P. C. (1994). Treating anxiety disorders in children: Results of a randomized clinical trial. *Journal of Consulting and Clinical Psychology, 62,* 100–110.

Kendall, P. C., Flannery-Schroeder, E., Panicelli-Mindel, S., Southam-Gerow, M., Henin, A., & Warman, M. (1997). Therapy for youths with anxiety disorders: A second randomized clinical trial. *Journal of Consulting and Clinical Psychology, 65,* 366–380.

Kendall, P. C., Brady, E. U., & Verduin, T. L. (2001). Comorbidity in childhood anxiety disorders and treatment outcome. *Journal of the American Academy of Child and Adolescent Psychiatry, 40,* 787–794.

Kendall, P. C., Safford, S., Flannery-Schroeder, E., & Webb, A. (2004). Child anxiety treatment: Outcomes in adolescence and impact on substance use and depression at 7.4-year follow-up. *Journal of Consulting and Clinical Psychology, 72,* 276–287.

Kessler, R. C., Berglund, P., Demler, O., Jin, R., Merikangas, K. R., & Walters, E. E. (2005). Lifetime prevalence and age-of-onset distributions of DSM-IV disorders in the national comorbidity survey replication. *Archives of General Psychiatry, 62,* 593–602.

King, N. J., Muris, P., & Ollendick, T. H. (2005). Childhood fears and phobias: Assessment and treatment. *Child and Adolescent Mental Health, 10,* 50–56.

Klein, D. F. (1993). False suffocation alarms, spontaneous panics, and related conditions. An integrative hypothesis. *Archives of General Psychiatry, 50,* 306–317.

Kolevzon, A., Mathewson, K. A., & Hollander, E. (2006). Selective serotonin reuptake inhibitors in autism: A review of efficacy and tolerability. *Journal of Clinical Psychiatry, 67,* 407–414.

Lewinsohn, P. M., Gotlib, I. H., Lewinsohn, M., Seeley, J. R., & Allen, N. B. (1998). Gender differences in anxiety disorders and anxiety symptoms in adolescents. *Journal of Abnormal Psychology, 107,* 109–117.

March, J. S. (2009). The future of psychotherapy for mentally ill children and adolescents. *Journal of Child Psychology and Psychiatry, 50,* 170–179.

March, J. S., & Ollendick, T. H. (2004). *Phobic and anxiety disorders in children and adolescents. A clinician's guide to effective psychosocial and pharmacological interventions.* New York: Oxford University Press.

Marks, I. M. (1987). *Fears, phobias, and rituals. Panic, anxiety, and their disorders.* New York: Oxford University Press.

Mowrer, O. H. (1960). *Learning theory and behavior.* New York: Wiley.

Muris, P. (2007). *Normal and abnormal fear and anxiety in children and adolescents.* Oxford: Elsevier.

Muris, P. (2012). Treatment of childhood anxiety disorders: What is the place for antidepressants? *Expert Opinion on Pharmacotherapy, 13,* 43–64.

Muris, P., & Field, A. (2008). Distorted cognition and pathological anxiety in children and adolescents. *Cognition and Emotion, 22,* 395–421.

Muris, P., & Field, A. P. (2010). The role of verbal threat information in the development of childhood fear. "Beware the Jabberwock!". *Clinical Child and Family Psychology Review, 13,* 129–150.

Muris, P., & Merckelbach, H. (2001). The etiology of childhood specific phobias: A multifactorial model. In M. W. Vasey & M. R. Dadds (Eds.), *The developmental psychopathology of anxiety* (pp. 355–385). New York: Oxford University Press.

Muris, P., & Ollendick, T. H. (2005). The role of temperament in the etiology of child psychopathology. *Clinical Child and Family Psychology Review, 8,* 271–289.

Muris, P., Steerneman, P., Merckelbach, H., & Meesters, C. (1996). The role of parental fearfulness and modeling in children's fear. *Behaviour Research and Therapy, 34,* 265–268.

Muris, P., Bos, A. E. R., Mayer, B., Verkade, R., Thewissen, V., & Dell'Avvento, V. (2009). Relations among behavioral inhibition, Big Five personality factors, and anxiety disorder symptoms in non-clinical children. *Personality and Individual Differences, 46,* 525–529.

Muris, P., Van Zwol, L., Huijding, J., & Mayer, B. (2010). Mom told me scary things about this animal! Parents installing fear beliefs in their children via the verbal information pathway. *Behaviour Research and Therapy, 48,* 341–346.

Nauta, M. H., Scholing, A., Emmelkamp, P., & Minderaa, R. B. (2003). Cognitive-behavioral therapy for children with anxiety disorders in a clinical setting: No additional effect of a cognitive parent training. *Journal of the American Academy of Child and Adolescent Psychiatry, 42,* 1270–1278.

Newman, D. L., Moffitt, T. E., Caspi, A., Magdol, L., Silva, P. A., & Stanton, W. R. (1996). Psychiatric disorder in a birth cohort of young adults: Prevalence, comorbidity, clinical significance, and new case incidence from ages 11 to 21. *Journal of Consulting and Clinical Psychology, 64,* 552–562.

Nigg, J. T. (2006). Temperament and developmental psychopathology. *Journal of Child Psychology and Psychiatry, 47,* 395–422.

Ollendick, T. H., King, N. J., & Frary, R. B. (1989). Fears in children and adolescents: Reliability and generalizability across gender, age, and nationality. *Behaviour Research and Therapy, 27,* 19–26.

Ollendick, T. H., Vasey, M. W., & King, N. J. (2001). Operant conditioning influences in childhood anxiety. In M. W. Vasey & M. R. Dadds (Eds.), *The developmental psychopathology of anxiety* (pp. 231–252). New York: Oxford University Press.

Ollendick, T. H., Öst, L. G., Reuterskiold, L., Costa, N., Cederlund, R., Sirbu, C., & Jarrett, M. A. (2009). One-session treatment of specific phobias in youth: A randomized clinical trial in the United States and Sweden. *Journal of Consulting and Clinical Psychology, 77,* 504–516.

Pine, D. S. (2007). A neuroscience framework for pediatric anxiety disorders. *Journal of Child Psychology and Psychiatry, 48,* 631–648.

Pine, D. S., Klein, R. G., Coplan, J. D., Papp, L. A., Hoven, C. W., Martinez, J., & Gorman, J. M. (2000). Differential carbon dioxide sensitivity in childhood anxiety disorders and non-ill comparison group. *Archives of General Psychiatry, 57,* 960–967.

Rapee, R. M., Schniering, C. A., & Hudson, J. L. (2009). Anxiety disorders during childhood and adolescence: Origins and treatment. *Annual Review of Clinical Psychology, 5,* 311–341.

Roy, A. K., Vasa, R. A., Bruck, M., Mogg, K., Bradley, B. P., Sweeney, M., & CAMS team (2008). Attention bias toward threat in pediatric anxiety disorders. *Journal of the American Academy of Child and Adolescent Psychiatry, 47,* 1189–1196.

RUPP Anxiety Study Group (2001). Fluvoxamine for the treatment of anxiety disorders in children and adolescents. *New England Journal of Medicine, 344,* 1279–1285.

Rynn, M. A., Siqueland, L., & Rickels, K. (2001). Placebo-controlled trial of sertraline in the treatment of children with generalized anxiety disorder. *American Journal of Psychiatry, 158,* 2008–2014.

Seligman, L. D., & Ollendick, T. H. (1998). Comorbidity of anxiety and depression in children and adolescents: An integrative review. *Clinical Child and Family Psychology Review, 1,* 125–144.

Seligman, L. D., & Ollendick, T. H. (2011). Cognitive behavior therapy for anxiety disorders in children and adolescents. *Psychiatric Clinics of North America, 20,* 217–238.

Tiet, Q. Q., Bird, H. R., Hoven, C. W., Moore, R., Wu, P., Wicks, J., & Cohen, P. (2001). Relationship between specific adverse life events and psychiatric disorders. *Journal of Abnormal Child Psychology, 29,* 153–164.

Trzaskowski, M., Zavos, H., Haworth, C., Plomin, R., & Eley, T. C. (2012). Stable genetic influence on anxiety-related behaviours across middle childhood. *Journal of Abnormal Child Psychology, 40,* 85–94.

Van Ameringen, M., Mancini, C., & Farvolden, P. (2003). The impact of anxiety disorders on educational achievement. *Journal of Anxiety Disorders, 17,* 561–571.

Vasey, M. W. (1993). Development and cognition in childhood anxiety: The example of worry. *Advances in Clinical Child Psychology, 15,* 1–39.

Vasey, M. W., & Dadds, M. R. (2001). *The developmental psychopathology of anxiety.* New York: Oxford University Press.

Vasey, M. W., & MacLeod, C. (2001). Information-processing factors in childhood anxiety: A review and developmental perspective. In M. W. Vasey & M. R. Dadds (Eds.), *The developmental psychopathology of anxiety* (pp. 253–277). New York: Oxford University Press.

Wagner, K. D., Berard, R., Stein, M. B., Wetherhold, E., Carpenter, D. J., Perera, P., & Machin, A. (2004). A multi-center, randomized, double-blind, placebo-controlled trial of paroxetine in children and adolescents with social anxiety disorder. *Archives of General Psychiatry, 61,* 1153–1162.

Walkup, J. T., Albano, A. M., Piacentini, J., Birmaher, B., Compton, S. N., Sherill, J. T., & Kendall, P. C. (2008). Cognitive behavioural therapy, sertraline, or a combination in childhood anxiety. *New England Journal of Medicine, 359,* 2753–2766.

Warren, S. L., Huston, L., Egeland, B., & Sroufe, L. A. (1997). Child and adolescent anxiety disorders and early attachment. *Journal of the American Academy of Child and Adolescent Psychiatry, 36,* 637–644.

Watson, J. B., & Rayner, R. (1920). Conditioned emotional reactions. *Journal of Experimental Psychology, 3,* 1–14.

Other Disorders Frequently Comorbid with Autism

Marie Nebel-Schwalm and Julie Worley

Introduction

A diagnosis of an autism spectrum disorder (ASD) carries with it developmental impairments that are the major focus of treatment; therefore, it is not difficult to understand why rates of comorbid conditions are often underestimated and overlooked (Moseley et al. 2011). When they are assessed, some of the more commonly reported co-occurring disorders include intellectual disability (ID), anxiety (e.g., phobias, obsessive-compulsive disorder—OCD, panic disorder), mood (depressive disorders, bipolar disorder), attention-deficit/hyperactivity disorder (ADHD), and disruptive behavior disorders (Abdallah et al. 2011; Lord and Jones 2012; Matson and Nebel-Schwalm 2007; Mazzone et al. 2012).

The ability to accurately assess comorbid conditions among individuals with ASD can be difficult for several reasons. Individuals on this spectrum may display cognitive deficits and these include verbal abilities in general and emotional expression in particular (Stewart et al. 2006). Further, some symptoms of ASD are nonspecific to this disorder, which creates a challenge for the clinician. For example, in depression, symptoms

such as poor eye contact, restricted affect, monotonous voice, and lethargy are often observed, but these can and do occur in ASD without the presence of depression (Ghaziuddin and Zafar 2008). Therefore, efforts to clarify the prevalence and features of comorbid disorders represent an important step toward more accurate assessment and treatment planning. In the following sections, we will consider general comorbidity rates and examine commonly reported comorbid conditions. Some of these categories have been renamed in the *Diagnostic and Statistical Manual of Mental Disorders, 5th edition* (DSM-5; American Psychiatric Association 2013); therefore, specific updates are noted in these instances. The information presented here emphasizes psychological and psychiatric disorders; however, medical conditions are also discussed where relevant.

General Comorbidity Prevalence Rates

Comorbidity rates across various psychological disorders among children and adolescents with autism range from approximately 40 (Moseley et al. 2011) to 70% (Brereton et al. 2006; Simonoff et al. 2008). These studies reveal an inverse relationship between the ages of participants and comorbidity levels. A similar comorbidity pattern is seen in those with high-functioning autism and Asperger syndrome. As one illustration, Mattila et al. (2010) found higher rates of comorbidity in the younger cohort (ages 7–12 years) from a community-based sample as

M. Nebel-Schwalm (✉)
Department of Psychology, Illinois Wesleyan University, P.O. Box 2900, Bloomington, IL 61702–2900, USA
e-mail: mnebelsc@iwu.edu

J. Worley
Center for Autism Research at the Children's Hospital of Philadelphia, Philadelphia, PA, USA

T. E. Davis III et al. (eds.), *Handbook of Autism and Anxiety,* Autism and Child Psychopathology Series, DOI 10.1007/978-3-319-06796-4_4, © Springer International Publishing Switzerland 2014

compared to an older, clinic-based cohort (ages 13–16 years).

Individuals with ASD yielded higher rates of comorbidity when compared with those with ID (Brereton et al. 2006), and those with ASD had higher rates when compared with a clinical comparison group matched on age and gender (Joshi et al. 2010). In the latter study, the ASD group had higher rates of encopresis, language disorders, and anxiety disorders, but lower rates of substance use disorders (Joshi et al. 2010).

In studies of adults with ASD, but not ID, comorbidity rates ranged from 63 to 80 % (Ryden and Bejerot 2008; Ghaziuddin and Zafar 2008, respectively). Common comorbidities reported in both studies were major depressive disorder (MDD), social anxiety disorder (SAD), OCD, and ADHD. Generalized anxiety disorder (GAD; Ghaziuddin and Zafar 2008) and panic disorder (Ryden and Bejerot 2008) were also reported.

Comorbidity rates in adults with ASD and ID range from 40 to 56 % (Lunsky et al. 2009; Melville et al. 2008; Tsakanikos et al. 2011). The differences in rates may be due to various sample settings (i.e., population-, community-, clinic-, and hospital-based), type of informant (i.e., caregiver, clinician, or both), and breadth of disorders being assessed.

As previously noted, comorbidity rates appear to be lower in older samples of children and adolescents. A simple explanation is that younger children experience higher rates of comorbidity when compared with older children and adolescents. However, others have pointed out that older adolescents and adults have had more time to learn how to cope with their symptoms, receive interventions, and are more likely to take psychotropic medication for comorbid issues, thus keeping these symptoms in check (Melville et al. 2008). A final consideration is that the developmental heterogeneity among younger children and adolescents, as compared to adults, reflects a more varied symptom presentation which can hamper accurate diagnoses. Thus, with older individuals, clinicians may be better able to discern and identify patterns of co-occurring disorders, but in younger samples, these diagnoses may be premature, provisional, less accurate, and more likely to change. However, once symptoms have been assessed, we have some evidence that they do persist over time. For example, according to a study of 12-year-olds with ASD, symptoms of comorbidity persisted 4 years later despite predictions that they would decline (Simonoff et al. 2013).

Intellectual Disability

ID (formerly referred to as mental retardation) is frequently concomitant with ASD. When considering the autism spectrum as a whole, epidemiological rates of ID comorbid with ASD range from 51 to 55 % (Centers for Disease Control 2009; Charman et al. 2011), but when considering only the more severe disorders on the autism spectrum (i.e., autistic disorder), rates have been reported to be as high as 75 % (Chakrabarti and Fombonne 2005; Lainhart 1999). With the publication of the *DSM-5* and the merging of the ASD into one-dimensional category (APA 2013), rates capturing the spectrum as a whole are more useful and follow in line with clinical practice.

While rates of ID comorbid with ASD are high, indicating both low intellectual and adaptive functioning, average or above-average intellectual functioning has also been reported, albeit a smaller percentage (Charman et al. 2011). Nonetheless, children with ASD most often have below-average adaptive skills, despite their level of cognitive functioning (Bölte and Poustka 2002; Charman et al. 2011; Kanne et al. 2011). Kanne et al. (2011) examined adaptive skills in children diagnosed with ASD and the relationship of these skills with ASD symptom severity. The mean adaptive scores for children and adolescents with ASD were low across all domains (i.e., socialization, communication, and daily living skills); no significant associations emerged between observations of ASD symptom severity and adaptive functioning. Thus, these results help to highlight that even though symptoms of ASD are quite heterogeneous, individuals with ASD often perform significantly below their age level with regard to adaptive functioning skills.

Although ID and ASD are frequently comorbid, differential diagnosis remains difficult for young children and individuals who are low functioning (de Bildt et al. 2004; see Chap. 3).

Behavioral overlap between the disorders makes the distinction difficult, and this overlap is most evident in the areas of social and communication impairments, which are core diagnostic criteria of ASD and are also skills indicative of adaptive functioning. However, research has shown that standardized measures of ASD can be useful in identifying ASD symptomatology in those diagnosed with ID or other developmental delays (de Bildt et al. 2004; Trillingsgaard et al. 2005).

Even though it can be difficult to assess for the presence of ID within ASD (or vice versa), it remains important to do so for a number of reasons. First, a comorbid diagnosis may have additive effects on functioning, resulting in greater impairment (Ben Itzchak et al. 2008; Matson et al. 2009). Second, high rates of ID comorbid with ASD may impress the need to assess for additional comorbidities. For example, epilepsy has been one of the most frequently reported co-occurring medical conditions in individuals diagnosed with ASD. While it is common in ASD, the probability of developing epilepsy increases for those diagnosed with both ASD and ID (Tuchman and Rapin 2002). As another example, challenging behaviors are often concomitant with ASD and emerge at a relatively young age (Fodstad et al. 2012), and individuals with ASD typically engage in more than one problem behavior (Emerson 2001; Murphy et al. 2009). Again, there is an increased risk of problem behaviors for individuals diagnosed with both ID and ASD (Murphy et al. 2009). Unfortunately, research shows that the additive effects of comorbid ID and ASD diagnoses lead to a poorer prognosis compared to individuals with an ASD diagnosis alone (Shattuck et al. 2007). Therefore, the high prevalence rates of ID comorbid with ASD highlight the need to accurately assess for the presence of ID in this population and will aid in selecting appropriate interventions.

Attention-Deficit/Hyperactivity Disorder

Among the most debated issues in ASD, as defined in the *Diagnostic and Statistical Manual of Mental Disorders (4th Edition, Text Revision;*

DSM-IV-TR), was the exclusion of a comorbid diagnosis of ADHD (American Psychiatric Association 2000). The debate was whether symptoms of ADHD were part of the ASD diathesis (Mayes, Calhoun, Mayes, & Molitoris 2012b) or a co-occurring disorder (Frazier et al. 2001; Goldstein and Schwebach 2004; Yoshida and Uchiyama 2004). Rates of ADHD within the ASD population have been assessed and are reported to range widely from about 17 to 83 % (Frazier et al. 2001; Hanson et al. 2012; Hartley and Sikora 2009; Lee and Ousley 2006; Leyfer et al. 2006; Yoshida and Uchiyama 2004), with some suggesting that ADHD is the most common comorbid disorder of ASD (Kaat et al. 2013). Thus, it is not surprising that the *DSM-5* now allows clinicians to diagnose ADHD as a comorbid condition (APA 2013).

Despite the *DSM-IV-TR* embargo on the dual diagnosis of ASD and ADHD, researchers continued to investigate overlapping features of the two disorders by comparing scores on measures assessing for symptoms of ASD and ADHD across groups. Results suggest that children diagnosed with ASD have more symptoms of ADHD compared to typically developing children and, conversely, that children diagnosed with ADHD have more symptoms of ASD compared to typically developing children (Hattori et al. 2006). While there is some overlapping phenotypic expression as noted above, differences also exist. Hartley and Sikora (2009) conducted a study to determine which symptoms of ASD distinguished between individuals diagnosed with ASD, ADHD, and anxiety disorders. Based on parental reports during a semi-structured interview, individuals with ASD had greater impairment in nonverbal behaviors, development of friendships, repetitive and idiosyncratic language, and make-believe/imaginative play compared to those with ADHD. However, there were no differences between symptoms of seeking to share enjoyment with others, restricted interests, adherences to nonfunctional routines, stereotyped motor mannerisms, and preoccupation with parts of objects. Thus, similar to other findings, symptoms within the restricted interests and repetitive behavior domain did not differ between children diagnosed with ADHD and children diagnosed with ASD.

Given these similarities, there is a concern regarding accurate phenotyping of these disorders. Different diagnostic methods have been employed across studies, and in some cases this results in a heterogeneous group of children that may include some false-positive ASD diagnoses. Hanson et al. (2012) utilized the Autism Diagnostic Observation Schedule (ADOS; Lord et al. 2000) and Autism Diagnostic Interview-Revised (ADI-R; Lord et al. 1994) to confirm ASD diagnoses and the Child Behavior Checklist (Achenbach and Rufle 2000) and the Teacher Report Form (Achenbach 1991) to measure ADHD symptoms. ADHD symptoms were much lower in this study compared to other studies, with approximately 17 % of the children having clinically elevated scores per parent report and just under 3 % with elevated scores according to parent and teacher report. However, the latter low rate may be due in part to lack of agreement among parents and teachers, rather than a lower incidence of clinically significant ADHD symptoms per se. In contrast to the aforementioned results of Mayes et al. (2012b), Hanson and colleagues found support for the notion that ADHD and ASD are distinct disorders and that ADHD can be diagnosed as a comorbid disorder.

Many researchers agree that ASD symptomology can be distinguished from that of ADHD (Frazier et al. 2001; Hanson et al. 2012) and that the phenotypic expression of ADHD is similar in children with and without ASD (Frazier et al. 2001). Accurate assessment is imperative because children diagnosed with ASD, who also have significant symptoms of ADHD, have also been found to have greater impairment in their executive functioning and adaptive skills, worse autism symptomatology, and more maladaptive behaviors compared to children with ASD and no ADHD (Yerys et al. 2009). Identifying these symptoms will enable a child to receive appropriate treatment designed to target symptoms of ADHD, which may then increase the effectiveness of treatments designed to target core deficits associated with the ASD diagnosis (Yoshida and Uchiyama 2004).

Oppositional Defiant Disorder and Conduct Disorder

In the *DSM-5,* oppositional defiant disorder (ODD) and conduct disorder (CD) have been grouped together in "Disruptive, Impulse-Control, and Conduct Disorders," (APA 2013). Because many studies discuss both disorders together we will report on evidence regarding both ODD and CD in this section. Some researchers have reported equal rates of ODD in typically developing children and children diagnosed with ASD (Gadow et al. 2008), while others have reported significantly higher rates in children diagnosed with ASD (Mayes et al. 2012a). The percentage of children diagnosed with ASD, who meet diagnostic criteria for ODD, has been reported to be as high as 20–40 % (Gadow et al. 2004; Mayes et al. 2012a). De Bruin et al. (2007) found that symptoms associated with disruptive behavior disorders (i.e., ADHD, ODD, and CD) were the most frequently endorsed symptoms in individuals with ASD when compared to symptoms of other psychiatric disorders.

While researchers have supported the ability to diagnose ODD in children with ASD (Gadow et al. 2008), it is important that problem behaviors (e.g., verbal and physical aggression), which are frequently concomitant with ASD, are not considered diagnostic of ODD or CD in isolation of other symptomatology. Mayes et al. (2012a) examined aggressive, oppositional, and explosive behaviors in children with ASD compared to typically developing children and five psychiatric control groups (i.e., children with ADHD-combined type, ADHD-inattentive type, depression, anxiety disorder, and acquired brain injury). Children diagnosed with ASD exhibited significantly more behaviors across all three disruptive behavioral categories compared to typically developing children, and comparable rates were reported between children with ASD and children with depression. Explosive and oppositional behaviors were reported for >67 % of children with ASD; however, rates of aggressive behaviors were significantly lower at 17 %. Thus, rates of ODD symptoms are high, despite lower rates of aggressive behavior, suggesting that children are not being captured under CD/ODD solely because they exhibit problem behaviors.

In another study, Guttmann-Steinmetz et al. (2009) compared symptoms of ODD and CD across five groups of boys including typically developing children, ADHD only, ASD only, ASD and ADHD, and chronic multiple tic disorder and ADHD. First, very few differences in CD symptomatology emerged across groups; however, this can be attributed to an overall low endorsement of these symptoms. Regarding ODD, according to both teacher and parent reports, symptoms were more prevalent in boys diagnosed with ASD compared to typically developing controls. Boys with both ASD and ADHD exhibited more symptoms of ODD compared to those with ASD only. Lastly, while parent report indicated no significant differences between boys with ASD and ADHD and those with ADHD only or chronic multiple tic disorder and ADHD, teachers reported more symptoms of ODD for boys with ASD and ADHD. While research to date has shown that some children with ASD also exhibit a pattern of symptoms consistent with a diagnosis of ODD, less research has been conducted on this topic compared to the comorbidity of other psychiatric disorders with ASD. Further research is needed to fully understand this relationship.

Tic Disorders

The primary tic disorders in *DSM-5* include Tourette's disorder, persistent (chronic) motor or vocal tic disorder, and provisional tic disorder (APA 2013). Tourette's disorder is the combination of motor and vocal tics persisting beyond 1 year, whereas persistent tic disorder is a single modality tic (either motor or vocal, but not both). Provisional tic disorder includes motor and/or vocal tics that have not been present for >1 year. Rates of tic disorders among those with ASD range from 8.1 (Baron-Cohen et al. 1999) to 22 % (Canitano and Vivanti 2007). Baron-Cohen et al. (1999) suggested their rate was likely an underestimate, given their small sample of 37 participants

and because the participants were from a special school rather than a clinic. Higher estimates were reported in the following study that utilized parent and teacher ratings, rather than clinical interview. According to parental report, preschool-aged children had lower rates of tic symptoms when compared with older children (25 and 60 %, respectively; Gadow and DeVincent 2005). Parent ratings of tics did not distinguish between different subtypes of ASD (e.g., autism, Asperger syndrome, or pervasive developmental disorder not otherwise specified—PDD-NOS); however, teacher ratings of preschoolers yielded higher rates of tics for children with autism as compared to those with Asperger syndrome or PDD-NOS (61 %, 36 %, and 33 %, respectively).

Much is unknown about the etiology of tics and their relationship to ASD, but researchers have proposed a common underlying neural circuitry for tics, stereotypies, self-injurious behaviors, and compulsive behaviors (Muehlmann and Lewis 2012). Differentiating between tics and stereotypies requires careful observation and assessment. Some important features to note are the age of onset, whether they can be suppressed, and how the movements are perceived by the individual (Freeman et al. 2010; Gilbert 2006). Tics typically emerge after 3 years of age (average age of onset is 5–7 years, p. 80; APA 2013), are non-rhythmic, can be suppressed with purposeful and voluntary movements, and they are usually not viewed favorably by the individual. By contrast, stereotypies usually begin before 3 years of age, are rhythmic, can break through voluntary movements when the individual is overwhelmed or excited (Gilbert 2006), are more likely to be viewed positively, and may occur while the individual is daydreaming or recalling a favorite movie scene or video game (Freeman et al. 2010). Of course, it is possible for the individual to present with both stereotypies and tics (e.g., Ringman and Jankovic 2000).

Tics can be very disturbing to older adolescents and adults who are aware of how they are being perceived by others. Clinicians warn against raising false hope for treatment of tic disorders and caution that, at best, 25–50 % of them will be successfully suppressed with medication (Gilbert 2006). Therefore, psychoeducation is an important component in treatment in order to set realistic expectations.

Sleep Disorders

Primary sleep disorders in the *DSM-5* include dyssomnias (i.e., insomnia, hypersomnia, narcolepsy, breathing-related sleep disorder, and circadian rhythm sleep disorder) and parasomnias (i.e., nightmares, sleep terrors, and sleepwalking disorders). Most of the studies presented in this section report on aspects of insomnia, including delayed sleep latency, night wakings, decreased sleep efficiency, and daytime sleepiness (APA 2013). Sleep disturbances in children with ASD have been well-documented and are consistently reported to be higher than in their typically developing peers (e.g., Krakowiak et al. 2008; Park et al. 2012; Sounders et al. 2009) and even higher than in developmentally delayed individuals (Krakowiak et al. 2008). In a population-based study of 2–5-year-olds, 53 % of children with ASD, 46 % of those with a developmental disability, and 32 % of typically developing children reported sleep problems (Krakowiak et al. 2008). Sounders et al. (2009) found a similar pattern of sleep problems with 4–10-year-olds using actigraphy (a wristwatch-like monitor of movement). The majority of children with an ASD (67 %) had sleep problems as compared to typically developing children (47 %). In an older sample whose age range was 4–15 years, rates of sleep problems were 47 and 20 % among those with an ASD and typically developing children, respectively (Park et al. 2012). A breakdown by diagnostic status revealed that 75 % of children with autism and Asperger syndrome had a sleep disturbance as compared to 52.4 % of those with PDD-NOS (Sounders et al. 2009). Overall, percentages of those on the autism spectrum with sleep problems typically range from 50 to 80 % (Richdale and Schreck 2009; Williams et al. 2004) and the pervasiveness of sleep problems has caused some to consider it part of the autism symptom complex (Mayes and Calhoun 2009).

Reliable assessment is an important part of diagnosing sleep disorders. The accuracy of parent reports of sleep problems is largely supported by objective measures such as actigraphy and polysomnography, but underestimations have been noted. For example, in one study with 59 children, parents reported sleep duration to be 9.8 hours on average as compared to an average of 7.8 hours according to the actigraphy results (Sounders et al. 2009). Even among adults with ASD who do not complain of sleep problems, laboratory measures (i.e., polysomnography) have documented qualitative sleep deficits (Limoges et al. 2013). A study on adolescents and young adults (ages 15–25 years) found that actigraphy results reported more sleep problems when compared with parent or caretaker report (Oyane and Bjorvatn 2005), suggesting that underreporting may be more a function of adaptation to sleep problems than an accurate portrayal of symptoms. This highlights the need for clinicians to carefully assess the quality of sleep even if the individual (or caretaker) is not spontaneously reporting difficulties.

Once identified, sleep problems have been shown to persist, although they may change with development (Goldman et al. 2012). Younger children are more likely to have difficulties with bedtime resistance (e.g., intense tantrums), sleep anxiety, and night wakings (Krakowiak et al. 2008; Goldman et al. 2012), whereas older children have more problems with falling sleep and daytime sleepiness (Goldman et al. 2012). Adults on the spectrum suffer from delayed sleep latency, daytime sleepiness, and frequent night wakings (Matson et al. 2008). When comparing adults who have comorbid ASD and ID with adults who have ID only, 45 % of those in the former group had sleep problems as compared to 14 % in the latter group.

The impact of poor sleep in children with an ASD on parents has been noted, particularly the adverse effects of children's sleep problems on maternal well-being (Park et al. 2012). Hodge et al. (2013) found that mothers of children with ASD reported more sleep problems for their children and themselves and parenting stress than mothers of typically developing children, and children's sleep problems were significantly correlated with maternal mental health. It follows, therefore, that the accurate assessment and treatment of sleep problems and sleep disorders has benefits beyond the targeted client and may reduce parental stress.

Feeding Disorders

Feeding disorders are not exclusive to children diagnosed with ASD; however, they tend to be reported at higher rates compared to typically developing children (TDC), with rates reported as high as 67–75 % (Martins et al. 2008; Schreck et al. 2004). Although symptoms related to feeding disorders are not inherent to the diagnostic definition of ASD, some researchers (e.g., Ahearn et al. 2001; Martins et al. 2008) have attempted to subsume feeding difficulties under the *DSM-IV-TR* diagnostic criterion for ASD (APA 2000). A new diagnostic criterion has been added to the *DSM-5* definition of ASD, hypersensitivity or hyposensitivity to sensory stimuli, which may capture feeding difficulties related to food texture or type sensitivities (APA 2013).

While children with ASD exhibit various feeding difficulties (e.g., low food acceptance, food selectivity), relatively few studies have included a control group of typically developing children for comparison (e.g., Ahearn et al. 2001). Schreck et al. (2004) conducted one of the first studies that included a control group of typically developing children, and results indicate that parents of children with ASD reported significantly more feeding problems compared to the reports of parents of children who were typically developing. Almost 75 % of children with ASD were reported to have a restricted diet, and they were more likely to refuse food, require specific utensils while eating, and to only accept foods that were prepared at a lower texture (i.e., pureed food).

Many potential explanations for the high comorbidity between ASD and feeding problems have been proposed. For example, feeding problems can be a manifestation of ASD diagnostic criteria (Ahearn et al. 2001; Martins et al. 2008),

be related to family eating habits (Martins et al. 2008; Schreck and Williams 2006), stem from aversions to different sensory stimuli (Martins et al. 2008), or develop from oral-motor difficulties or medical problems such as reflux, eosinophilic esophagitis, or dysphagia (Manikam and Perman 2000; Nadon et al. 2011). Aside from the etiological theories, parents often respond in a way that perpetuates mealtime problem behavior through reinforcement (e.g., coaxing their children to take a bite, removing unwanted food from the child's plate; Borrero et al. 2010) and by exhibiting emotional reactions to problems during mealtimes (Martins et al. 2008).

Some researchers have looked at the potential environmental influences on the child's mealtime behaviors. For example, Nadon et al. (2011) utilized a comparison group comprised of typically developing siblings in an effort to control for environmental factors on problematic eating behaviors. Results indicated that children with ASD as a group had significantly more mealtime problems compared to the group of typically developing siblings, with food selectivity being the most commonly reported problem. Other mealtime problems rated as significantly worse compared to their siblings included staying in their seat during mealtimes, eating at the family table, eating an adequate number of meals, tolerating novel foods on their plate, refusing previously accepted foods, refusal to try novel foods, texture selectivity, and temperature selectivity. Thus, results suggested no significant familial impact on feeding problems.

With regard to potential medical causes, feeding difficulties may emerge and serve as an indicator of underlying gastrointestinal (GI) problems or disorders such as reflux, aspiration, or dysphagia (Manikam and Perman 2000). GI problems have been reported in a high number of children with ASD (Horvath and Perman 2002; Kuddo and Nelson 2003), and they have the potential to cause mealtime problems, which may result in conflict between parent and child. For example, reflux may lead to vomiting or gagging, and in an effort to avoid these consequences, children may begin to refuse food. Mealtime problem behaviors exacerbate following continued efforts (e.g., coaxing) by parents to get their child to accept food (Manikam and Perman 2000). This highlights the fact that medical factors should be assessed prior to initiating treatment of food refusal or selectivity.

The impact of feeding disorders can be substantial. They often emerge at a very young age, frequently when transitioning from pureed to higher textured foods, and can continue without sufficient intervention (Williams et al. 2005). Researchers have reported that many children with ASD will not eat outside of their home environment (e.g., at school), which can be stressful for parents and present nutritional concerns (Nadon et al. 2011). Families often have to make multiple meals in an effort to satisfy the nutritional needs of the family while satisfying the selective requests of the child (Nadon et al. 2011). Thus, intervention is not only beneficial for the child but also for the family unit as a whole.

Elimination Disorders

Self-care skills are critical when considering quality of life issues, and among these, toileting skills rank very high. Thus, comorbid elimination disorders can present significant barriers to quality of life for individuals and their caretakers (Rinald and Mirenda 2012). Elimination disorders in the *DSM-5* form their own category and include enuresis, encopresis, other specified elimination disorder and unspecified elimination disorder (APA 2013). In a medical clinic-based study of children and adolescents in general, prevalence estimates for enuresis (nocturnal, diurnal, or both) was 10.5% and encopresis (with or without constipation) was 4.4% (Loening-Baucke 2007). This is comparable to the rates cited in the *DSM-IV-TR* and *DSM-5* for enuresis (5–10% among 5-year-olds with lower rates for older children) and higher than the rate of 1% for encopresis (APA 2000, 2013). When comparing children with ASD with typically developing children, in one study, 18.4% of those with ASD and 2.5% of those without ASD had enuresis (van Tongerloo et al. 2012). Among encopretic individuals in general, it is estimated that 80%

or more have constipation (also called retentive subtype); however, some argue that the subtype without accompanying constipation (called nonretentive) is more common among those with ASD (Radford and Anderson 2003). Although both subtypes of voiding can be involuntary or intentional, nonretentive encopresis may more often be associated with oppositionality (APA 2013). Successful toileting requires many skills such as proper bodily sensory perception, fine motor skills, communication skills, social awareness, and complex behavioral sequencing. For individuals with ASD, each of these areas can present a significant challenge (Radford and Anderson 2003). In addition to these, fear, anxiety, and pain may contribute to difficulties in obtaining appropriate toileting skills (Dalrymple and Ruble 1992; Radford and Anderson 2003). Some have noted that given the myriad requirements needed for these skills, it is a wonder that more individuals do not have problems (Radford and Anderson 2003). Among individuals with ASD, greater verbal impairments and lower cognitive abilities were correlated with later age of onset of toilet training and longer length of time needed for successful completion (Dalrymple and Ruble 1992). The average duration of urine training (1.6 years) and bowel training (2.1 years) for these individuals extended for such a long period of time that researchers suggested parents wait until 4 years of age to begin urine training and 4.5 years of age to begin bowel training (except when a child shows interest at an earlier age; Dalrymple and Ruble 1992).

Depressive Disorders

Mood disorders have been separated into two categories in the *DSM-5*: depressive disorders and bipolar and related disorders (APA 2013). Changes made to depressive disorders in the *DSM-5* include the addition of disruptive mood dysregulation disorder and premenstrual dysphoric disorder, a revised persistent depressive disorder (which includes dysthymia and chronic major depression), and the elimination of the bereavement exclusion when diagnosing MDD

(Wakefield 2013). In this section, we will focus on MDD and dysthymic disorder (as previously defined in the *DSM-IV-TR*; APA 2000).

Across the age span, older individuals with ASD have higher rates of depression when compared with younger individuals (Simonoff et al. 2012). Prevalence rates among adults range from 37 to 70 % (Ghaziuddin and Greden 1998; Lugnegard et al. 2011). Diagnostic rates of depressive disorders among children range from 1.4 (Simonoff et al. 2008) to 10 % (Leyfer et al. 2006).

Individuals with less severe symptoms of social impairment and higher cognitive ability are at greater risk for developing depression (Sterling et al. 2008). In school-aged children, higher-functioning youth are more likely to have mainstream classroom experiences and face more frequent and difficult social demands (Mayes et al. 2011). Also, higher-functioning individuals perceive more social rejection and negative peer interactions and report more victimization, more conflict with friends, and more interpersonal conflict with family members (Magnuson and Constantino 2011).

It is challenging to accurately assess depression in the ASD population because core deficits of ASD often lend themselves to impaired abilities of expression. These include verbal abilities in general and emotional expression in particular (Perry et al. 2001). Also, lower-functioning individuals may lack insight; thus, the assessment of a mood disorder may depend on observable and behavioral symptoms. Unfortunately, clinicians may misattribute these symptoms to behavioral rather than mood-disordered etiologies (Lainhart and Folstein 1994).

A complicating issue is that behaviors associated with depression can occur at higher rates in the ASD population (e.g., changes in mood, sleep, and activity levels). These higher base rates make the detection of actual depressive symptoms more difficult because the observer must notice change in intensity rather than the emergence of a symptom. Thus, having an accurate sense of the individual's baseline functioning is critical for an accurate diagnosis of depression (Lainhart and Folstein 1994).

Some of the noted observable symptoms that could indicate depression in this population include increases in aggression, irritability, and stereotypies (Perry et al. 2001); screaming and social isolation (Clarke and Gomez 1999); and self-injurious behaviors (Magnuson and Constantino 2011). Also, decreases in certain behaviors, such as decreased involvement in a restricted interest (Perry et al. 2001), reduced communication, reduced mobility, and a decline in self-care skills (Clarke and Gomez 1999; Magnuson and Constantino 2011), may point to a mood disorder. Unfortunately, depressive disorders can be extremely impairing for the individual and his or her family members. Kim et al. (2000) found that individuals with ASD and comorbid depressive symptoms had poorer relationships with teachers, peers, and family members. Further, families of these individuals report lower quality of life and higher rates of depression among parents (Kim et al. 2000; van Tongerloo et al. 2012). Thus, proper assessment and an accurate understanding of how depressive disorders are manifested in this population could improve the quality of life for the individual and his or her family members.

Bipolar and Related Disorders

Information about prevalence rates of bipolar and related disorders as compared to depressive disorders among those with ASD is lacking. Some studies with clinic-referred samples of children and adolescents with ASD have reported rates ranging from 21 (Wozniak et al. 1997) to 27 % (Munesue et al. 2008). In both cases, typically developing control groups were used, and bipolar disorders were higher for individuals with an ASD compared to those without. A lower estimate was reported in an epidemiological survey that assessed mood problems among those with ID (Bradley and Bolton 2006). They identified 36 matched pairs of teenagers (one with ASD and the other without) who were matched on sex, age, and IQ. Two individuals with ASD and none without ASD had a bipolar disorder diagnosis. This translates to a 5.5 % comorbidity rate, which is significantly lower than previously mentioned estimates. Differences in estimates could be due to sample characteristics (i.e., epidemiological vs. clinic-referred samples) and diagnostic methodology (i.e., standardized methods, such as the ADI-R, vs. less standardized methods). More information is needed to clarify the prevalence of bipolar disorders and whether ASD increases the risk of comorbidity (Simonoff et al. 2012).

Varied ways of conceptualizing mania in this population have led to assessment difficulties. Also, it is possible that clinicians are overlooking manic symptoms to a large degree (Munesue et al. 2008). Many of the studies previously mentioned reported cases with hypomania; thus, a more subtle presentation requires careful assessment and may be more likely to escape recognition or be attributed to other causes. There are important treatment implications when clinicians misattribute mood disturbances to a depressive disorder rather than a bipolar disorder; antidepressants can trigger a manic episode and are not the first line of treatment for bipolar disorders (Henry et al. 2001).

Suicidality

Suicide is one of the most disconcerting circumstances highly correlated with mood disorders in the typically developing population. Although it is not currently considered a disorder per se, suicidal behavior disorder has been included in conditions for further study in the *DSM-5* (APA 2013). Underreporting of suicide is a common problem, but even less is known about how this risk is manifested in those with ASD. Some studies have attempted to determine the prevalence of suicidality among developmentally delayed individuals. One such study on hospitalized developmentally delayed children found 20% reported suicidal ideation, behavior, or attempts; however, having an ASD lowered the prevalence of these symptoms to 12.5% (Hardan and Sahl 1999). Differences were also noted depending on the ASD diagnosis one had. Those with an autism diagnosis had a lower incidence of ideation and behaviors than those with a PDD-NOS diagnosis (8 vs. 15%, respectively). The authors in that

case concluded that a diagnosis of autism was associated with a lower risk of suicide.

By contrast, a much higher rate was reported in a study of clinic-referred adults with ASD. In this case, 46% of the sample had suicidal ideation, attempts, or, in a few cases, completed suicides (Raja et al. 2011). The authors cautioned that the presence of ASD can make evaluation of comorbidity more difficult, particularly when verbal delays are present. The lack of adequate language for communication can mask emotional turmoil and make suicidal risk more difficult to assess. The individual may be portraying a calmer demeanor than is actually the case. Further, issues of self-harm and self-injury can be difficult to tease apart from suicidal behaviors because the intent of the behavior can be hard to discern. These obstacles highlight the need for clinicians to remain vigilant for signs of suicide in those with ASD.

Conclusions

Unfortunately, individuals with ASD experience significant distress due to core features of their disorder and, in many cases, co-occurring disorders. Underreporting of comorbidities in this population is common, yet, when they have been reported, prevalence rates are higher as compared to typically developing peers and, in some cases, psychiatric control groups. Our relatively poor understanding of comorbidities in this population has been aided by the phenotypic heterogeneity of ASD and the varied manifestations of comorbid conditions as compared to typically developing individuals. This further complicates the clinical picture and heightens the need for clarity and rigor regarding assessment. In some cases, we have seen attempts to clarify how various comorbid disorders may be uniquely expressed among those with ASD, but more work is needed. Our efforts in these areas will not only improve our ability to accurately identify comorbidities but will also aid efforts toward developing and implementing effective treatments for the betterment of these individuals and their families.

References

Abdallah, M. W., Greaves-Lord, K., Grove, J., Norgaard-Pedersen, B., Hougaard, D. M., & Mortensen, E. L. (2011). Psychiatric comorbidities in autism spectrum disorders: Findings from a Danish historic birth cohort. *European Child & Adolescent Psychiatry, 20,* 599–601. doi:10.1007/200787-011-0220-2.

Achenbach, T. (1991). *Manual for teacher's report form and 1991 profile.* Burlington: University of Vermont, Department of Psychiatry.

Achenbach, T. M., & Rufle, T. M. (2000). The child behavior checklist and related forms for assessing behavioral/emotional problems and competencies. *Pediatrics in Review, 21,* 265–271.

Ahearn, W. H., Castine, T., Nault, K., & Green, G. (2001). An assessment of food acceptance in children with autism or pervasive developmental disorders-not otherwise specified. *Journal of Autism and Developmental Disorders, 31,* 505–511.

American Psychiatric Association. (2000). *Diagnostic and statistical manual of mental disorders-text revision* (4th ed.). Washington, DC: American Psychiatric Association.

American Psychiatric Association. (2013). *Diagnostic and statistical manual of mental disorders* (5th ed.). Washington, DC: American Psychiatric Association.

Baron-Cohen, S., Mortimore, C., Moriarty, J., Izaguirre, J., & Robertson, M. (1999). The prevalence of Gilles de la Tourette's syndrome in children and adolescents with autism. *Journal of Child Psychology and Psychiatry, 40,* 213–218.

Ben Itzchak, E., Lahat, E., Burgin, R., & Zachor, A. D. (2008). Cognitive, behavior, and intervention outcome in young children with autism. *Research in Developmental Disabilities, 29,* 447–458.

Bölte, S., & Poustka, F. (2002). The relation between general cognitive level and adaptive behavior domains in individuals with autism with and without comorbid mental retardation. *Child Psychiatry and Human Development, 33,* 165–172.

Borrero, C. S. W., Woods, J. N., Borrero, J. C., Masler, E. A., & Lesser, A. D. (2010). Descriptive analysis of pediatric food refusal and acceptance. *Journal of Applied Behavior Analysis, 43,* 71–88.

Bradley, E., & Bolton, P. (2006). Episodic psychiatric disorders in teenagers with learning disabilities with and without autism. *British Journal of Psychiatry, 189,* 361–366. doi:10.1192/bjp.bp.105.018127.

Brereton, A. V., Tonge, B. J., & Einfeld, S. L. (2006). Psychopathology in children and adolescents with autism compared to young people with intellectual disability. *Journal of Autism and Developmental Disorders, 36,* 863–870. doi:10.1007/s10803-006-0125-y.

Canitano, R., & Vivanti, G. (2007). Tics and Tourette syndrome in autism spectrum disorders. *Autism: The International Journal of Research and Practice, 11,* 19–28. doi:10.1177/1362361307070992.

Centers for Disease Control (2009). Prevalence of autism spectrum disorders: Autism and developmental disabilities monitoring network, United States, 2006. *MMWR Surveillance Summaries, 58,* 1–20.

Chakrabarti, S., & Fombonne, E. (2005). Pervasive developmental disorders in preschool children: Confirmation of high prevalence. *American Journal of Psychiatry, 162,* 1133–1141.

Charman, T., Pickles, A., Simonoff, E., Chandler, S., Loucas, T., & Baird, G. (2011). IQ in children with autism spectrum disorders: Data from the Special Needs and Autism Project (SNAP). *Psychological Medicine, 41,* 619–627. doi:10.1017/S0033291710000991.

Clarke, D. J., & Gomez, G. A. (1999). Utility of modified DCR-10 criteria in the diagnosis of depression associated with intellectual disability. *Journal of Intellectual Disability Research, 43,* 413–420.

Dalrymple, N. J., & Ruble, L. A. (1992). Toilet training and behaviors of people with autism: Parent views. *Journal of Autism and Developmental Disorders, 22,* 265–275.

de Bildt, A., Sytema, S., Ketelaars, C., Kraijer, D., Mulder, E., Volkmar, F., & Minderaa, R. (2004). Interrelationship between Autism Diagnostic Observation Schedule-Generic (ADOS-G), Autism Diagnostic Interview-Revised (ADI-R), and the Diagnostic and Statistical Manual of Mental Disorders (DSM-IV-TR) classification in children and adolescents with mental retardation. *Journal of Autism and Developmental Disorders, 34,* 129–137.

De Bruin, E. L., Ferdinand, R. F., Meester, S., De Nijs, P., & Verheij, F. (2007). High rates of psychiatric comorbidity in PDD-NOS. *Journal of Autism and Developmental Disorders, 37,* 877–886.

Emerson, E. (2001). *Challenging behavior: Analysis and intervention in people with severe intellectual disabilities* (2nd ed.). Cambridge: Cambridge University Press.

Fodstad, J. C., Rojahn, J., & Matson, J. L. (2012). Emergence of challenging behaviors in at-risk toddlers with and without autism spectrum disorder: A cross-sectional study. *Journal of Developmental and Physical Disabilities, 24,* 217–234.

Frazier, J. A., Biederman, J., Bellordre, C. A., Garfield, S. B., Geller, D. A., Coffey, B. J., & Faraone, S. V. (2001). Should the diagnosis of attention-deficit/hyperactivity disorder be considered in children with pervasive developmental disorder? *Journal of Attention Disorders, 4,* 203–211.

Freeman, R. D., Soltanifar, A., & Baer, S. (2010). Stereotypic movement disorder: Easily missed. *Developmental Medicine & Child Neurology, 52,* 733–738. doi:10.1111/j.1469-8749.2010.03627.x.

Gadow, K. D., & DeVincent, C. J. (2005). Clinical significance of tics and attention-deficit hyperactivity disorder (ADHD) in children with pervasive developmental disorder. *Journal of Child Neurology, 20,* 481–488.

Gadow, K. D., DeVincent, C. J., Pomeroy, J., & Azazian, A. (2004). Psychiatric symptoms in preschool children with PDD and clinic comparison samples. *Journal of Autism and Developmental Disorders, 34,* 379–393.

Gadow, K. D., DeVincent, C. J., & Drabick, D. A. G. (2008). Oppositional defiant disorder as a clinical phenotype on children with autism spectrum disorders.

Journal of Autism and Developmental Disorders, 38, 1302–1310.

Ghaziuddin, M., & Greden, J. (1998). Depression in children with autism/pervasive developmental disorders: A case-control family history study. *Journal of Autism and Developmental Disorders, 28,* 111–115.

Ghaziuddin, M., & Zafar, S. (2008). Psychiatric comorbidity of adults with autism spectrum disorders. *Clinical Neuropsychiatry, 5,* 9–12.

Gilbert, D. (2006). Treatment of children and adolescents with tics and Tourette syndrome. *Journal of Child Neurology, 21,* 690–700. doi:10.2310/7010.2006.00161.

Goldman, S. E., Richdale, A. L., Clemons, T., & Malow, B. A. (2012). Parental sleep concerns in autism spectrum disorders: Variations from childhood to adolescence. *Journal of Autism and Developmental Disorders, 42,* 531–538. doi:10.1007/s10803-011-1270-5.

Goldstein, S., & Schwebach, A. (2004). The comorbidity of pervasive developmental disorder and attention deficit hyperactivity disorder: Results of a retrospective chart review. *Journal of Autism and Developmental Disorders, 34,* 329–339.

Guttmann-Steinmetz, S., Gadow, K. D., & DeVincent, C. J. (2009). Oppositional defiant and conduct disorder behaviors in boys with autism spectrum disorder with and without attention-deficit hyperactivity disorder versus several comparison samples. *Journal with Autism and Developmental Disorders, 39,* 976–985.

Hanson, E., Cerban, B. M., Slater, C. M., Caccamo, L. M., Bacic, J., & Chan, E. (2012). Brief report: Prevalence of attention deficit/hyperactivity disorder among individuals with an autism spectrum disorder. *Journal of Autism and Developmental Disorders, 43,* 1459–1464.

Hardan, A., & Sahl, R. (1999). Suicidal behavior in children and adoelscents with developmental disorders. *Research in Developmental Disabilities, 20,* 287–296.

Hartley, S. L., & Sikora, D. M. (2009). Which DSM-IV-TR criteria best differentiate high-functioning autism spectrum disorder from ADHD and anxiety disorders in older children? *Autism: The International Journal of Research and Practice, 13,* 485–509.

Hattori, J., Ogino, T., Abiru, K., Nakano, K., Oka, M., & Ohtsuka, Y. (2006). Are pervasive developmental disorders and attention-deficit/hyperactivity disorder distinct disorders. *Brain & Development, 28,* 371–374.

Henry, C., Sorbara, F., Lacoste, J., Gindre, C., & Leboyer, M. (2001). Antidepressant-induced mania in bipolar patients: Identification of risk factors. *Journal of Clinical Psychiatry, 62,* 249–255.

Hodge, D., Hoffman, C. D., Sweeney, D. P., & Riggs, M. L. (2013). Relationship between children's sleep and mental health in mothers of children with and without autism. *Journal of Autism and Developmental Disorders, 43,* 956–963. doi:10.1007/s10803-012-1639-0.

Horvath, K., & Perman, J. A. (2002). Autism and gastrointestinal symptoms. *Current Gastroenterology Reports, 4,* 251–258.

Joshi, G., Petty, C., Wozniak, J., Henin, A., Fried, R., Galdo, M., et al. (2010). The heavy burden of psychiatric comorbidity in youth with autism spectrum disorders: A large comparative study of psychiatrically

referred population. *Journal of Autism and Developmental Disorders, 40,* 1361–1370. doi:10.1007/s10803-010-0996-9.

Kaat, A. J., Gadow, K. D., & Lecavalier, L. (2013). Psychiatric symptom impairment in children with autism spectrum disorders. *Journal of Abnormal Child Psychology.* Advance Online Publication. doi:10.1007/s10802-013-9739-7.

Kanne, S. M., Gerber, A. J., Quirmbach, L. M., Sparrow, S. S., Cicchetti, D. V., & Saulnier, C. A. (2011). The role of adaptive behavior in autism spectrum disorders: Implications for functional outcome. *Journal of Autism and Developmental Disorders, 41,* 1007–1018.

Kim, J. A., Szatmari, P., Bryson, S. E., Streiner, D. L., & Wilson, F. J. (2000). The prevalence of anxiety and mood problems among children with autism and Asperger syndrome. *Autism: The International Journal of Research and Practice, 4,* 117–132.

Krakowiak, P., Goodlin-Jones, B., Hertz-Picciotto, I., Croen, L. A., & Hansen, R. L. (2008). Sleep problems in children with autism spectrum disorders, developmental delays, and typical development: A population-based study. *Journal of Sleep Research, 17,* 197–206. doi:10.1111/j.1365-2869.2008.00650.x.

Kuddo, T., & Nelson, K. B. (2003). How common are gastrointestinal disorders in children with autism? *Current Opinions in Pediatrics, 15,* 339–343.

Lainhart, J. E. (1999). Psychiatric problems in individuals with autism, their parents and siblings. *International Review of Psychiatry, 11,* 278–298.

Lainhart, J. E., & Folstein, S. E. (1994). Affective disorders in people with autism: A review of published cases. *Journal of Autism and Developmental Disorders, 24,* 587–601.

Lee, D. O., & Ousley, O. Y. (2006). Attention-deficit hyperactivity disorder symptoms in a clinic sample of children and adolescents with pervasive developmental disorders. *Journal of Child and Adolescent Psychopharmacology, 16,* 737–746.

Leyfer, O. T., Folstein, S. E., Bacalman, S., Davis, N. O., Dihn, E., Morgan, J., et al. (2006). Comorbid psychiatric disorders in children with autism: Interview development and rates of disorders. *Journal of Autism and Developmental Disorders, 36,* 849–861. doi:10.1007/s10803-006-0123-0.

Limoges, E., Bolduc, C., Berthiaume, C., Mottron, L., & Godbout, R. (2013). Relationship between poor sleep and daytime cognitive performance in young adults with autism. *Research in Developmental Disabilities, 34,* 1322–1335. doi:10.1016/j.ridd.2013.01.013.

Loening-Baucke, V. (2007). Prevalence rates for constipation and fecal and urinary incontinence. *Archives of Disease in Childhood, 92,* 486–489. doi:10.1136/adc.2006.098335.

Lord, C., & Jones, R. M. (2012). Annual research review: Re-thinking the classification of autism spectrum disorders. *Journal of Child Psychology and Psychiatry, 53,* 490–509. doi:10.1111/j.1469-7610.2012.02547.x.

Lord, C., Rutter, M., & Le Couteur, A. (1994). Autism diagnostic interview-revised: A revised version of a diagnostic interview for caregivers of individuals with possible pervasive developmental disorders. *Journal of Autism and Developmental Disorders, 24,* 659–685.

Lord, C., Risi, S., Lambrecht, L., Cook, E. H., Leventhal, B. L., DiLavore, P. C., et al. (2000). The Autism diagnostic observation schedule-generic: A standard measure of social and communication deficits associated with the spectrum of autism. *Journal of Autism and Developmental Disorders, 30,* 205–223.

Lugnegard, T., Hallerback, M. U., & Gillberg, C. (2011). Psychiatric comorbidity in young adults with a clinical diagnosis of Asperger syndrome. *Research in Developmental Disabilities, 32,* 1910–1917. doi:10.1016/j.ridd.2011.03.025.

Lunsky, Y., Gracey, C., & Bradley, E. (2009). Adults with autism spectrum disorders using psychiatric hospitals in Ontario: Clinical profile and service needs. *Research in Autism Spectrum Disorders, 3,* 1006–1013. doi:10.1016/j.rasd.2009.06.005.

Magnuson, K. M., & Constantino, J. N. (2011). Characterization of depression in children with autism spectrum disorders. *Journal of Developmental & Behavioral Pediatrics, 32,* 332–340. doi:10.1097/DBP.0b013e318213f56c.

Manikam, R., & Perman, J. (2000). Pediatric feeding disorders. *Journal of Clinical Gastroenterology, 30,* 34–46.

Martins, Y., Young, R. L., & Robson, D. C. (2008). Feeding and eating behaviors in children with autism and typically developing children. *Journal of Autism and Developmental Disorders, 38,* 1878–1887.

Matson, J. L., & Nebel-Schwalm, M. S. (2007). Comorbid psychopathology with autism spectrum disorder in children: An overview. *Research in Developmental Disabilities, 28,* 341–352. doi:10.1016/j.ridd/2005.12.004.

Matson, J. L., Ancona, M. N., & Wilkins, J. (2008). Sleep disturbances in adults with autism spectrum disorders and severe intellectual impairments. *Journal of Mental Health Research, 1,* 129–139. doi:10.1080/19315860801988210.

Matson, J. L., Dempsey, T., & Fodstad, J. C. (2009). The effect of autism spectrum disorders on adaptive independent living skills in adults with severe intellectual disability. *Research in Developmental Disabilities, 30,* 1203–1211.

Mattila, M., Hurtig, T., Haapsamo, H., Jussila, K., Kuusikko-Gauffin, S., Kielinin, M., et al. (2010). Comorbid psychiatric disorders associated with Asperger Syndrome/high-functioning autism: A community- and clinic-based study. *Journal of Autism and Developmental Disorders, 40,* 1080–1093. doi:10.1007/s10803-010-0958-2.

Mayes, S. D., & Calhoun, S. L. (2009). Variables related to sleep problems in children with autism. *Research in Autism Spectrum Disorders, 3,* 931–941. doi:10.1016/j.rasd.2009.04.002.

Mayes, S. D., Calhoun, S. L., Murray, M. J., & Zahid, J. (2011). Variables associated with anxiety and depression in children with autism. *Journal of Developmental and Physical Disabilities, 23,* 325–337. doi:10.1007/s10882-011-9231-7.

Mayes, S. D., Calhoun, S. L., Aggarwal, R., Baker, C., Mathapati, S., Anderson, R., & Petersen, C. (2012a). Explosive, oppositional, and aggressive behavior in children with autism compared to other clinical disorders and typical children. *Research in. Autism: the international journal of research and practice Spectrum Disorders, 6,* 1–10.

Mayes, S. D., Calhoun, S. L., Mayes, R. D., & Molitoris, S. (2012b). Autism and ADHD: Overlapping and discriminating symptoms. *Research in Autism Spectrum Disorders, 6,* 277–285.

Mazzone, L., Ruta, L., & Reale, L. (2012). Psychiatric comorbidities in Asperger Syndrome and high functioning autism: Diagnostic challenges. *Annals of General Psychiatry, 32,* 237–251.

Melville, C. A., Cooper, S., Morrison, J., Smiley, E., Allan, L., Jackson, A., et al. (2008). The prevalence and incidence of mental ill-health in adults with autism and intellectual disabilities. *Journal of Autism and Developmental Disorders, 38,* 1676–1688. doi:10.1007/s10803-008-0549-7.

Moseley, D. S., Tonge, B. J., Brereton, A. V., & Einfeld, S. (2011). Psychiatric comorbidity in adolescents and young adults with autism. *Journal of Mental health Research in Intellectual Disabilities, 4,* 229–243. doi:10.1080/19315864.2011.595535.

Muehlmann, A. M., & Lewis, M. H. (2012). Abnormal repetitive behaviors: Shared phenomenology and pathophysiology. *Journal of Intellectual Disability Research, 56,* 427–440. doi:10.1111/j.1365-2788.2011.01519.x.

Munesue, T., Ono, Y., Mutoh, K., Shimoda, K., Nakatani, H., & Kikuchi, M. (2008). High prevalence of bipolar disorder comorbidity in adolescents and young adults with high-functioning autism spectrum disorder: A preliminary study of 44 outpatients. *Journal of Affective Disorders, 111,* 170–175. doi:10.1016/j.jad.2008.02.015.

Murphy, O., Healy, O., & Leader, G. (2009). Risk factors for challenging behaviors among 157 children with autism spectrum disorder in Ireland. *Research in Autism , 3,* 474–482.

Nadon, G., Feldman, D. E., Dunn, W., & Gisel, E. (2011). Mealtime problems in children with autism spectrum disorder and their typically developing siblings: A comparison study. *Autism: The International Journal of Research and Practice, 15,* 98–113.

Oyane, N. M. F., & Bjorvatn, B. (2005). Sleep disturbances in adolescents and young adults with autism and Asperger syndrome. *Autism: The International Journal of Research and Practice, 9,* 83–94. doi:10.1177/1362361305049031.

Park, S., Cho, S., Cho, I. H., Kim, B., Kim, J., Shin, M., et al. (2012). Sleep problems and their correlates and comorbid psychopathology of children with autism spectrum disorders. *Research in Autism Spectrum Disorders, 6,* 1068–1072. doi:10.1016/j.rasd.2012.02.004.

Perry, D. W., Marston, G. M., Hinder, S. A. J., Munden, A. C., & Roy, A. (2001). The phenomenology of depressive illness in people with a learning disability and autism. *Autism: The International Journal of Research and Practice, 5,* 265–275.

Radford, J., & Anderson, M. (2003). Encopresis in children on the autistic spectrum. *Early Child Development and Care, 173,* 375–382. doi:10.1080/0300443032000 079069.

Raja, M., Azzoni, A., & Frustaci, A. (2011). Autism spectrum disorders and suicidality. *Clinical Practice & Epidemiology in Mental Health, 7,* 97–105.

Richdale, A. L., & Schreck, K. A. (2009). Sleep problems in autism spectrum disorders: Prevalence, nature, & possible biopsychological etiologies. *Sleep Medicine Reviews, 13,* 403–411. doi:10.1016/j.smrv.2009.02.003.

Rinald, K., & Mirenda, P. (2012). Effectiveness of a modified rapid toilet training workshop for parents of children with developmental disabilities. *Research in Developmental Disabilities, 33,* 933–943. doi:10.1016/j.ridd.2012.01.003.

Ringman, J. M., & Jankovic, J. (2000). Occurrence of tics in Asperger's syndrome and autistic disorder. *Journal of Child Neurology, 15,* 394–400.

Ryden, E., & Bejerot, S. (2008). Autism spectrum disorders in an adult psychiatric population. A naturalistic cross-sectional controlled study. *Clinical Neuropsychiatry, 5,* 13–21.

Schreck, K. A., & Williams, K. (2006). Food preferences and factors influencing food selectivity for children with autism spectrum disorders. *Research in Developmental Disabilities, 27,* 353–363.

Schreck, K. A., Williams, K., & Smith, A. F. (2004). A comparison of eating behaviors between children with and without autism. *Journal of Autism and Developmental Disabilities, 34,* 433–438.

Shattuck, P. T., Seltzer, M. M., Greenberg, J. S., Orsmond, G. I., Bolt, D., Kring, S., et al. (2007). Change in autism symptoms and maladaptive behaviors in adolescents and adults with an autism spectrum disorder. *Journal of Autism and Developmental Disorders, 37,* 1735–1747.

Simonoff, E., Pickles, A., Charman, T., Chandler, S., Loucas, T., & Baird, G. (2008). Psychiatric disorders in children with autism spectrum disorders: Prevalence, comorbidity, and associated factors in a population-derived sample. *Journal of the American Academy of Child and Adolescent Psychiatry, 47,* 921–929.

Simonoff, E., Jones, C. R. G., Pickles, A., Happe, F., Baird, G., & Charman, T. (2012). Severe mood problems in adolescents with autism spectrum disorder. *Journal of Child Psychology and Psychiatry, 53,* 1157–1166. doi:10.1111/j.1469-7610.2012.02600.x.

Simonoff, E., Jones, C. R. G., Baird, G., Pickles, A., Happe, F., & Charman, T. (2013). The persistence and stability of psychiatric problems in adolescents with autism spectrum disorders. *Journal of Child Psychology and Psychiatry, 54,* 186–194. doi:10.1111/j.1469-7610.2012.02606.x.

Sounders, M. C., Mason, T. B. A., Valladares, O., Bucan, M., Levy, S. E., Mandell, D. S., et al. (2009). Sleep behaviors and sleep quality in children with autism spectrum disorders. *Sleep: Journal of Sleep and Sleep Disorders Research, 32,* 1566–1578.

Sterling, L., Dawson, G., Estes, A., & Greenson, J. (2008). Characteristics associated with presence of depressive symptoms in adults with autism spectrum disorder. *Journal of Autism and Developmental Disorders, 38,* 1011–1018. doi:10.1007/s10803-007-0477-y.

Stewart, M. E., Barnard, L., Pearson, J., Hasan, R., & O'Brien, G. (2006). Presentation of depression in autism and Asperger syndrome: A review. *Autism: The International Journal of Research and Practice, 10,* 103–116. doi:10.1177/1362361306062013.

Trillingsgaard, A., Sørensen, E. U., Němec, G., & Jørgensen, M. (2005). What distinguishes autism spectrum disorders from other developmental disorders before the age of four years? *European Child & Adolescent Psychiatry, 14,* 65–72.

Tsakanikos, E., Underwood, L., Kravariti, E., Bouras, N., & McCarthy, J. (2011). Gender differences in comorbid psychopathology and clinical management in adults with autism spectrum disorders. *Research in Autism Spectrum Disorders, 5,* 803–808. doi:10.1016/j.rasd.2010.09.009.

Tuchman, R., & Rapin, I. (2002). Epilepsy in autism. *The Lancet Neurology, 1,* 352–358.

van Tongerloo, M. A. M. M., Bor, H. H. J., & Lagro-Janssen, A. L. M. (2012). Detecting autism spectrum disorders in the general practitioner's practice. *Journal of Autism and Developmental Disorders, 42,* 1531–1538. doi:10.1007/s10803-011-1384-9.

Wakefield, J. (2013). DSM-5: An overview of changes and controversies. *Clinical Social Work Journal, 41,* 139–154. doi:10.1007/s10615-013-0445-2.

Williams, P. G., Sears, L. L., & Allard, A. (2004). Sleep problems in children with autism. *Journal of Sleep Research, 13,* 265–268.

Williams, K. E., Gibbons, B. G., & Schreck, K. A. (2005). Comparing selective eaters with and without developmental disabilities. *Journal of Developmental and Physical Disabilities, 17,* 299–309.

Wozniak, J., Biederman, J., Faraone, S. V., Frazier, J., Kim, J., Millstein, R., et al. (1997). Mania in children with pervasive developmental disorder revisited. *Journal of the American Academy of Child and Adolescent Psychiatry, 36,* 1552–1559. doi:10.1016/s0890-8567(09)66564-3.

Yerys, B. E., Wallace, G. L., Sokoloff, J. L., Shook, D. A., James, J. D., & Kenworthy, L. (2009). Attention deficit/hyperactivity disorder symptoms moderate cognition and behavior in children with autism spectrum disorders. *Autism Research, 2,* 322–333.

Yoshida, Y., & Uchiyama, T. (2004). The clinical necessity for assessing Attention deficit/hyperactivity disorder (AD/HD) symptoms in children with high-functioning pervasive developmental disorder (PDD). *European Child & Adolescent Psychiatry, 13,* 307–314.

Laura D. Seligman, Erin F. Swedish
and Ellen Flannery-Schroeder

Anxiety Assessment and Treatment in Typically Developing Children

Increasingly, children's mental health is attracting significant attention. Numerous sources of information point to the importance of the topic. The American Psychological Association notes that an estimated 15 million US children and adolescents can currently be diagnosed with a mental health disorder (American Psychological Association, n.d.); yet, only approximately 7% of these youth ever receive mental health services (US Public Health Service 2000). Prevalence estimates for emotional and behavioral disorders in our nation's youth range from 16 to 22% (Costello et al. 1996; Roberts et al. 1998). In addition, childhood disorders have been linked to problems in adjustment in adolescence and adulthood (e.g., Colman et al. 2007). Childhood mental disorders persist into adulthood with 74% of 21-year-olds with mental disorders reporting prior problems (US Public Health Service 2000).

The authors have nothing to disclose

L. D. Seligman (✉)
Department of Psychology, University of Texas Pan American, Edinburg, TX, USA
e-mail: laura.seligman@utoledo.edu

E. F. Swedish
Department of Psychology, University of Toledo, 2801 West Bancroft St., Toledo, OH 43606-3390, USA

E. Flannery-Schroeder
Department of Psychology, University of Rhode Island, Kingston, RI, USA

It is widely purported that anxiety disorders represent the most common disorders of childhood and adolescence (Cartwright-Hatton et al. 2006; Kessler et al. 2005) and, therefore, may represent the earliest form of psychopathology. While the prevalence rates for childhood anxiety disorders vary by study, the majority report lifetime prevalence rates between 15 and 32% (Beesdo et al. 2009; Merikangas et al. 2010). Childhood anxiety disorders often overlap in symptoms and are highly comorbid with each other (Kendall et al. 2010), with 40–75% of anxious children meeting criteria for more than one anxiety disorder (Rapee et al. 2009; Seligman and Ollendick 2011). Additionally, childhood anxiety disorders are highly comorbid with other affective disorders, such as depression (Angold et al. 1999; Seligman and Ollendick 1998), and moderately comorbid with externalizing disorders (Russo and Beidel 1994). Therefore, the assessment and treatment of childhood anxiety disorders must necessarily take into account the presence of comorbid conditions.

Evidence exists suggesting that childhood anxiety is associated with moderate-to-severe disruptions in child development and later adjustment (Mattison 1992). Negative consequences associated with anxiety disorders in youth include intellectual difficulties and academic underachievement (Davis et al. 2008), underemployment, substance use, lower levels of social support, and high comorbidity with other psychiatric disorders (Velting et al. 2004). Unsurprisingly, the social and economic burdens of anxiety disorders are extremely high. In 1990, the costs associated with anxiety disorders were US\$ 46.6 billion, just over 30% of total expenditures for mental illness (DuPont et al. 1996). While less than 25% of these costs were associated with medical treatment, more than 75% were the result of lost or reduced productivity. Epidemiological studies suggest that over half of adults with anxiety disorders first manifest the disorder in youth (e.g., Newman et al. 1996), suggesting the effective treatment of anxiety disorders in children and adolescents has the potential to significantly impact the long-term costs associated with anxiety disorders in adulthood.

Hence, there is tremendous need for easily accessible, consumer-friendly, and effective interventions for childhood anxiety disorders. In recent years, the field of clinical child psychology has recognized this need and responded with an abundance of empirical examinations of assessment instruments and interventions for anxiety disorders in youth.

Assessment

The assessment of anxiety disorders in youth can be a complex endeavor. First, as noted above, the high rate of comorbidity between anxiety disorders and depression and some externalizing disorders (Brady and Kendall 1992; Essau et al. 2002; Seligman and Ollendick 1998; Woodward and Fergusson 2001) requires one to go beyond the assessment of anxiety in order to get a full clinical picture. Second, assessment of anxiety in youth must be developmentally sensitive; anxieties and fears considered developmentally normative and desirable at one stage of development (e.g., a toddler's fear of separation from a parent) could be symptomatic of a disorder at a later developmental stage (Ollendick et al. 1989). Moreover, assessment of anxious symptoms in youth often requires multiple methods and multiple informants, as research suggests that different types of instruments are best suited for different tasks (i.e., screening, diagnosis, treatment planning, monitoring of change) and different information is obtained from different informants (Achenbach et al. 1987; Grills and Ollendick 2002, 2003; Silverman and Ollendick 2005; Verhulst

and Van der Ende 1991). Given the complexities of the issues involved in assessing anxiety disorders in youth and the many measures that are currently available for these purposes, our goal here is to distill this vast literature to provide the reader with an introduction to some of the most widely used methods and measures used to assess anxiety in youth. Further, while past efforts have focused primarily, although not exclusively, on the assessment of the signs and symptoms of anxiety disorders in youth, without regard to the underlying processes that give rise to these symptoms, this has started to change and we fully expect these efforts to grow exponentially as the field continues to move beyond efforts to define anxiety disorders in youth toward more sophisticated models that identify the social, cultural, biological, and psychological processes that cause pathological anxiety and maintain or disrupt pathological anxiety processes. Therefore, we briefly review some of the measures that have been developed to assess constructs relevant to such models.

Diagnostic Interviews Diagnostic interviews represent the gold standard for diagnosis of anxiety disorders in youth. Additionally, they are often used to assess treatment outcome (i.e., whether the child is diagnosis free after treatment) and, when done correctly, a thorough diagnostic interview can yield the necessary information—such as feared stimuli, avoidance patterns, disturbed cognitions, and environmental contingences—that allow for effective treatment planning. Although unstructured diagnostic interviews are often used for the assessment of anxiety disorders in youth, such methods are prone to flaws inherent with clinical bias and evidence suggests that the unstructured interview, although frequently used in clinical practice, is of questionable validity (McLeod et al. 2013; Miller et al. 2001; Zimmerman and Mattia 1999). Therefore, the use of structured or semi-structured diagnostic interviews is highly desirable. Fortunately, there are several options available. These interviews generally evidence good psychometric properties when used for the identification of the most commonly occurring anxiety disorders in youth; however, it should be noted that less is known about the performance of these interviews when they are used to diagnose anxiety disorders with low base rates in pediatric populations (i.e., disorders that are relatively rare in youth, such as panic disorder in preadolescent children; Silverman and Ollendick 2005) or when they are used for purposes other than diagnosis (e.g., case conceptualization).

Although several widely available structured and semi-structured diagnostic interviews for children and adolescents can be used for the assessment of anxiety disorders in youth, the Anxiety Disorders Interview Schedule for Children for *Diagnostic and Statistical Manual of Mental Disorders-IV* (*DSM-IV*): Child and Parent Versions (ADIS-IV: C/P; Silverman and Albano 1996; Silverman et al. 2001) is the only one that was designed specifically for the assessment of anxiety disorders in children and adolescents. The ADIS-IV and its predecessor are also the most widely used diagnostic interviews in the child anxiety treatment research literature. Parent and child versions of the interview are available and are often used in combination to arrive at a diagnosis. In addition to providing thorough modules for the assessment of anxiety disorders as well as questions that can help with treatment planning, the ADIS-IV provides modules for a thorough assessment of those disorders most commonly associated with anxiety disorders and screening questions for several less common disorders or syndromes (e.g., schizophrenia and somatoform disorders). However, of particular interest for the reader of the current volume, there is limited research on the use of the ADIS-IV on children with developmental disabilities and the ADIS-IV provides only screener questions for developmental disorders in the parent interview. The ADIS-IV was designed, however, as a semi-structured interview, allowing for the clinician to follow standard queries for symptoms with probing questions for clarification. This may be particularly important in using the ADIS-IV, or any diagnostic interview, when assessing for anxiety in youth with developmental disorders in that structured diagnostic interviews may yield some false positives in this population due to

the similarity of some symptoms (e.g., repetitive behaviors such as hand flapping could cause a parent to endorse compulsive behaviors when asked about obsessive–compulsive disorder, OCD; Kerns and Kendall 2012; Mazefsky et al. 2012). Therefore, while we endorse the use of structured and semi-structured diagnostic interviews in the assessment of anxiety disorders in youth, we contend that the validity of these interviews is dependent on the user having a broad-based knowledge of childhood psychopathology.

Rating Scales Numerous rating scales exist for the purpose of quantifying the symptoms of anxiety disorders and several are emerging to help with the assessment of the hypothesized processes underlying the anxiety disorders (e.g., attributional biases). In this section, however, we focus primarily on rating scales that assess the signs and symptoms of anxiety disorders in youth. These types of rating scales have been designed to be completed by the child, parent, clinician, and/or significant others such as teachers. The interested reader is referred to Silverman and Ollendick (2005) for a thorough review of available scales for anxiety assessment in youth. We do note that, in terms of symptom measures, there are generally two types of rating scales currently in use. One kind, typified by the Revised Children's Manifest Anxiety Scale (RCMAS; Reynolds and Richmond 1985), the State Trait Anxiety Inventory for Children (STAIC; Spielberger 1973), and the Child Behavior Checklist (CBCL; Achenbach 1991), aims to assess anxiety (or negative affect) as a more holistic construct. The second type of measure, best exemplified by measures such as the Spence Children's Anxiety Scale (SCAS; Spence 1998) and the Screen for Child Anxiety Related Emotional Disorders (SCARED; Birmaher et al. 1997), assesses anxiety symptoms that map directly onto the *DSM* anxiety disorders and result in subscale scores that more closely mirror these disorders.

Evidence supports the use of rating scales for the assessment of anxiety disorders in youth and for monitoring treatment outcome (Seligman et al. 2004); however, it should be noted that, as with diagnostic interviews, rating scales completed by different informants often yield different results (e.g., Muris et al. 1999) and that self-report rating scales may be particularly sensitive to changes unrelated to treatment (e.g., demand characteristics), calling into question their use for monitoring of change throughout treatment (Seligman et al. 2014).

Although rating scales are best used for screening and treatment monitoring rather than diagnosis, a strength of rating scales is that they often provide age-based norms, allowing for a more developmentally sensitive assessment. However, one must proceed with caution when inferring the benefits of such norms, as there has been little research investigating whether relative standing on rating scale measures is related to clinical severity or day-to-day impairment in functioning (Silverman and Ollendick 2005). Additionally, the somewhat arbitrary scoring systems almost ubiquitously used would seem to call into question such a presumption. Rating scales are typically scored by simply summing up the individual item scores that comprise the measure or its subscales. This is true despite the fact that factor analyses of these scales rarely suggest that all items equally reflect the underlying construct they are purported to measure (e.g., negative affect and physiological arousal). In other words, some items on a rating scale may be very good indicators of the presence or absence of the construct of interest while others may be only weakly related; however, both weak and strong indicators usually figure equally when determining a child's score. Moreover, it may be that some symptoms are more clinically meaningful than others, though little research has attended to such questions. For example, it could be that stomach upset is more related to disruptions to a child's life (i.e., distress, school attendance, and medical visits) than muscle aches but a rating scale that assesses physiological anxiety symptoms would typically include items related to both types of symptoms, and both would weigh equally in the calculation of a physiological anxiety score regardless of how well they tap the underlying construct of physiological anxiety or how related each symptom is to clinically meaningful "real-world" criteria.

In addition to these concerns, the high face validity of many rating scales intended for use with children and adolescents may be problematic in that youth with anxiety disorders may be reluctant to reveal their symptoms. Although there has been little research into how anxious youth view the social desirability of the symptoms assessed by such rating scales, it stands to reason that children with significant anxiety may be anxious about revealing their symptoms. For instance, the hallmark of a fairly common anxiety disorder in youth, social anxiety disorder, is a fear of negative evaluation by others. As such it may be that anxiety symptoms themselves can sometimes lead to a reluctance to report these symptoms. Again, although there has been little research to address such issues, research on the social desirability or "lie scale" of the RCMAS does suggest that social desirability can play a role in children and adolescents' self-reports of anxiety and that this may be particularly true for younger children and African-American and Hispanic and Latino/a youth (Dadds et al. 1998; Pina et al. 2001).

In sum, rating scales can be very useful in the assessment of anxiety in children and adolescents; they offer a relatively inexpensive and quick way to screen for the signs and symptoms of anxiety disorders and provide a dimensional evaluation that can be useful in monitoring treatment outcome. Moreover, many rating scales offer norms that allow a clinician to assess a youth's relative standing compared to same-age and same-sex peers. However, clinicians using rating scales for the assessment of anxiety in youth must also be cognizant of the limitations of such measures. These limitations include lack of validation with clinically meaningful criteria, questions about the validity of the scoring algorithms used by most rating scales, and the potential impact of social desirability, particularly for young children and minority youth.

Assessment of Anxiety in Youth: Moving Beyond Signs and Symptoms Up until recently, most of the efforts to assess anxiety in children and adolescents have focused on assessing the signs and symptoms of anxiety disorders in youth. This phenomenological and theory-free approach is consistent with the *DSM* model.

There are many strengths to such an approach and it is clear that there has been much benefit for the field of anxiety disorders. In fact, anxiety disorders represent an area in our field that has been able to progress toward well-established links between diagnosis, theory, and treatment; this research base and the connections between theory and application in the anxiety disorders could arguably be a model for the field. These successes have enabled us to begin to address new and more sophisticated questions such as what really changes when a child undergoes successful treatment for an anxiety disorder. Why do some children benefit from treatment while others do not? Do some children benefit more from one type of intervention (e.g., exposure) than others (e.g., cognitive restructuring), and, if so, is there a way to match children to the most effective type of intervention (i.e., to personalize and streamline treatment)? These types of questions require a different approach to the assessment of anxiety in youth—one that focuses more on the underlying processes that are hypothesized to cause and maintain anxiety disorders in youth and one that can measure potential mechanisms or mediators of treatment.

Fortunately, newer measures, including both rating scales and laboratory tasks, have begun to focus on assessing such relevant constructs. For example, the Children's Automatic Thoughts Scale (Schniering and Rapee 2002) assesses the cognitive content (i.e., thoughts about physical threat, failure, and hostility) that could give rise to or maintain anxiety disorders in youth as does the Anxiety Control Questionnaire for Children (Weems et al. 2003). Additionally, performance tasks such as the Stroop and dot probe as well as rating scales such as the Effortful Control Scale (Muris et al. 2008) allow for the measurement of cognitive processes hypothesized to be relevant to anxiety disorders in youth. Moreover, the repeated use of such measures can aide in determining the mediators of treatment outcome. Whether these measures can be used to accurately identify youth with clinically significant anxiety or discriminate between youth with anxiety disorders and other clinically significant problems remains to be seen. In addition, the feasibility of using such measures, particularly performance measures, outside research settings is questionable at this time and transportability of such technology is an area in need of further development.

Empirically Supported Treatments for Anxiety Disorders in Youth

A preponderance of evidence supports the use of cognitive-behavioral therapy (CBT) for the treatment of childhood anxiety disorders (Kendall et al. 1997; Silverman 2008). Numerous randomized clinical trials have demonstrated its efficacy (e.g., Kendall et al. 2009; Kendall et al. 1997). Taken together, these studies provide the empirical support to identify CBT as an evidence-based treatment for childhood anxiety (Ollendick et al. 2006). Based on Chambless and Hollon's (1998) criteria for empirically supported treatments, CBT for children with anxiety disorders is designated as "probably efficacious" (Davis et al. 2011; Ollendick et al. 2006).

Although more than 100 evidence-based treatment programs for child and adolescent anxiety have been identified in the literature (Chorpita et al. 2011), these treatments share seven common elements: psychoeducation, exposure, cognitive restructuring, parent training or parent psychoeducation, relaxation, modeling, and self-monitoring (Rotheram-Borus et al. 2012). Moreover, modular treatments (i.e., those in which the clinician selects and implements evidence-based practice elements) may result in better outcomes than the use of treatment manuals (Weisz et al. 2012). Therefore, we provide a brief description of each of these evidence-based treatment elements below.

Psychoeducation

Psychoeducation typically occurs at the beginning of treatment in order to provide families a treatment rationale and to develop a shared understanding of the processes that maintain the problem or disorder. Although psychoeducation is often a relatively brief component of the overall intervention, lasting only one or two sessions, it can be a pivotal one in that evidence-based treatments for child anxiety disorders are typically collaborative in nature and require the child and his or her family to be active participants. This requires that they both understand the treatment plan and the reasoning behind the plan. Psychoeducation allows the family to gain a more fact-based understanding of the nature of anxiety and the CBT model. The CBT model is introduced to help families understand interactions among thoughts, feelings, and behaviors. Maintaining factors are also discussed, typically with a particular focus on accommodation, avoidance, and the types of cognitive errors commonly found in youth with anxiety disorders.

Exposure

Most anxious children have developed avoidant ways of dealing with anxiety-provoking situations. While families often view such a strategy as one that makes sense because it results in a decrease of distress in the short term, in the long term this results in negative reinforcement of the avoidance behavior which ultimately increases restriction of the child's activities and impairs daily functioning. Moreover, avoidance does not allow the child to learn that the feared event or stimulus is not realistically dangerous. Therefore, to overcome anxiety, exposure is a critical component of treatment. Exposure addresses avoidant behavior by having the child experience distress in real or imagined anxiety-provoking situations. Exposures can be conducted either by flooding or in a graduated method. In flooding, the child completes a prolonged exposure to the feared stimulus at full intensity and would remain in the anxiety-provoking situation until his or her self-reported levels of anxiety reduce. In the graduated approach, children rank their fears to generate a fear hierarchy and then work their way up to experiencing the most intense stimuli or situations. For example, a child with a snake phobia might first complete an exposure session

viewing a picture of a snake and ultimately work his or her way up to being in the room with a snake. Both graduated exposures and flooding help children learn that by exposing themselves to the anxiety-provoking situation their anxiety decreases and they are able to cope with their fear. Moreover, the child is able to see that feared catastrophic consequences do not occur. Of note, however, while research supports the efficacy of flooding as a treatment for anxiety (Zoellner et al. 2009), children and parents tend to view graduated methods of exposure more favorably (King and Gullone 1990).

Cognitive Restructuring

An anxious child may believe that his or her feelings and emotions are directly caused by events or situations without realizing that it is in fact her *interpretation* of those external events that give rise to anxiety. Therefore, learning to think more realistically is a common strategy for helping children overcome anxiety. To address this issue, the child is introduced to cognitive restructuring, a process of identifying, challenging, and changing cognitive distortions. During this process, children identify and replace maladaptive thoughts with more adaptive beliefs, which helps promote more accurate and useful thinking. This allows the child to approach anxiety-provoking situations with more confidence. In general, cognitive restructuring for anxiety typically addresses two common cognitive distortions: overestimation of the probability of threat and overestimation of the probability of negative consequences of an event. However, the concept of cognitive restructuring and actually changing cognitive distortions is challenging, even for adults. Therefore, cognitive restructuring may be most useful for older children and youth with more advanced cognitive skills. When working with anxious youth, cognitive restructuring is often introduced as a game; for example, the child may be asked to become a detective to identify anxious thoughts and then find clues to determine whether their anxious thought is accurate.

Parent Psychoeducation and Parent-Training

Research suggests that parental psychopathology may lead to the development or maintenance of child anxiety (e.g., Beidel and Turner 1997). Parental over-control, negative family interactions, and inconsistent parenting have also been associated with anxiety disorders in youth (Hudson and Rapee 2001, 2002; Muris and Merckelbach 1998). For example, parents may model or verbally communicate information related to their own biased beliefs about likely threat or harm, which may lead to an increase in anxious symptomology in their children. Through the CBT model, parents are provided examples and strategies to address their own anxiety. These strategies may be very similar to those the child is learning throughout the course of treatment (e.g., cognitive restructuring). In order to combat inconsistent parenting, parenting strategies focused on reinforcing approach behavior, removing reinforcement for anxious behavior (i.e., planned ignoring), and decreasing parental modeling of anxious behavior are introduced. Negative communication patterns are also addressed and adaptive communication is encouraged. For example, parents would be introduced to problem-solving skills; caregivers may also work together on conflict negotiation to decrease disputes around child rearing and increase consistency (Barrett et al. 1996).

Relaxation

Relaxation techniques are introduced to help anxious youth develop awareness and control over physiological responses to anxiety. The most common techniques include diaphragmatic breathing and progressive muscle relaxation. Diaphragmatic, or deep, breathing consists of taking slow deep breaths that expand the stomach rather than the chest. Progressive muscle relaxation involves systematically relaxing muscle groups through the use of a tension-release procedure. The more the child practices relaxation the more confident they become in using the techniques to help them relax. However, although relaxation training and instruction in deep breathing are common components of treatment for child anxiety, it is unclear whether these interventions are necessary or even helpful (e.g., Meuret et al. 2009; Meuret et al. 2003). When they are used, it is important for the clinician to introduce these skills as tools to help the child engage in approach behavior, not a necessity for controlling "dangerous" bodily sensations. In this way, the clinician can prevent the child from engaging in relaxation or breathing exercises as a safety behavior or from interpreting relaxation and breathing training as the therapist's implied agreement that physiological symptoms of anxiety are dangerous.

Modeling

Research suggests that children observe and emulate the attitudes, emotions, and behaviors modeled by others (Bandura and McClelland 1977). Therefore, an important component of therapy is modeling nonanxious behavior to help youth with anxiety learn more adaptive and approach oriented ways to cope with their anxiety. In session, therapists can model how to regulate their own emotions, thoughts, and behavior, especially in anxiety-provoking situations, which helps the child learn that they can face their fears and use approach behaviors. By modeling strategies such as effective regulation of negative emotions, successfully handling anxiety-provoking situations, and active problem solving, the child can develop more effective coping strategies. Parents are often actively encouraged to use such modeling strategies at home—modeling approach behavior and adaptive problem solving while refraining from modeling avoidant behavior or anxious thinking.

Self-Monitoring

Observing and recording a target behavior, or self-monitoring, is a skill introduced at the beginning of treatment as a way for the child and therapist to better understand the nature of the problem. More specifically, the child collects "data" outside of therapy sessions to help gather information to guide treatment. Self-monitoring helps facilitate the child's understanding of the interaction between his or her thoughts, feelings, and behaviors. Additionally, self-monitoring involves teaching the child to identify and differentiate feelings and to increase awareness of his or her emotions. This can help children begin to recognize the triggers for their anxiety and can help prepare them to monitor anxious cognitions as well as to use coping strategies between therapy sessions. Self-monitoring exercises include tracking changes in mood, dysfunctional thoughts, and anxious behaviors.

Evidence for the Efficacy of CBT for the Treatment of Childhood Anxiety Disorders

Treatment outcome studies have typically examined outcomes for youth diagnosed with generalized anxiety disorder (GAD), separation anxiety disorder (SAD), and social phobia together, whereas specific phobias (SPs), OCD, and post-traumatic stress disorder (PTSD) have typically been the focus of more specific treatments. Given that OCD and PTSD have historically been considered anxiety disorders but are not included in the anxiety disorders chapter of the *DSM* (5th ed.; *DSM-5,* American Psychiatric Associaton 2013), the research on treatments for these disorders will be reviewed briefly. Additionally, we review the treatment literature separately for SPs and provide an overview of the studies that have investigated outcomes for the heterogeneous group of children diagnosed with GAD, SAD, and/or social phobia. However, given the high rates of comorbidity within the anxiety disorders, it should be noted that these may be somewhat artificial distinctions as many of the youth in these trials had more than one anxiety disorder.

Obsessive–Compulsive Disorder

The core components of treatment for OCD are similar to those listed previously; however, a main component in CBT for OCD in youth is exposure and response prevention (ERP), in which the child is exposed to an obsession and refrains from engaging in the compulsion that was previously used to mitigate the anxiety or feared consequences. Although the phrase "ERP" is typically used in the literature on OCD, these exposures are not unlike the exposure treatments used for other anxiety disorders in that the child is exposed to the anxiety-provoking stimulus (e.g., germs, a social interaction, the scene of a traumatic event) and refrains from engaging in the response designed to decrease the anxiety (e.g., the compulsion avoidance). Research suggests that CBT can be an efficacious treatment for addressing the symptoms of OCD in children when it is delivered either in an individual format, family-focused format, or group format (e.g., Barrett et al. 2005; POTS 2004). Moreover, CBT treatment has been shown to be superior to medication treatments (i.e., selective serotonin reuptake inhibitor; SSRIs; for review see Barrett et al. 2008).

Post-Traumatic Stress Disorder

For the treatment of PTSD, trauma-focused CBT (TF-CBT) is the most well-researched and supported treatment (e.g., Cohen and Mannarino 1996, 1998; Cohen et al. 2004, 2005). TF-CBT typically involves training in relaxation techniques and exposing children to their traumatic event either by writing, drawing, or using other imaginational methods. In general, TF-CBT can be completed in 12–18 sessions with children as young as 3 years of age (Cohen and Mannarino 1996). Across several studies, TF-CBT was more effective at decreasing symptoms related to post-traumatic stress, anxiety, depression, and externalizing problems compared to non-CBT treatments (Cohen and Mannarino 1996).

Specific Phobias

Evidence also indicates that CBT is effective for the treatment of SPs in children (Davis et al. 2009). More specifically, evidence suggests that exposure to the phobic stimulus is critical in the treatment of SPs (Cornwall et al. 1996; Silverman et al. 1999a). For example, Silverman and colleagues found exposure therapy to be superior to a control group for the treatment of specific phobias. Children aged 6–16 with a phobic disorder were assigned to exposure with self-control, exposure plus a contingency management, or education support. Eighty-eight percent of children who received exposure therapy with self-control were diagnosis free at posttreatment compared to 56 % of the youth who received education support (Silverman et al. 1999b). Furthermore, positive treatment gains were maintained at 3, 6, and 12-month follow-up assessments (Silverman et al. 1999b). Additionally, one-session CBT has been shown to be effective for youth with SPs (Davis et al. 2009). For example, in a study by Ollendick et al. (2009), youth evidenced significant improvements in phobic symptoms after only one session of behavioral exposure treatment.

GAD, SAD, and Social Phobia

Empirical evidence from randomized controlled trials (RCTs) provides strong support for CBT in the treatment of GAD, SAD, and social phobia for children and adolescents (Barrett et al. 2008; Kendall 1994; Minde 2010). More specifically, group cognitive therapy (GCBT) with or without parental involvement and individual cognitive behavioral therapy (ICBT) have both been shown to be effective therapeutic options (Davis et al. 2011). Overall, research indicates that CBT with or without parental involvement is comparable, as is ICBT and GCBT; however, some evidence suggests that girls and children under 10 years of age may do better with CBT with parent involvement (Barrett 1998; Barrett et al. 1996; Flannery-Schroeder and Kendall 2000).

As many as 65–70 % of youth are diagnosis free immediately after treatment (Barrett et al. 1996; Flannery-Schroeder and Kendall 2000). For example, early trials of the Coping Cat Program (Kendall 1994), a manual for children aged 8–13 with GAD, SAD, and social phobia, have shown the Coping Cat to be effective compared to a wait-list group, with 64 % of youth in remission at the end of treatment (Kendall 1994). Positive treatment gains were maintained across time, with follow-up studies suggesting that gains are maintained at least 7 years after the completion of the active treatment phase (Kendall et al. 2004). Importantly, this suggests that the benefits of CBT treatment can be maintained across developmental periods.

Conclusions

As can be seen from the previous review, significant advances have been made in the assessment and treatment of child anxiety disorders and effective treatment options exist for youth suffering with a variety of anxiety disorders. Dissemination and accessibility to these treatments is another hurdle (e.g., Borntrager et al. 2013). While children with an anxiety disorder seeking treatment in an academic medical center or urban environment may receive an evidence-based approach to treatment, the same quality of care may not be routinely available outside research settings (Borntrager et al. 2013) or in more rural settings, particularly for lower income and minority youth. Therefore, while evidence-based treatments will certainly be refined in the upcoming years, with more attention to the mediators and moderators of treatment outcome, increased effort needs to focus on understanding effective methods of treatment dissemination (e.g., self-help and computer augmented therapies) and the barriers to effective interventions (e.g., clinician attitudes). In this way the full promise of the progress made in the treatment of child anxiety can be realized.

References

Achenbach, T. M. (1991). *Manual for the child behavior checklist/4–18 and 1991 profile*. Burlington: University of Vermont, Department of Psychiatry.

Achenbach, T. M., McConaughy, S. H., & Howell, C. T. (1987). Child/adolescent behavioral and emotional problems: Implications of cross-informant correlations for situational specificity. *Psychological Bulletin, 101*(2), 213–232.

American Psychiatric Associaton. (2013). Diagnostic and statistical manual of mental disorders (5thed.). Arlington, VA: American Psychiatric Publishing.

American Psychological Association. (n.d.). Children's mental health. Public interest directorate. http://www.apa.org/pi/families/children-mental-health.aspx. Accessed 11 July 2013

Angold, A., Costello, E. J., & Erkanli, A. (1999). Comorbidity. *Journal of Child Psychology and Psychiatry, 40*(1), 57–87. doi:10.1111/1469-7610.00424.

Bandura, A. (1977). Social learning theory. Oxford, England: Prentice-Hall.

Barrett, P. M. (1998). Evaluation of cognitive-behavioral group treatments for childhood anxiety disorders. *Journal of Clinical Child Psychology, 27*(4), 459–468.

Barrett, P. M., Dadds, M. R., & Rapee, R. M. (1996). Family treatment of childhood anxiety: A controlled trial. *Journal of Consulting & Clinical Psychology, 64*(2), 333–342.

Barrett, P., Farrell, L., Dadds, M., & Boulter, N. (2005). Cognitive-behavioral family treatment of childhood obsessive-compulsive disorder: Long-term follow-up and predictors of outcome. *Journal of the American Academy of Child & Adolescent Psychiatry, 44*(10), 1005–1014.

Barrett, P., Farrell, L., Pina, A., Peris, T., & Piacentini, J. C. (2008). Evidence-based psychosocial treatments for child and adolescent obsessive-compulsive disorder. *Journal of Clinical Child & Adolescent Psychology, 37*(1), 131–155.

Beesdo, K., Knappe, S., & Pine, D. S. (2009). Anxiety and anxiety disorders in children and adolescents: Developmental issues and implications for DSM-V. *The Psychiatric Clinics of North America, 32*(3), 483.

Beidel, D. C., & Turner, S. M. (1997). At risk for anxiety: I. Psychopathology in the offspring of anxious parents. *Journal of the American Academy of Child & Adolescent Psychiatry, 36*, 918–924.

Birmaher, B., Khetarpal, S., Brent, D., Cully, M., Balach, L., Kaufman, J., et al. (1997). The screen for child anxiety related emotional disorders (SCARED): Scale construction and psychometric characteristics. *Journal of the American Academy of Child and Adolescent Psychiatry, 36*(4), 545–553.

Borntrager, C., Chorpita, B. F., Higa-McMillan, C. K., Daleiden, E. L., & Starace, N. (2013). Usual care for trauma-exposed youth: Are clinician-reported therapy techniques evidence-based? *Children and Youth Services Review, 35*(1), 133–141. doi:10.1016/j.childyouth.2012.09.018.

Brady, E. U., & Kendall, P. C. (1992). Comorbidity of anxiety and depression in children and adolescents. *Psychological Bulletin, 111*(2), 244–255.

Cartwright-Hatton, S., McNicol, K., & Doubleday, E. (2006). Anxiety in a neglected population: Prevalence of anxiety disorders in pre-adolescent children. *Clinical Psychology Review, 26*(7), 817–833.

Chambless, D. L., & Hollon, S. D. (1998). Defining empirically supported therapies. *Journal of Consulting and Clinical Psychology, 66*(1), 7.

Chorpita, B. F., Bernstein, A., & Daleiden, E. L. (2011). Empirically guided coordination of multiple evidence-based treatments: An illustration of relevance mapping in children's mental health services. *Journal of Consulting and Clinical Psychology, 79*(4), 470–480. doi:10.1037/a0023982.

Cohen, J., & Mannarino, A. (1996). A treatment outcome study for sexually abused preschool children: Initial findings. *Journal of the American Academy of Child & Adolescent Psychiatry, 35*(1), 42–50.

Cohen, J., & Mannarino, A. (1998). Interventions for sexually abused children: Initial treatment outcome findings. *Child Maltreatment, 3*(1), 17–26.

Cohen, J., Deblinger, E., Mannarino, A., & Steer, R. (2004). A multisite, randomized controlled trial for children with sexual abuse-related PTSD symptoms. *Journal of the American Academy of Child & Adolescent Psychiatry, 43*(4), 393–402.

Cohen, J., Mannarinio, A., & Knudsen, K. (2005). Treating sexually abused children: 1 year follow-up of a randomized controlled trial. *Child Abuse & Neglect, 29*, 135–145.

Colman, I., Wadsworth, M., Croudace, T., & Jones, P. (2007). Forty-year psychiatric outcomes following assessment for internalizing disorder in adolescence. *American Journal of Psychiatry, 164*(1), 126–133.

Cornwall, E., Spence, S. H., & Schotte, D. (1996). The effectiveness of emotive imagery in the treatment of darkness phobia in children. *Behaviour Change, 13*(4), 223–229.

Costello, E. J., Angold, A., Burns, B. J., Stangl, D. K., Tweed, D. L., Erkanli, A., et al. (1996). The great Smoky Mountains study of youth: Goals, design, methods, and the prevalence of DSM-III-R disorders. *Archives of general psychiatry, 53*(12), 1129.

Dadds, M. R., Perrin, S., & Yule, W. (1998). Social desirability and self-reported anxiety in children: An analysis of the RCMAS lie scale. *Journal of Abnormal Child Psychology, 26*(4), 311–317.

Davis, T. E., Ollendick, T. H., & Nebel-Schwalm, M. (2008). Intellectual ability and achievement in anxiety-disordered children: A clarification and extension of the literature. *Journal of Psychopathology and Behavioral Assessment, 30*(1), 43–51.

Davis, T., Ollendick, T., & Öst, L.-G. (2009). Intensive treatment of specific phobias in children and adolescents. *Cognitive and Behavioral Practice, 16*(3), 294–303. doi:10.1016/j.cbpra.2008.12.008.

Davis, T. E. III, May, A. C., & Whiting, S. E. (2011). Evidence-based treatment of anxiety and phobia in children and adolescents: Current status and effects on the emotional response. *Clinical Psychology Review, 31,* 592–602. doi:10.1016/j.cpr.2011.01.001.

DuPont, R. L., Rice, D. P., Miller, L. S., Shiraki, S. S., Rowland, C. R., & Harwood, H. J. (1996). Economic costs of anxiety disorders. *Anxiety, 2*(4), 167–172.

Essau, C. A., Conradt, J., & Petermann, F. (2002). Course and outcome of anxiety disorders in adolescents. *Journal of Anxiety Disorders, 16*(1), 67–81.

Flannery-Schroeder, E. C., & Kendall, P. C. (2000). Group and individual cognitive-behavioral treatments for youth with anxiety disorders: A randomized clinical trial. *Cognitive Therapy and Research, 24*(3), 251–278.

Grills, A. E., & Ollendick, T. H. (2002). Issues in parent-child agreement: The case of structured diagnostic interviews. *Clinical Child and Family Psychology Review, 5,* 57–83.

Grills, A. E., & Ollendick, T. H. (2003). Multiple informant agreement and the anxiety disorders interview schedule for parents and children. *Journal of the American Academy of Child & Adolescent Psychiatry, 42*(1), 30–40.

Hudson, J. L., & Rapee, R. M. (2001). Parent-child interactions and anxiety disorders: An observational study. *Behaviour Research & Therapy, 39*(12), 1411–1427.

Hudson, J. L., & Rapee, R. M. (2002). Parent-child interactions in clinically anxious children and their siblings. *Journal of Clinical Child and Adolescent Psychology, 31*(4), 548–555.

Kendall, P. C. (1994). Treating anxiety disorders in children: Results of a randomized clinical trial. *Journal of Consulting & Clinical Psychology, 62*(1), 100–110.

Kendall, P. C., FlannerySchroeder, E., PanichelliMindel, S. M., SouthamGerow, M., Henin, A., & Warman, M. (1997). Therapy for youths with anxiety disorders: A second randomized clinical trial. *Journal of Consulting and Clinical Psychology, 65*(3), 366–380.

Kendall, P. C., Safford, S., Flannery-Schroeder, E., & Webb, A. (2004). Child anxiety treatment: Outcomes in adolescence and impact on substance use and depression at 7.4-year follow-up. *Journal of Consulting and Clinical Psychology, 72*(2), 276–287. doi:10.1037/0022-006x.72.2.276.

Kendall, P. C., Comer, J. S., Marker, C. D., Creed, T. A., Puliafico, A. C., Hughes, A. A., Hudson, J., et al. (2009). In-session exposure tasks and therapeutic alliance across the treatment of childhood anxiety disorders. *Journal of Consulting and Clinical Psychology, 77*(3), 517.

Kendall, P. C., Compton, S. N., Walkup, J. T., Birmaher, B., Albano, A. M., Sherrill, J., Gosch, E., et al. (2010). Clinical characteristics of anxiety disordered youth. *Journal of Anxiety Disorders, 24*(3), 360–365.

Kerns, C. M., & Kendall, P. C. (2012). The presentation and classification of anxiety in autism spectrum disorder. *Clinical Psychology: Science and Practice, 19*(4), 323–347. doi:10.1111/cpsp.12009.

Kessler, R. C., Berglund, P., Demler, O., Jin, R., Merikangas, K. R., & Walters, E. E. (2005). Lifetime prevalence and age-of-onset distributions of DSM-IV disorders in the National Comorbidity Survey Replication. *Archives of general psychiatry, 62*(6), 593.

King, N. J., & Gullone, E. (1990). Acceptability of fear reduction procedures with children. *Journal of Behavior Therapy and Experimental Psychiatry, 21*(1), 1–8. doi:10.1016/0005-7916(90)90042-J.

Mattison, R. E. (1992). Anxiety Disorders. In R. Hooper, G. W. Hynd, & R. E. Mattison (Eds.), *Child psychopathology: Diagnostic criteria and clinical assessment.* Hillsdale: Lawrence Erlbaum Associates.

Mazefsky, C. A., Oswald, D. P., Day, T. N., Eack, S. M., Minshew, N. J., & Lainhart, J. E. (2012). ASD, a psychiatric disorder, or both? Psychiatric diagnoses in adolescents with high-functioning ASD. *Journal of Clinical Child and Adolescent Psychology, 41*(4), 516–523.

McLeod, B. D., Jensen-Doss, A., Wheat, E., & Becker, E. M. (2013). Evidence-based assessment and case formulation for childhood anxiety disorders. In C. A. Essau & T. H. Ollendick (Eds.), *The Wiley-Blackwell handbook of the treatment of childhood and adolescent anxiety* (pp. 177–206). West Sussex: Wiley-Blackwell.

Merikangas, K. R., He, J.-P., Burstein, M., Swanson, S. A., Avenevoli, S., Cui, L., et al. (2010). Lifetime prevalence of mental disorders in US adolescents: Results from the National Comorbidity Survey Replication-Adolescent Supplement (NCS-A). *Journal of the American Academy of Child & Adolescent Psychiatry, 49*(10), 980–989.

Meuret, A. E., Wilhelm, F. H., Ritz, T., & Roth, W. T. (2003). Breathing training for treating panic disorder: Useful intervention or impediment? *Behavior Modification, 27*(5), 731–754. doi:10.1177/0145445503256324.

Meuret, A. E., Rosenfield, D., Hofmann, S. G., Suvak, M. K., & Roth, W. T. (2009). Changes in respiration mediate changes in fear of bodily sensations in panic disorder. *Journal of Psychiatric Research, 43*(6), 634–641. doi:10.1016/j.jpsychires.2008.08.003.

Miller, P. R., Dasher, R., Collins, R., Griffiths, P., & Brown, F. (2001). Inpatient diagnostic assessments: 1. Accuracy of structured vs. unstructured interviews. *Psychiatry Research, 105*(3), 255–264. doi:10.1016/S0165-1781(01)00317-1.

Minde, K., Roy, J., Bezonsky, R., & Hashemi, A. (2010). The effectiveness of CBT in 3–7 year old anxious children: Preliminary data. *Journal of the Canadian Academy of Child & Adolescent Psychiatry, 19*(2), 19–115.

Muris, P., & Merckelbach, H. (1998). Perceived parental rearing behaviour and anxiety disorders symptoms in normal children. *Personality & Individual Differences, 25*(6), 1199–1206.

Muris, P., Merckelbach, H., van Brakel, A., & Mayer, B. (1999). The revised version of the screen for child anxiety related emotional disorders (SCARED-R): Further evidence for its reliability and validity. *Anxiety, Stress & Coping: An International Journal, 12*(4), 411–425.

Muris, P., van der Pennen, E., Sigmond, R., & Mayer, B. (2008). Symptoms of anxiety, depression, and aggression in non-clinical children: Relationships with self-report and performance-based measures of attention and effortful control. *Child Psychiatry and Human Development, 39*(4), 455–467. doi:10.1007/s10578-008-0101-1.

Newman, D. L., Moffitt, T. E., Caspi, A., Magdol, L., Silva, P. A., & Stanton, W. R. (1996). Psychiatric disorder in a birth cohort of young adults: Prevalence, comorbidity, clinical significance, and new case incidence from ages 11–21. *Journal of Consulting and Clinical Psychology, 64*(3), 552–562. doi:10.1037/0022-006x.64.3.552.

Ollendick, T. H., King, N. J., & Frary, R. B. (1989). Fears in children and adolescents: Reliability and generalizability across gender, age, and nationality. *Behavior Reseach Therapy, 27*(1), 19–26.

Ollendick, T. H., King, N. J., & Chorpita, B. F. (2006). Empirically supported treatments for children and adolescents. In P. C. Kendall (Ed.), *Child and adolescent therapy: Cognitive-behavioral procedures* (3rd ed., pp. 492–520). New York: Guilford.

Ollendick, T. H., Öst, L. G., Reuterskiöld, L., Costa, N., Cederlund, R., Sirbu, C., Jarrett, M., et al. (2009). One-session treatment of specific phobias in youth: A randomized clinical trial in the USA and Sweden. *Journal of Consulting and Clinical Psychology, 77*, 504–516. doi:10.1037/a0015158.

Pina, A. A., Silverman, W. K., Saavedra, L. M., & Weems, C. F. (2001). An analysis of the RCMAS lie scale in a clinic sample of anxious children. *Journal of Anxiety Disorders, 15*(5), 443–457.

POTS, T. P. O. S. (2004). Cognitive-behavioral therapy, sertraline, and their combination for children and adolescents with obsessive-compulsive disorder. *Journal of the American Medical Association, 292*, 1969–1976.

Rapee, R. M., Schniering, C. A., & Hudson, J. L. (2009). Anxiety disorders during childhood and adolescence: Origins and treatment. *Annual Review of Clinical Psychology, 5*, 311–341.

Reynolds, C. R., & Richmond, B. O. (1985). *Manual for the revised children's manifest anxiety scale*. Los Angeles: Western Psychological Services.

Roberts, R. E., Attkisson, C. C., & Rosenblatt, A. (1998). Prevalence of psychopathology among children and adolescents. *American Journal of Psychiatry, 155*(6), 715–725.

Rotheram-Borus, M. J., Swendeman, D., & Chorpita, B. F. (2012). Disruptive innovations for designing and diffusing evidence-based interventions. *American Psychologist, 67*(6), 463–476. doi:10.1037/a0028180.

Russo, M. F., & Beidel, D. C. (1994). Comorbidity of childhood anxiety and externalizing disorders: Prevalence, associated characteristics, and validation issues. *Clinical Psychology Review, 14*(3), 199–221.

Schniering, C. A., & Rapee, R. M. (2002). Development and validation of a measure of children's automatic thoughts: The children's automatic thoughts scale. *Behaviour Research and Therapy, 40*(9), 1091–1109. doi:10.1016/S0005-7967(02)00022-0.

Seligman, L. D., & Ollendick, T. H. (1998). Comorbidity of anxiety and depression in children and adolescents: An integrative review. *Clinical Child and Family Psychology Review, 1*(2), 125–144.

Seligman, L., & Ollendick, T. (2011). Cognitive behavioral therapy for anxiety disorders in youth. *Child and adolescent psychiatric clinics of North America, 20*(2), 217.

Seligman, L. D., Ollendick, T. H., Langley, A. K., & Bechtoldt Baldacci, H. (2004). The utility of measures of child and adolescent anxiety: A meta-analytic review of the revised children's anxiety scale, the state-trait anxiety inventory for children, and the child behavior checklist. *Journal of Clinical Child and Adolescent Psychology, 33*(3), 557–565.

Seligman, L. D., Swedish, E. F., & Ollendick, T. H. (2014). Anxiety disorders. In C. A. Alfano & D. C. Beidel (Eds.), Comprehensive Evidence Based Interventions for Children and Adolescents (pp. 93–110). New York: Wiley.

Silverman, W., Pina, A., & Viswesvaran, C. (2008). Evidence-based psychosocial treatments for phobic and anxiety disorders in children and adolescents. *Journal of Clinical Child & Adolescent Psychology, 37*(1), 105–130.

Silverman, W. K., & Albano, A. M. (1996). *Anxiety disorders interview schedule for DSM-IV, child version*. San Antonio: The Psychological Corporation.

Silverman, W. K., & Ollendick, T. H. (2005). Evidence-based assessment of anxiety and its disorders in children and adolescents. *Journal of Clinical Child and Adolescent Psychology, 34*(3), 380–411.

Silverman, W. K., Kurtines, W. M., Ginsburg, G. S., Weems, C. F., Lumpkin, P. W., & Carmichael, D. H. (1999a). Treating anxiety disorders in children with group cognitive-behaviorial therapy: A randomized clinical trial. *Journal of Consulting and Clinical Psychology, 67*(6), 995–1003.

Silverman, W. K., Kurtines, W. M., Ginsburg, G. S., Weems, C. F., Rabian, B., & Serafini, L. T. (1999b). Contingency management, self-control, and education support in the treatment of childhood phobic disorders: A randomized clinical trial. *Journal of Consulting and Clinical Psychology, 67*(5), 675–687.

Silverman, W. K., Saavedra, L. M., & Pina, A. A. (2001). Test-retest reliability of anxiety symptoms and diagnoses with anxiety disorders interview schedule for DSM-IV: Child and parent versions. *Journal of the American Academy of Child & Adolescent Psychiatry, 40*(8), 937–944. doi:10.1097/00004583-200108000-00016.

Spence, S. H. (1998). A measure of anxiety symptoms among children. *Behaviour Research & Therapy, 36*(5), 545–566.

Spielberger, C. D. (1973). *Manual for the state-trait anxiety inventory for children*. Palo Alto: Consulting Psychologists.

U.S. Public Health Service. (2000). *Report of the surgeon general's conference on children's mental health: A national action agenda*. Washington, DC: Department of Health and Human Services.

Velting, O. N., Setzer, N. J., & Albano, A. M. (2004). Update on and advances in assessment and cognitive-behavioral treatment of anxiety disorders in children and adolescents. *Professional Psychology: Research and Practice, 35*(1), 42.

Verhulst, F. C., & Van der Ende, J. (1991). Assessment of child psychopathology: Relationships between different methods, different informants and clinical judgment of severity. *Acta Psychiatrica Scandinavica, 84*(2), 155–159.

Weems, C. F., Silverman, W. K., Rapee, R. M., & Pina, A. A. (2003). The role of control in childhood anxiety disorders. *Cognitive Therapy and Research, 27*(5), 557–568. doi:10.1023/A:1026307121386.

Weisz, J. R., Chorpita, B. F., Palinkas, L. A., Schoenwald, S. K., Miranda, J., Bearman, S. K., Gibbons, R. D., et al. (2012). Testing standard and modular designs for psychotherapy treating depression, anxiety, and conduct problems in youth: A randomized effectiveness trial. *Archives of General Psychiatry, 69*(3), 274–282. doi:10.1001/archgenpsychiatry.2011.147.

Woodward, L. J., & Fergusson, D. M. (2001). Life course outcomes of young people with anxiety disorders in adolescence. *Journal of the American Academy of Child & Adolescent Psychiatry, 40*(9), 1086–1093. doi:10.1097/00004583-200109000-00018.

Zimmerman, M., & Mattia, J. I. (1999). Psychiatric diagnosis in clinical practice: Is comorbidity being missed? *Comprehensive Psychiatry, 40*(3), 182–191. doi:10.1016/S0010-440X(99)90001-9.

Zoellner, L. A., Abramowitz, J. S., Moore, S. A., & Slagle, D. M. (2009). Flooding. In W. T. O'Donohue & J. E. Fisher (Eds.), *General principles and empirically supported techniques of cognitive behavior therapy* (pp. 300–308). Hoboken: Wiley.

Autism and Anxiety: Overlap, Similarities, and Differences

Connor Morrow Kerns and Philip C. Kendall

Autism and Anxiety: Overlap, Similarities, and Differences

Anxiety has historically been associated with cases of autism spectrum disorders (ASD). In their seminal articles of 1943 and 1944, both Kanner and Asperger, respectively, described symptoms of anxiety in their efforts to carve out the defining features of the autism spectrum. In *Autistic Disturbances of Affective Contact* (1943), Kanner described symptoms of anxiety in 6 of his original 11 case studies, reporting social fear, "…a good deal of worrying," unusual obsessiveness, a compulsive need for sameness, and phobias of both common and uncommon focus (e.g., fears of storms, loud sounds, and animals, as well as fears of running water, spinning tops, and mechanical noise). In Kanner's and Asperger's accounts, the anxiety of their patients is both clearly apparent and qualitatively different. Anxiety is depicted as not only a prevalent but also an auxiliary feature of the autism spectrum.

So the treatment of anxiety in ASD was anecdotally predetermined and perpetuated for several decades. Accordingly, whether symptoms in

ASD such as anxiety are inextricably intertwined with the core features of ASD or reflective of a distinct vulnerability remains a complex issue for both clinicians and researchers alike. Clarification of this issue has been long deferred, potentially due to the tendency for co-occurring mental health issues to be both attributed to and minimized by a more salient disability, such as ASD (MacNeil et al. 2009; Mason and Scior 2004). This propensity, often referred to as *diagnostic overshadowing* (Mason and Scior 2004), has likely contributed to both the limited amount of research on anxiety in ASD prior to the late 1990s and as the unresolved measurement and theoretical challenges apparent in current empirical investigations (Davis 2012; Kerns and Kendall 2012; Scahill 2012). Though relatively recent, efforts to study and better understand the occurrence and presentation of anxiety in ASD are now burgeoning, suggesting a potential change in perspective and renewed interest in the relationship of these syndromes. The number of studies assessing prevalence of anxiety in ASD alone has increased almost sevenfold in the last decade, from only three studies published in the 1990s to 23 published from 2000 to 2010 (van Steensel et al. 2011). Additional studies have explored predictors and characteristics of anxiety in ASD (Kerns and Kendall 2012; White et al. 2009), and still more have evaluated the effectiveness of cognitive–behavioral therapy (CBT) and modified CBT in reducing anxiety symptoms in this population (MacNeil et al. 2009; McNally et al. 2013; Puleo and Kendall 2011).

C. M. Kerns (✉)
AJ Drexel Autism Institute, Drexel University,
3020 Market Street, Suite 560,
Philadelphia, PA 19104–3734, USA
e-mail: cmk352@drexel.edu

P. C. Kendall
Temple University, Philadelphia, PA, USA

T. E. Davis III et al. (eds.), *Handbook of Autism and Anxiety,* Autism and Child Psychopathology Series,
DOI 10.1007/978-3-319-06796-4_6, © Springer International Publishing Switzerland 2014

Despite this growing recognition and investigation, questions regarding the prevalence, presentation, and appropriate classification of anxiety in ASD persist. As reviewed later, studies of anxiety in ASD have resulted in a range of inconsistent, sometimes contradictory, findings. This dilemma may be attributable to confusion regarding the role and potential atypical presentation of anxiety in ASD (Kerns et al. 2013), or reflect the related dearth of anxiety measures designed or validated for use with ASD youth (for a more detailed review, see Kerns and Kendall 2012).

Past and Present Challenges

The challenges of elucidating and studying the role of anxiety in ASD are multifold and reflective of both past inattention to the issue and difficulties related to the comorbidity of psychopathology generally (Lilienfeld et al. 1994; Regier et al. 2009). Categorical diagnostic systems, such as the Diagnostic Statistical Manual, Fourth Edition, Revised (DSM-IV-TR; American Psychiatric Association 2000) and Fifth Edition (DSM-5; American Psychiatric Association 2013), are characterized by a "plethora of comorbidity" that may challenge the validity of a categorical approach (p. 645; Regier et al. 2009). The pervasiveness of comorbidity may reflect a problem of dichotomous classification rather than a meaningful relationship between pathologies (Angold et al. 1999; Regier et al. 2009). Whereas medical disciplines look to organic processes to inform differential diagnosis, the definition of comorbidity in psychopathology is highly reliant on observable symptoms and behaviors (Lilienfeld et al. 1994). Comorbidity may be an artifact of symptom overlap, chance, sampling bias, or heterogeneous symptom expression (Drabick and Kendall 2010). These confounds are exemplified in the case of anxiety and ASD, which share symptoms, frequently co-occur, and manifest heterogeneously (White et al. 2009; Wood and Gadow 2010). The difficulties associated with comorbidity provide a rationale for the development of dimensional approaches to classification, wherein behavioral (or other) continua are emphasized (Regier et al. 2009).

Differential diagnosis of anxiety and ASD is inherently challenging due to the overlap and unusual presentation of some anxiety and ASD symptoms (Wood and Gadow 2010). Social awkwardness and avoidance, compulsive and ritualistic behavior, as well as some communication deficits may be particularly problematic areas of overlap. Studies comparing youth with anxiety disorders with youth with ASD without intellectual disability suggest that communication, and to a lesser degree, social deficits, may differentiate the disorders (Baron-Cohen and Belmonte 2005; Hartley and Sikora 2009). In a study of youth (6–16 years) with high-functioning ASD (IQ $\geq$ 70; $n=55$), anxiety disorders ($n=23$) or attention deficit/hyperactivity disorders (ADHD; $n=27$), Hartley and Sikora (2009) found that deficits in social and emotional reciprocity did not reliably distinguish between youth with ASD versus anxiety disorders, perhaps due to the reduced social reciprocity that may result from severe anxiety. Symptoms in the repetitive and restrictive interests domain appear even less discriminating (Baron-Cohen and Belmonte 2005; Cath et al. 2008; Hartley and Sikora 2009). Several studies report a positive association between anxiety and perseverative behavior in youth with ASD (Gadow et al. 2005; Guttmann-Steinmetz et al. 2010) as well as between anxiety and social deficits (Bellini 2004, 2006), illustrating the complexity of determining when such symptoms reflect anxiety, ASD, or both.

The reliable differentiation of anxiety and autism spectrum symptoms is further complicated by the possibility that symptoms of anxiety in ASD may manifest in an atypical fashion (Kerns and Kendall 2012; Kerns et al. 2013; Scahill 2012). Whereas some studies describe anxiety symptoms in individuals with ASD that appear consistent with DSM-IV-TR and DSM-5 criteria, others describe more unusual fears, worries, and rituals, whose proper classification as anxiety or autism is less clear (Kerns et al. 2013). These descriptions are apparent in both historical accounts (Asperger 1944; Kanner 1943) and recent empirical studies (Leyfer et al. 2006; Mayes et al.

2013; Muris et al. 1998). In one of the few studies to directly measure these atypical symptoms, Kerns et al. (2013) found that although 48% of youth ($N=59$; ages 7–17 years) with ASD presented with DSM-IV-TR-consistent anxiety disorders, 55% of those with DSM-IV-TR anxiety also presented with atypical or ambiguous anxiety symptoms, such as social fear without a fear of negative social evaluation, unusual specific phobias, or circumscribed fears of change or novelty. Further, 15% of youth presented with only these atypical or ambiguous symptoms, highlighting how different views of these symptoms may substantially influence anxiety prevalence estimates in ASD. Whether atypical symptoms reflect an aspect of ASD or potentially overlook symptoms of a co-occurring anxiety disorder remains unclear.

The lack of a unified approach for differentiating anxiety and ASD is notable, given these challenges, and reflects a significant limitation of much of the extant literature. The majority of studies on anxiety and ASD have relied on anxiety measures developed and psychometrically validated for youth *without* ASD (Kerns and Kendall 2012). Initial research in this area has been strongly influenced by theories and approaches developed in typically developing youth and adults with anxiety disorders, though such "downward or lateral extensions" to research have long been criticized as overly general and developmentally uninformed in child anxiety research (Davis 2012). The use of existing anxiety measures—albeit a necessary first step—does not ensure that these measures discriminate and capture the full range of anxiety symptoms that may occur in ASD. This concern may be particularly true when considering the results of informant or self-report measures, which rely on inexperienced raters and lack the flexibility of a semi-structured diagnostic interview. The limitations of current self-report and informant-report measures as well as semi-structured diagnostic interviews are particularly a concern, given that individuals with ASD may struggle to correctly identify and communicate their emotions (Scahill 2012).

Only a few studies have modified rating scales to assess anxiety in ASD. Adaptations consist predominantly of eliminating items that might overlap with the core features of ASD, an encouraging but likely insufficient strategy (Bakken et al. 2010; Brereton et al. 2006; Helverschou and Martinsen 2010; Kuusikko et al. 2008; Sukhodolsky et al. 2008). Kuusikko et al. (2008) found significantly higher levels of social anxiety in youth with ASD ($N=54$; IQ$\geq$80, 8–15 years) when compared with youth recruited from mainstream classrooms in the same community ($n=305$) both before and after removing potential ASD symptoms from self-report measures of general and social anxiety. This study did not assess whether the questionnaires provided a valid measure of social phobia (SocP) in ASD, however. In a sample of 171 youth (ages 5–17 years) with pervasive developmental disorders, an inclusive term used to describe DSM-IV-TR Asperger syndrome, autistic disorder, and pervasive developmental disorder, not otherwise specified (American Psychiatric Association 2000), Sukhodolsky et al. (2008) found good internal consistency in a modified version of the Child and Adolescent Symptom Inventory, Fourth Edition in a sample of youth with ASD. Additionally, Lecavalier (2006) found support for an anxiety cluster based on parent and teacher reports of behavioral issues in 487 youth with ASD. Again, these studies did not attempt to validate these instruments by establishing their association with an external criterion for anxiety disorders in each sample.

The lack of consensus regarding the operationalization and assessment of anxiety in ASD is perhaps most apparent in studies employing semi-structured diagnostic interviews. Variable strategies for differential diagnosis have been described (Kerns et al. 2013; Leyfer et al. 2006; Muris et al. 1998; Simonoff et al. 2008), but approaches generally lack full validation and have yielded discrepant results. Without consensus on how to differentiate the symptoms of anxiety in ASD, even semi-structured interviews have produced highly variable rates of the anxiety disorder, including obsessive-compulsive disorder (OCD): 6–37%, SocP: 8–29%, and generalized anxiety disorder: 2–35% (GAD; Kerns and Kendall 2012). In their efforts to differentiate anxiety and autism spectrum symptoms with a semi-structured diagnostic interview, Muris et al. (1998) noted that though 73% of their sample displayed ritualistic behavior, OCD was diagnosed only in those 11% of cases where parents identified ritual-related distress. Similarly, in developing the Autism Comorbidities Interview (ACI), one of the few instruments expressly designed to differentiate anxiety and ASD, Leyfer et al. (2006) noted relatively low rates of SocP (8%) and GAD (2%) in their sample after differentiating these conditions from pure social avoidance and routine-related agitation. These results are consistent with the suggestion that atypical anxiety presentations are relatively common in ASD and may substantially influence study outcomes depending on how they are conceptualized (Kerns et al. 2013).

Psychometric data supporting the use of existing diagnostic interviews in individuals with ASD are limited. Storch et al. (2012) reported good-to-excellent diagnostic agreement between parents and clinical consensus ratings on the Anxiety Disorders Interview Schedule-Child/ Parent (ADIS-C/P; Silverman and Albano 1996), but poor agreement between child and parent ratings, a pattern also apparent for typically developing youth with anxiety disorders (Benjamin et al. 2011). Acceptable inter-rater reliability for the ADIS-C/P in youth with ASD has been reported in several studies (Kerns et al. 2013; Ung et al. 2013; Wood et al. 2009). Additionally, Leyfer et al. (2006) found that the ACI delivered reliable (inter-rater) DSM diagnoses, which were consistent with a child's prior treatment history and community diagnoses in 109 youth with ASD. By contrast, Mazefsky et al. (2012) found that 60% of community psychiatric diagnoses in 35 youth (10–17 years) with ASD and unimpaired intellect were not supported by the ACI, illustrating the challenge of accurately diagnosing psychiatric comorbidities within the context of ASD. The majority of existing anxiety measures have yet to be validated in youth with ASD, that is, whether such measures adequately capture the construct of anxiety in ASD (content validity) and correlate

with theoretically related constructs (convergent validity) and measures of anxiety in ASD (concurrent validity), while being poorly associated with unrelated constructs (discriminant validity) is unclear and has yet to be sufficiently studied (Ollendick and White 2012).

How best to validate such instruments without clarification, theoretically and operationally, of the construct of anxiety in ASD is a looming question (Ollendick and White 2012). With this limitation in mind, Renno and Wood (2013) recently examined the discriminant and convergent validity of anxiety symptoms in youth with ASD and unimpaired intelligence ($N = 88$, 7–11 years) using a compilation of autism and anxiety-focused semi-structured diagnostic interviews and parent questionnaires. Results supported both the independence of anxiety and ASD constructs (i.e., youth with greater anxiety symptoms were no more likely to have greater ASD severity when compared with those with lower anxiety symptoms or vice versa) and the convergence of anxiety measures in this sample, though not for all anxiety subtypes. Whereas measures of separation and total anxiety appeared to converge, there was no evidence of convergent validity for social anxiety. Though this study reflects an encouraging first step, much further work is needed.

A history of inconsistent diagnostic standards and lack of validated measurement instruments has both tempered what conclusions can be drawn from existing research and prolonged confusion regarding the appropriate classification of anxiety in ASD. Whether anxiety symptoms in ASD are best conceptualized as core features of ASD, comorbid anxiety disorders, or another variant of anxiety in ASD remains unclear (Kerns and Kendall 2012; Wood and Gadow 2010). Kerns and Kendall (2012) suggested that a single model (e.g., core feature or comorbid disorder) may not be sufficient to characterize the relationship between these disorders. Further, Ollendick and White (2012) suggested that anxiety in youth with and without ASD is characterized by a set of both shared and unique features that must be considered when attempting to assess the construct of anxiety in this population. Consistent with this approach, comparisons of anxiety in youth with and without ASD suggest areas of both similarity and divergence.

In summary, findings regarding anxiety in ASD are substantially varied and limited by a lack of consensus regarding the differentiation and role of anxiety in ASD as well as by a nearly unanimous reliance on subjective anxiety measures, the validity of which is uncertain, given the communication and emotion recognition deficits that characterize ASD. Nevertheless, understanding these limitations as well as the potentially varied phenomenology of anxiety in ASD may provide some guidance for the wide variety of findings presented below.

Prevalence of Anxiety in ASD

Reviews of the empirical literature suggest that impairing anxiety presents in anywhere from 11–84 % of ASD youth, a range reflecting the results of 24 national and international studies from both clinical and community-based samples (Kerns and Kendall 2012; White et al. 2009). Sampling methods likely influence prevalence rates. Community and epidemiological studies estimate the prevalence of anxiety disorders in ASD to be between 40 and 50 % (Leyfer et al. 2006; Mattila et al. 2010; Simonoff et al. 2008), a range that is consistent with a recent meta-analysis (40 %; van Steensel et al. 2011). Estimates of problematic anxiety appear slightly higher in samples recruited from treatment settings, where anxiety symptom prevalence ranges from 14 to 59 % and anxiety disorder prevalence ranges from 35 to 55 % across studies. The highest prevalence estimates (e.g., 50–84 %) are apparent in projects that were more transparent and did not obscure their interest in anxiety during recruitment (Bellini 2004; Muris et al. 1998).

Some variation in prevalence may be attributable to the broad range of assessment measures employed across studies and, particularly, the inconsistent use of informant report measures versus semi-structured diagnostic interviews. Whereas a semi-structured interview identified anxiety disorders in 42 % of ASD youth ($N = 112$)

recruited from a population-derived cohort in the UK (Simonoff et al. 2008), a parent questionnaire identified significant anxiety symptoms in 25 % of youth in a Finnish epidemiological sample (Hurtig et al. 2009). This comparison may reflect the tendency for studies employing questionnaires to report generally lower rates (range 11–40 %; Hurtig et al. 2009; Kim et al. 2000, Lecavalier 2006; Ooi et al. 2011; Sukhodolsky et al. 2008) of problematic anxiety in ASD when compared with those utilizing semi-structured diagnostic interviews (range 42–84 %; de Bruin et al. 2007; Mattila et al. 2010; Muris et al. 1998; Simonoff et al. 2008).

Studies examining the prevalence of anxiety in ASD have been conducted in various countries, such as the USA (Gadow et al. 2004), UK (Simonoff et al. 2008), Finland (Mattila et al. 2010), Norway (Bakken et al. 2010), and Singapore (Ooi et al. 2011). They have included individuals of varying age ranges (Hofvander et al. 2009; Sukhodolsky et al. 2008), DSM-IV-TR autism spectrum diagnoses (Gadow et al. 2004), and intellectual impairment levels (Bradley et al. 2004; Hurtig et al. 2009; Sukhodolsky et al. 2008). The lack of anxiety assessments validated for individuals with ASD may contribute to the underestimation (e.g., true anxiety symptoms are dismissed as symptoms of ASD) or overestimation (e.g., symptoms of ASD are misconstrued as anxiety) of prevalence. However, the range of anxiety disorder rates suggested by epidemiological and community-based studies (i.e., 40–50 %) is generally consistent with that reported in two studies that employed comprehensive assessment approaches (44 %—Leyfer et al. 2006; 46 %—Kerns et al. 2013). Moreover, it is of interest that studies find anxiety symptoms to be distinct from ASD severity (Renno and Wood 2013; Kerns et al. 2013) and apparent in many, but often not the majority of individuals with ASD (Bellini 2006; Gadow and Wood 2010; Helverschou and Martinsen 2010; Leyfer et al. 2006).

Similarities and Differences

Occurrence

Anxiety disorders occur in approximately 18% of adults (Kessler et al. 2005) and 15% of children (Beesdo et al. 2009) in the population (see also Muris, Chap. 3, this volume). As noted previously, estimates of anxiety disorder prevalence in individuals with ASD are substantially higher when compared with those apparent in the general population. Studies comparing the rate of anxiety problems in youth with ASD relative to other groups of youth suggest that anxiety difficulties are significantly more common in youth with ASD than typically developing children (Gadow et al. 2005; Hurtig et al. 2009; Kim et al. 2000) as well as youth with learning disabilities (Burnette et al. 2005), specific language impairments (Gillott et al. 2001), Down syndrome (Evans et al. 2005), and Williams syndrome (Rodgers et al. 2012).

There are multiple anxiety disorders, but the most common anxiety disorder in ASD is unclear. However, like youth without ASD, specific phobia, GAD, SocP, and Separation Anxiety Disorder (SAD) are among the most common anxiety disorders overall. Though OCD and post-traumatic stress disorder (PTSD) have been separated from the anxiety disorders in the DSM-5, they have been historically considered to have a strong anxiety component and studied as anxiety disorders prior to this recent DSM revision, including in many samples of youth with ASD. As such, we will include a review of this research herein. Compulsive behaviors generally appear more frequently (6–37%; Bakken et al. 2010; Gillott et al. 2001) in ASD when compared with typically developing youth (1%; Rapee et al. 2009). By comparison, rates of PTSD are rarely reported in youth with ASD, though youth with developmental disabilities appear at increased risk for abuse (Mandell et al. 2005). In one of the few studies to assess rates of PTSD in 69 (53 male) children and adolescents with ASD, Mehtar and Mukaddes (2011) reported PTSD in 17% of their sample, suggesting that PTSD may

be relatively common in youth with ASD and requires further study.

Anxiety Presentation

Though comorbidity may often be associated with a more severe presentation and course (Cerdá et al. 2008), one study did not find anxiety disorders in youth with ASD to be associated with more severe outcomes when compared with those in youth without ASD (Cath et al. 2008). Whereas differences were not apparent in overall anxiety scores per child report, Russell and Sofronoff (2005) reported greater severity of parent-reported general anxiety, obsessive-compulsive symptoms, and physical injury concerns in 65 adolescents with Asperger's syndrome relative to an anxious sample without ASD. Similarly, Farrugia and Hudson (2006) found more negative automatic thoughts in adolescents with Asperger's syndrome compared to anxious youth without ASD, despite equivalent overall anxiety symptom severity, suggesting the potential for symptom-level differences that are not immediately apparent when examining overall severity scores.

Studies suggest some notable similarities in the presentation of anxiety disorders and symptoms in youth with ASD versus youth without ASD and also some notable differences. As in youth with anxiety disorder, but not ASD (Kendall et al. 2010), the presentation and prevalence of anxiety symptoms in males versus females with ASD appear similar, though only one study has directly considered this issue (Worley et al. 2010). Gadow et al. (2005) observed that, with the exception of compulsions, specific and social phobias, the distribution of co-occurring mental health problems was similar in a sample of children (ages 6–12 years) with ASD ($n=284$) and non-ASD disorders ($n=189$). Similarly, Farrugia and Hudson (2006) found that adolescents with Asperger's syndrome and adolescents with anxiety disorders (but not Asperger's syndrome) both frequently reported symptoms of GAD, SocP, and OCD; however, only the Asperger group reported more thoughts of physical injury and social threat. Russell and Sofronoff (2005) observed significantly more obsessive-compulsive symptoms and physical injury fears but fewer social evaluation concerns in adolescents with Asperger's syndrome and anxiety disorder versus those with anxiety disorder alone. In summary, whereas studies note many similarities in the anxiety symptoms of youth with and without ASD, a pattern of increased obsessive-compulsive symptoms and fears of physical injury and social avoidance, despite reduced social evaluation concerns, is also apparent. This pattern supports the potential distinctiveness of these symptoms from other anxieties, and is supported by variation in the symptom profiles of specific phobia, SocP, and OCD in ASD youth.

Studies suggest that specific phobias are present in as many as 44–63 % of ASD youth (Leyfer et al. 2006; Muris et al. 1998), across various levels of intellectual functioning (Sukhodolsky et al. 2008). Yet, phobias in this population may have an unusual focus. In 109 youth with autism and IQ greater than 65, Leyfer et al. (2006) found that fears of shots/needles and crowds were most common, whereas phobias typical in normative samples, such as tunnels, flying, and bridges, were rare. Additionally, 10 % of ASD youth reported a fear of loud noises, a relatively uncommon fear in the general population. Evans et al. (2005) also reported a distinct pattern of phobias, including more medical, situational (e.g. dark, large crowds, closed spaces), and animal fears in youth with ASD versus youth with Down Syndrome, or two groups of typically developing, chronological and mental-age-matched participants, suggesting that observed differences in phobia focus were not attributable to youth's intellectual or developmental level. Finally, in a sample of 1,033 children with autism studied by Mayes at al. (2013), 42 % of parents reported unusual fears, including fears of mechanical things, swings, weather, and toilets, in addition to many common fears in children with ASD. In short, whereas many youth present with common specific phobias, at least a portion also present with more unusual fears, which may or may not be unique to this population.

The expression of SocP in ASD may be different from its expression in typically developing youth. Gillott et al. (2001) found that fears of negative social evaluation (e.g., fears of appearing foolish or becoming embarrassed), a defining feature of SocP, were fewer in children with autism (and no intellectual disability) compared to typically developing youth or youth with specific language impairment. By comparison, Russell and Sofronoff (2005) found equal rates of parent-reported self-consciousness and avoidance in adolescents with anxiety disorders and those with Asperger's syndrome. Though ASD-related social avoidance may be mistaken for SocP, Kuusikko et al. (2008) observed elevated rates of other, distinct social anxiety symptoms in youth with high-functioning ASD after removing potentially ambiguous symptoms from a parent report measure. Further, interfering social anxiety, sensitive to increased social pressures (Kuusikko et al. 2008), and social skills deficits (Bellini 2004, 2006) have been found despite stringent diagnostic evaluation in several studies (Kerns et al. 2013; Leyfer et al. 2006). Cumulatively, results support both the presence of traditional social anxiety, including a fear of negative evaluation or rejection, and a qualitatively distinct pattern of social avoidance and agitation which lacks this core feature in youth with ASD.

As mentioned previously, OCD has been separated from the anxiety disorders in DSM-5; nonetheless, it has long been understood to have a strong anxiety component, warranting its inclusion in the present chapter. The differentiation of OCD symptoms in ASD from ASD-related rituals, perseverations, or other repetitive behaviors is daunting. Research suggests that restricted and repetitive behaviors in ASD can be subdivided into repetitive sensory motor and insistence on sameness behaviors, which may be particularly difficult to distinguish from OCD (Bishop et al. 2013). As a result, many studies have opted to measure repetitive behaviors generally as opposed to attempting differential diagnosis. Zandt et al. (2007; $N = 54$) found a hierarchy of repetitive behaviors in community-recruited youth with ASD (without intellectual disability), OCD, and typical development (i.e., the control group), with obsessions, routines, and rituals being most pronounced and complex in youth with OCD, followed by youth with ASD and then controls. Though age influenced repetitive behavior presentation in the OCD group, it was unrelated to the presentation of obsessions, compulsions, repetitive movements, or rigidity in ASD youth. Notably, rates of OCD symptoms in ASD also appear substantially lower when evidence of premonitory distress or a purposeful quality to compulsions is required (Muris et al. 1998; Simonoff et al. 2008). These results support the presence of compulsive, ritualistic behaviors in ASD that are somewhat distinct from OCD symptoms.

Studies support a different presentation of obsessions and compulsions in ASD. In their study of 109 youth (ages 5–17 years) with ASD and ranging intellectual abilities, Leyfer et al. (2006) observed that urges to tell/ask and verbal or behavioral rituals involving another person were the most common compulsions. McDougle et al. (1995) found that adults with ASD demonstrated significantly more repeating, touching, tapping, and hoarding compulsions and less cleaning, checking, counting, and aggressive obsessions when compared with adults with OCD (but not ASD); however, this study did not control for significantly different intellectual levels between groups. Two studies comparing OCD in intellectually average adults with and without ASD suggest more similarities than differences in symptom presentation (Cath et al. 2008; Russell and Sofronoff 2005). Cath et al. (2008) reported no differences in compulsive symptoms or egodystonia (i.e., the feeling that one's symptoms are unwanted and in conflict with one's self and personal goals), but less obsessions in ASD/OCD versus OCD only groups. Similarly, Russell et al. (2005) noted few differences in symptom presentation between adults with ASD, OCD, and both disorders (25% of ASD sample) after carefully distinguishing between stereotypic behaviors and interests and OCD symptoms.

In summary, the data support both similarity and divergence in the distribution, severity, and quality of anxiety symptoms apparent in youth with ASD versus youth without anxiety disorders. Key areas of divergence arise in disorders and symptoms that are both more aligned with the core deficits of ASD and likely to be altered by them. For example, whereas compulsive behavior, social avoidance, and unusual specific phobias appear more common in ASD youth, fears of social evaluation and obsessions appear less frequent. These preliminary results are in keeping with the notion that both typical and atypical expressions of anxiety may arise in ASD.

Onset and Trajectory

Research investigating the onset and trajectory of anxiety symptoms in youth with and without ASD has produced varied results. Some studies report no relationship between age and anxiety severity (Sukhodoksy et al. 2008; White and Robertson-Nay 2009), whereas others note a developmental fluctuation in anxiety risk (Davis et al. 2011a). Though some symptoms of anxiety, specifically compulsions and specific and social phobia symptoms, appear elevated in youth with ASD very early in life (i.e., ages 3–5 years; Gadow et al. 2004, 2005), such studies of anxiety in very young children have relied rather fully on parent and teacher reports of potentially ambiguous behaviors (e.g., social avoidance) on screening measures rather than comprehensive anxiety scales. As such, these findings should be interpreted with caution. Further, the anxiety referenced in these very young age groups, and that found to be unrelated to age or intellectual ability (Sukhodolsky et al. 2008; White and Roberson-Nay 2009), may be distinct from that shown to fluctuate with time, child awareness, and age in other studies (Davis et al. 2011a).

Consideration of similar and dissimilar varieties of anxiety presentation in ASD may reconcile findings from studies that do report a relationship between age and anxiety with those that do not. Whereas teachers, but not parents, report anxiety problems in 3–5-year-olds with ASD, anxiety problems appear evident to both parents and teachers by age 6–12 years (Weisbrot et al. 2005). In two studies of youth with ASD, Gadow et al. (2004, 2005) noted over twice as many anxiety symptoms in school-aged children (12%) as preschoolers (5%). This pattern may reflect an increase in social evaluation concerns (as is typical developmentally) or the ability to express them with increasing age for youth with ASD. It may also reflect the particular difficulty of differentiating anxiety and ASD symptoms in very young children. Kuusikko et al. (2008) reported an increase in social anxiety concerns and social avoidance with age in a study of 359, 8–15-year-old youth (54 intellectually average ASD youth vs. 305 community controls). Parent-reported social avoidance and fears of negative evaluation were elevated in youth with ASD relative to typically developing youth after removing potentially overlapping symptoms and increased with age, an inverse pattern from that observed in typically developing youth, whose fears reduced over time. Specifically, adolescents with ASD displayed significantly more social avoidance, inhibition, and social discomfort when compared with children with ASD. Consistent with the notion that anxiety changes developmentally, Davis et al. (2011a), in their cross sectional study of toddlers (17–36 months), children (3–16 years), young adults (20–48 years), and older adults (49–65 years) with ASD, found a waxing and waning pattern of anxiety symptoms with age. Anxiety increased in childhood and adolescence, diminished in adulthood, and rebounded again in later life (49–65 years), a trajectory that resembles that seen in typically developing youth, though illness onset and severity may be delayed by the presence of ASD. Specifically, the development of higher cognitive abilities appears to predate anxiety symptoms in both ASD and typically developing samples; however, given that these abilities are often delayed or deficient in individuals with ASD, abstract anxieties appear to arise later and to a diminished degree.

Though tempered by measurement limitations, studies suggest many similarities in the distribution, severity, symptom presentation, and developmental course of anxiety in youth with and without ASD. These similarities are consistent with the notion that anxiety disorders may present similarly in ASD as they do in youth without ASD or other comorbidities

IQ, Language, and ASD subtype

Dissimilarity in the expression and presentation of anxiety in ASD may in part be a reflection of developmental and cognitive differences inherent to this disorder (Ollendick and White 2012). Studies have explored relationships between anxiety and intellectual ability, language skill, and, prior to DSM-5, specific DSM-IV-TR ASD diagnoses (e.g., Asperger syndrome, autistic disorder, pervasive developmental disorder, not otherwise specified or PDD-NOS) with mixed results.

Where some studies support a positive relationship between anxiety and IQ (Lecavalier 2006; Sukhodolsky et al. 2008; Weisbrot et al. 2005), others report no relationship (Brereton et al. 2006; Simonoff et al. 2008). In a sample of 172 youth with PDD-NOS and a broad range of cognitive abilities (profound disability to average intelligence), Sukhodolsky et al. (2008) found that individuals with IQs above rather than below 70 were significantly more likely to present with an anxiety disorder. Mayes et al. (2011) observed parent-reported impairing anxiety in 67 versus 79% of ASD youth with ($n=117$, IQ<80) and without ($n=233$, IQ$\geq$80) significant intellectual impairment, with unimpaired youth demonstrating significantly more overall anxiety symptoms (e.g., worry, self-consciousness, "sick with worry"), but not more behavior problems (e.g., oppositional behavior, avoidance). Consistently, anxiety symptoms in youth with ASD, particularly GAD symptoms, appear related to increased intellectual ability in several studies (Gadow et al. 2005; Weisbrot et al. 2005). Further, Lecavalier (2006) found that very severe intellectual deficits were associated with fewer anxiety symptoms in a study of youth with ASD and varied intellectual disability (i.e., mild, moderate, and severe).

Notably, the diagnosis of anxiety problems in youth with ASD and intellectual disability via solely subjective or observer report measures is inherently problematic, limiting confidence in the conclusions that can be drawn. Still, impairing anxiety symptoms, measured via parent and teacher questionnaires of children's stressed or agitated behavior, have been reported in 11–42% of youth with ASD across a broad range of intellectual abilities (Bakken et al. 2010; Bradley et al. 2004; Lecavalier 2006; Sukhodolsky et al. 2008). Additionally, anxiety symptoms appear more common in intellectually impaired individuals with, rather than without, ASD (Bradley et al. 2004). Some studies suggest that anxiety severity is unrelated to IQ; others suggest that IQ differentially predicts certain anxiety symptoms. For example, in their study, Sukhodolsky et al. (2008) found that parent reports of certain anxieties, such as specific and social phobias, were equally prevalent in ASD individuals with and without intellectual disability, whereas generalized and separation- and panic-related worries as well as total anxiety symptoms were greater in those with higher IQ. Intellectual abilities may thus be more predictive of the form of anxiety symptoms, than the frequency of this psychopathology.

Prior to the introduction of a single ASD category in the DSM-5, studies explored differences in anxiety presentation in youth with autistic disorder, Asperger's Syndrome and PDD-NOS. Several studies report no differences in the number of parent- and self-reported anxiety problems of youth with Asperger disorder versus high-functioning autism (Hurtig et al. 2009; Kim et al. 2000; Kuusikko et al. 2008). Gadow et al. (2004) also found no variation in the anxiety symptoms of preschoolers with varied DSM-IV-TR ASD diagnoses, and Simonoff et al. (2008) found no relationship between ASD symptoms and anxiety disorder severity in 112 adolescents with ASD. By comparison, some studies suggest significantly more GAD worries and overall anxiety symptoms, after controlling for age and intellectual level in youth with Asperger's syndrome versus high-functioning autism (Thede and Coolidge 2007; Tonge et al. 1999). Other studies report more anxiety disorders (Muris et al. 1998) and symptoms (Weisbrot et al. 2005) in children with Asperger's syndrome and PDD-NOS versus autistic disorder; however, these studies did not control for IQ. In a study of children with autistic disorder (but no intellectual disability) and PDD-NOS (IQ $\geq$ 70), Kanai et al. (2004) found better social relatedness and predicted more separation anxiety in PDD-NOS youth. Finally, behavioral

indicators of anxiety in ASD (e.g., avoidance, restricted, ritualistic behavior) appear to present more frequently in young children (17–36 months) with autism as opposed to PDD-NOS (Davis et al. 2011a; Matson et al. 2010).

These contradictory results may reflect the questionable reliability and validity of DSM-IV-TR ASD subtypes. Moreover, differences in anxiety by ASD type, when present, may be attributable to the variable cognitive and verbal functioning of youth. In a sample of 66 ASD children (ages 2–14 years), Davis et al. (2011b) noted an interaction between ASD diagnosis and communication deficits, such that more communication difficulties were associated with more anxiety in youth with PDD-NOS ($n=33$), but less anxiety in those with autism ($n=33$). By contrast, in a sample of 735 infants and toddlers, Davis et al. (2012) found that greater expressive and receptive language skills predicted more anxiety symptoms in youth with PDD-NOS and autism, but not atypical development (i.e., developmental delays not amounting to ASD). Though these results should be considered preliminary, they suggest that poorer language skills may minimize anxiety or the report of anxiety in infants with ASD, while mild to moderate, but not severe language deficits, may result in greater anxiety in older youth. The association between anxiety and higher-functioning youth with PDD-NOS and Asperger's syndrome in some studies is notable, given that these same youth are at greatest risk of being excluded from new ASD DSM-5 criteria, a diagnostic shift with potentially important ramifications for the future study of anxiety in ASD (Davis et al. 2012). Given this risk, it will be important to assess how new ASD severity levels, now specified when diagnosing ASD according to DSM-5 criteria, may influence the prevalence and presentation of anxiety in this potentially modified population. For example, whether more traditional (as opposed to atypical or ambiguous) symptoms of anxiety will be more consistently and robustly associated with less severe ASD (i.e., Severity Level 1 vs. 2 or 3) is of interest.

Conclusions

Anxiety, a long noted but relatively neglected difficulty in youth with ASD, has recently gained research and clinical attention. Future work will need to shed additional light on the prevalence and presentation of anxiety in ASD, while also addressing concerns about how best to conceptualize and assess these conditions. Though efforts to understand the anxiety of individuals with ASD via existing measures reflect an essential first step, the successes and challenges of these early ventures must now inform and shape our next steps. Research suggests that anxiety problems commonly occur in youth with ASD with ranging intellectual and verbal abilities. Moreover, findings suggest that the anxiety of individuals with ASD shares many features with the anxiety of typical developing youth. Similarities are apparent in symptom expression, severity, trajectory, and sensitivity to developmental factors. Variations in the expression, presentation, and course of anxiety in youth with ASD versus without ASD are also apparent. These distinctive features of anxiety in ASD challenge existing anxiety measures, obfuscate findings, and may reflect ongoing confusion regarding the differentiation and role of anxiety in ASD.

Diagnostic confusion is not unique to anxiety and ASD, but rather appears to be an issue within mental health nosology in general (Regier et al. 2009). Similarly, an overreliance on subjective anxiety measures, as seen in the current literature on anxiety in ASD, is a frequently cited limitation in anxiety disorder research (Davis 2012; Davis and Ollendick 2005; Scahill 2012). Consensus regarding the differential diagnosis and role of anxiety disorders in ASD is needed, but may take time and patience to achieve. A critical initial step includes studying the properties of anxiety measures in samples of ASD youth. Future steps may involve designing novel, developmentally informed measures of anxiety for this population. How biologically based measurements (e.g., electrophysiological or neurobiological indicators) of anxiety may add to these efforts should also be considered, given that alternative assessments may help address the inherent challenge of recognizing and reporting emotional states for individuals with ASD. Empirically based assessment of both typical anxiety symptoms and the atypical, potentially unique features of anxiety in ASD will also help elucidate whether atypical symptoms should be conceptualized as aspects of ASD, as comorbid anxiety, or as a novel behavioral dimension common to both disorders.

A comprehensive understanding of anxiety and ASD may call for a willingness to (a) consider common, underlying behavioral and neurobiological dimensions of functioning (e.g., emotion dysregulation, executive dysfunction) and (b) develop a clearer theoretical model of anxiety in ASD to inform measurement development and validation. Downward or lateral extensions of adult and child anxiety research are likely to be insufficient, given the unique developmental and neurobiological facets of ASD and its complex relationship with anxiety (Davis 2012). Clarification of the origins, phenomenology, and differentiation of anxiety in youth with ASD will thus be instrumental in progressing the future study, understanding, and successful treatment of these disorders. It may also provide a novel, potentially generalizable model of psychological comorbidity.

References

American Psychiatric Association. (2000). *Diagnostic and statistical manual of mental disorders* (4th ed.). Arlington: American Psychiatric Publishing.

American Psychiatric Association. (2013). *Diagnostic and statistical manual of mental disorders* (5th ed.). Arlington: American Psychiatric Publishing.

Angold, A., Costello, E. J., & Erkanli, A. (1999). Comorbidity. *Journal of Child Psychology and Psychiatry, 40*, 57–87.

Asperger, H. (1944). "Die "Autistischen Psychopathen" im Kindesalter [Autistic psychopaths in childhood]". *Archiv für Psychiatrie und Nervenkrankheiten, 177*, 76–136. doi:10.1007/BF01837709 (in German).

Bakken, T. L., Helverschou, S. B., Eilertsen, D. E., Heggelund, T., Myrbakk, E., & Martinsen, H. (2010). Psychiatric disorders in adolescents and adults with autism and intellectual disability: A representative study in one county in Norway. *Research in Developmental Disabilities, 31*, 1669–1677. doi:10.1016/j.ridd.2010.04.009.

Baron-Cohen, S., & Belmonte, M. K. (2005). Autism: A window onto the development of the social and the analytic brain. *Annual Review of Neuroscience, 28,* 109–126. doi:10.1146/annurev.neuro.27.070203.144137.

Bellini, S. (2004). Social skill deficits and anxiety in high-functioning adolescents with autism spectrum disorders. *Focus on Autism and Other Developmental Disabilities, 19,* 78–86. doi:10.1177/10883576040190 020201.

Bellini, S. (2006). The development of social anxiety in adolescents with autism spectrum disorders. *Focus on Autism and Other Developmental Disabilities, 21,* 138–145. doi:10.1177/1088357606021003020.

Benjamin, C. L., Puleo, C. M., & Kendall, P. C. (2011). Informant agreement in treatment gains for child anxiety. *Child & Family Behavior Therapy, 33*(3), 199–216. doi:10.1080/07317107.2011.595987.

Beesdo, K., Knappe, S., & Pine, D. S. (2009). Anxiety and anxiety disorders in children and adolescents: Developmental issues and implications for DSM-V. *The Psychiatric Clinics of North America, 32*(3), 483. doi:10.1016/j.psc.2009.06.002.

Bishop, S. L., Hus, V., Duncan, A., Huerta, M., Gotham, K., Pickles, A., & Lord, C. (2013). Subcategories of restricted and repetitive behaviors in children with autism spectrum disorders. *Journal of autism and developmental disorders, 43,* 1287–1297.

Bradley, E. A., Summers, J. A., Wood, H. L., & Bryson, S. E. (2004). Comparing rates of psychiatric and behavior disorders in adolescents and young adults with severe intellectual disability with and without autism. *Journal of Autism and Developmental Disorders, 34,* 151–161. doi:10.1023/B:JADD.0000022606.97580.19.

Brereton, A. V., Tonge, B. J., & Einfeld, S. L. (2006). Psychopathology in children and adolescents with autism compared to young people with intellectual disability. *Journal of Autism and Developmental Disorders, 36,* 863–870. doi:10.1007/s10803-006-0125-y.

Burnette, C. P., Mundy, P. C., Meyer, J. A., Sutton, S. K., Vaughan, A. E., & Charak, D. (2005). Weak central coherence and its relations to theory of mind and anxiety in autism. *Journal of Autism and Developmental Disorders, 35,* 63–73. doi:10.1007/s10803-004-1035-5.

Cath, D. C., Ran, N., Smit, J. H., Van Balkom, A., & Comijs, H. C. (2008). Symptom overlap between autism spectrum disorders, generalized social anxiety disorder and obsessive-compulsive disorder in adults: A preliminary case-controlled study. *Psychopathology, 41,* 101–110. doi:10.1159/000111555.

Cerdá, M., Sagdeo, A., & Galea, S. (2008). Comorbid forms of psychopathology: Key patterns and future research directions. *Epidemiologic Reviews, 30,* 155–177. doi:10.1093/epirev/mxn003.

Davis, T. E. III, Hess, J. A., Moree, B. N., Fodstad, J. C., Dempsey, T., Jenkins, W. S., & Matson, J. L. (2011a). Anxiety symptoms across the lifespan in people diagnosed with autistic disorder. *Research in Autism Spectrum Disorders, 5,* 112–118. doi:10.1016/j.rasd.2010.02.006.

Davis, T. E. III, Moree, B. N., Dempsey, T., Reuther, E. T., Fodstad, J. C., Hess, J. A., & Matson, J. L. (2011b). The relationship between autism spectrum disorders and anxiety: The moderating effect of communication. *Research in Autism Spectrum Disorders, 5,* 324–329. doi:10.1016/j.rasd.2010.04.015.

Davis, T. E. (2012). Where to from here for ASD and Anxiety? Lessons Learned from Child anxiety and the Issue of DSM-5. *Clinical Psychology: Science and Practice, 19,* 358–363.

Davis, T. E., & Ollendick, T. H. (2005). Empirically supported treatments for specific phobia in children: Do efficacious treatments address the components of a phobic response?. *Clinical Psychology: Science and Practice, 12*(2), 144-160.

Davis, T. E., Moree, B. N., Dempsey, T., Hess, J. A., Jenkins, W. S., Fodstad, J. C., & Matson, J. L. (2012). The effect of communication deficits on anxiety symptoms in infants and toddlers with autism spectrum disorders. *Behavior Therapy, 43*(1), 142–152. doi:10.1016/j.beth.2011.05.003.

de Bruin, E. I., Ferdinand, R. F., Meester, S., de Nijs, P. F. A., & Verheij, F. (2007). High rates of psychiatric comorbidity in PDD-NOS. *Journal of Autism and Developmental Disorders, 37,* 877–886. doi:10.1007/s10803-006-0215-x.

Drabick, D. A. G., & Kendall, P. C. (2010). Developmental psychopathology and the diagnosis of mental health problems among youth. *Clinical Psychology: Science and Practice, 17,* 272–280. doi:10.1111/j.1468-2850.2010.01219.x.

Evans, D. W., Canavera, K., Kleinpeter, F. L., Maccubbin, E., & Taga, K. (2005). The fears, phobias and anxieties of children with autism spectrum disorders and Down syndrome: Comparisons with developmentally and chronologically age matched children. *Child Psychiatry and Human Development, 36,* 3–26. doi:10.1007/s10578-004-3619-x.

Farrugia, S., & Hudson, J. (2006). Anxiety in adolescents with Asperger syndrome: Negative thoughts, behavioral problems, and life interference. *Focus on Autism and Other Developmental Disabilities, 21,* 25–35. doi:10.1177/10883576060210010401.

Gadow, K. D., DeVincent, C. J., Pomeroy, J., & Azizian, A. (2004). Psychiatric symptoms in preschool children with PDD and clinic and comparison samples. *Journal of Autism and Developmental Disorders, 34,* 379–393. doi:10.1023/B:JADD.0000037415.21458.93.

Gadow, K. D., DeVincent, C. J., Pomeroy, J., & Azizian, A. (2005). Comparison of DSM-IV symptoms in elementary school-age children with PDD versus clinic and community samples. *Autism: The International Journal of Research and Practice, 9,* 392–415. doi:10.1177/1362361305056079.

Gillott, A., Furniss, F., & Walter, A. (2001). Anxiety in high-functioning children with autism. *Autism: The International Journal of Research and Practice, 5*(3), 277–286. doi:10.1177/1362361301005003005.

Guttmann-Steinmetz, S., Gadow, K. D., DeVincent, C. J., & Crowell, J. (2010). Anxiety symptoms in boys with autism spectrum disorder, attention-deficit hyperactivity disorder, or chronic multiple tic disorder and community controls. *Journal of Autism and Developmental Disorders, 40*, 1006–1016. doi:10.1007/s10803-010-0950-x.

Hartley, S. L., & Sikora, D. M. (2009). Which DSM-IV-TR criteria best differentiate high-functioning autism spectrum disorder from ADHD and anxiety disorders in older children? *Autism: The International Journal of Research and Practice, 13*, 485–509. doi:10.1177/1362361309335717.

Helverschou, S. B., & Martinsen, H. (2010). Anxiety in people diagnosed with autism and intellectual disability: Recognition and phenomenology. *Research in Autism Spectrum Disorders, 5*, 377–387. doi:10.1016/j.rasd.2010.05.003.

Hofvander, B., Delorme, R., Chaste, P., Nyden, A., Wentz, E., Stahlberg, O., et al. (2009). Psychiatric and psychosocial problems in adults with normal-intelligence autism spectrum disorders. *BMC psychiatry, 9*, 35. doi:10.1186/1471-244X-9-35.

Hurtig, T., Kuusikko, S., Mattila, M. L., Haapsamo, H., Ebeling, H., Jussila, K., et al. (2009). Multi-informant reports of psychiatric symptoms among high-functioning adolescents with Asperger or autism. *Autism: The International Journal of Research and Practice, 13*, 583–598. doi:10.1177/1362361309335719..

Kanai, C., Koyama, T., Kato, S., Miyamoto, Y., Osada, H., & Kurita, H. (2004). Comparison of high-functioning atypical autism and childhood autism by childhood autism rating scale-Tokyo version. *Psychiatry and Clinical Neurosciences, 58*, 217–221. doi:10.1111/j.1440-1819.2003.01220.x.

Kanner, L. (1943). Autistic disturbances of affective contact. *Nervous Child, 2*, 217–250.

Kendall, P. C., Compton, S. N., Walkup, J. T., Birmaher, B., Albano, A. M., Sherrill, J., et al. (2010). Clinical characteristics of anxiety disordered youth. *Journal of Anxiety Disorders, 24*, 360–365. doi:10.1016/j.janxdis.2010.01.009.

Kerns, C. M., & Kendall, P. C. (2012). The presentation and classification of anxiety in autism spectrum disorder. *Clinical Psychology: Science & Practice, 19*, 323–347. doi:10.1111/cpsp.12009.

Kerns, C. M., Kendall, P.C., Berry, L., Souders, M. C., Franklin, M. E., Schultz, R. T., Miller, J., Herrington, J. (in press). Traditional and atypical presentations of anxiety in youth with autism spectrum disorder. *Journal of Autism and Developmental Disorders*.

Kessler, R. C., Chiu, W. T., Demler, O., & Walters, E. E. (2005). Prevalence, severity, and comorbidity of 12-month DSM-IV disorders in the National Comorbidity Survey Replication. *Archives of General Psychiatry, 62*(6), 617. doi:10.1001/archpsyc.62.6.617.

Kim, J. A., Szatmari, P., Bryson, S. E., Streiner, D. L., & Wilson, F. J. (2000). The prevalence of anxiety and mood problems among children with autism and Asperger syndrome. *Autism: The International Journal of Research and Practice, 4*, 117–132. doi:10.1177/1362361300004002002.

Kuusikko, S., Pollock-Wurman, R., Jussila, K., Carter, A. S., Mattila, M. L., Ebeling, H., et al. (2008). Social anxiety in high-functioning children and adolescents with autism and Asperger syndrome. *Journal of Autism and Developmental Disorders, 38*, 1697–1709. doi:10.1007/s10803-008-0555-9.

Lecavalier, L. (2006). Behavioral and emotional problems in young people with pervasive developmental disorders: Relative prevalence, effects of subject characteristics, and empirical classification. *Journal of Autism and Developmental Disorders, 36*, 1101–1114. doi:10.1007/s10803-006-0147-5.

Leyfer, O. T., Folstein, S. E., Bacalman, S., Davis, N. O., Dinh, E., Morgan, J., & Lainhart, J. E. (2006). Comorbid psychiatric disorders in children with autism: Interview development and rates of disorders. *Journal of Autism and Developmental Disorders, 36*, 849–861. doi:10.1007/s10803-006-0123-0.

Lilienfeld, S. O., Waldman, I. D., & Israel, A. C. (1994). The critical examination of the use of the term and concept of *comorbidity* in psychopathology research. *Clinical Psychology: Science and Practice, 1*, 71–83. doi:10.1111/j.1468-2850.1994.tb00007.x.

MacNeil, B. M., Lopes, V. A., & Minnes, P. M. (2009). Anxiety in children and adolescents with autism spectrum disorders. *Research in Autism Spectrum Disorders, 3*(1), 1–21.doi:10.1016/j.rasd.2008.06.001.

Mandell, D. S., Walrath, C. M., Manteuffel, B., Sgro, G., & Pinto-Martin, J. A. (2005). The prevalence and correlates of abuse among children with autism served in comprehensive community-based mental health settings. *Child Abuse & Neglect, 29*(12), 1359–1372. doi:10.1016/j.chiabu.2005.06.006.

Mason, J. S., & Scior, K. (2004). 'Diagnostic Overshadowing' amongst clinicians working with people with intellectual disability in the UK. *Journal of Applied Research in Intellectual Abilities, 17*, 85–90. doi:10.1111/j.1360-2322.2004.00184.x.

Matson, J. L., Hess, J. A., & Boisjoli, J. A. (2010). Comorbid psychopathology in infants and toddlers with autism and pervasive developmental disorders-not otherwise specified (PDD-NOS). *Research in Autism Spectrum Disorders, 4*, 300–304. doi:10.1016/j.rasd.2009.10.001.

Mattila, M. L., Hurtig, T., Haapsamo, H., Jussila, K., Kuusikko-Gauffin, S., Kielinen, M., & Joskitt, L. (2010). Comorbid psychiatric disorders associated with Asperger syndrome/high-functioning autism: A community- and clinic-based study. *Journal of Autism and Developmental Disorders, 40*, 1080–1093. doi:10.1007/s10803-010-0958-2.

Mayes, S. D., Calhoun, S. L., Murray, M. J., Ahuja, M., & Smith, L. A. (2011). Anxiety, depression, and irritability in children with autism relative to other neuropsychiatric disorders and typical development. *Research in Autism Spectrum Disorders, 5*(1), 474–485. doi:10.1016/j.rasd.2010.06.012.

Mayes, S. D., Calhoun, S. L., Aggarwal, R., Baker, C., Mathapati, S., Molitoris, S., & Mayes, R. D. (2013). Unusual fears in children with autism. *Research in*

Autism Spectrum Disorders, 7, 151–158. doi:10.1016/j.rasd.2012.08.002.

Mazefsky, C. A., Oswald, D. P., Day, T. N., Eack, S. M., Minshew, N. J., & Lainhart, J. E. (2012). ASD, a psychiatric disorder, or both? Psychiatric diagnoses in adolescents with high-functioning ASD. *Journal of Clinical Child & Adolescent Psychology, 41,* 516–523.

McDougle, C. J., Kresch, L. E., Goodman, W. K., Naylor, S. T., Volkmar, F. R., Cohen, D. J., & Price, L. H. (1995). A case-controlled study of repetitive thoughts and behavior in adults with autistic disorder and obsessive-compulsive disorder. *American Journal of Psychiatry, 152,* 772–777.

McNally, K. R. H., Lincoln, A. J., Brown, M. Z., & Chavira, D. A. (2013). The Coping Cat program for children with anxiety and autism spectrum disorder: A pilot randomized controlled trial. *Journal of Autism and Developmental Disabilities, 43,* 57–67. doi:10.1007/s10803-012-1541.

Mehtar, M., & Mukaddes, N. M. (2011). Posttraumatic stress disorder in individuals with diagnosis of autistic spectrum disorders. *Research in Autism Spectrum Disorders, 5*(1), 539–546. doi:10.1016/j.rasd.2010.06.020.

Muris, P., Steerneman, P., Merckelbach, H., Holdrinet, I., & Meesters, C. (1998). Comorbid anxiety symptoms in children with pervasive developmental disorders. *Journal of Anxiety Disorders, 12,* 387–393.doi:10.1016/S0887-6185(98)00022–X.

Ollendick, T. H., & White, S. W. (2012). The presentation and classification of anxiety in autism spectrum disorder: Where to from here? *Clinical Psychology: Science and Practice, 19*(4), 352–355. doi:10.1111/cpsp.12013.

Ooi, Y., Tan, W., Lim, C., Goh, T., & Sung, M. (2011). Prevalence of emotional and behavioral problems in children with high functioning autism spectrum disorders. *Australian and New Zealand Journal of Psychiatry, 44,* 370–375. doi:10.3109/00048674.2010.534071.

Puleo, C. M., & Kendall, P. C. (2011). Anxiety disorders in typically developing youth: Autism spectrum symptoms as a predictor of cognitive-behavioral treatment. *Journal of Autism and Developmental Disorders, 41,* 275–286. doi:10.1007/s10803-010-1047-2.

Rapee, R. M., Schniering, C. A., & Hudson, J. L. (2009). Anxiety disorders during childhood and adolescence: Origins and treatment. *Annual Review of Clinical Psychology, 5,* 311–341. doi:10.1146/annurev.clinpsy.032408.153628.

Regier, D. A., Narrow, W. E., Kuhl, E. A., & Kupfer, D. J. (2009). The conceptual development of DSM-V. *American Journal of Psychiatry, 166,* 645–650. doi:10.1176/appi.ajp.2009.09020279.

Renno, P., & Wood, J. J. (2013). Discriminant and convergent validity of the anxiety construct in children with autism spectrum disorders. *Journal of Autism and Developmental Disorders, 43,* 1–12. doi:10.1007/s10803-013-1767-1.

Rodgers, J., Riby, D. M., Janes, E., Connolly, B., & McConachie, H. (2012). Anxiety and repetitive behaviours in autism spectrum disorders and Williams syndrome: A cross-syndrome comparison. *Journal of Autism and Developmental Disorders, 42*(2), 175–180. doi:10.1007/s10803-011-1225-x.

Russell, A. J., Mataix-Cols, D., Anson, M., & Murphy, D. G. (2005). Obsessions and compulsions in Asperger syndrome and high-functioning autism. *The British Journal of Psychiatry, 186*(6), 525–528. doi:10.1192/bjp.186.6.525.

Russell, E., & Sofronoff, K. (2005). Anxiety and social worries in children with Asperger syndrome. *Australian and New Zealand Journal of Psychiatry, 39,* 633–638. doi:10.1111/j.1440-1614.2005.01637.x.

Scahill, L. (2012). Commentary on Kerns and Kendall. *Clinical Psychology: Science and Practice, 19,* 348–351. doi:10.1111/cpsp.12018.

Silverman, W. K., & Albano, A. M. (1996). *Guide to the use of the Anxiety Disorders Interview Schedule for DSM-IV-Child and Parent Versions.* London: Oxford University Press.

Simonoff, E., Pickles, A., Charman, T., Chandler, S., Loucas, T., & Baird, G. (2008). Psychiatric disorders in children with autism spectrum disorders: Prevalence, comorbidity, and associated factors in a population-derived sample. *Journal of the American Academy of Child & Adolescent Psychiatry, 47,* 921–929. doi:10.1097/CHI.0b013e318179964f.

Storch, E. A., Ehrenreich, J. M., Wood, J. L., Jones, A. M., De Nadai, A. A., Lewin, A. B., et al. (2012). *Journal of Child and Adolescent Psychopharmacology, 22,* 292–299. doi:10.1089/cap.2011.0114.

Sukhodolsky, D. G., Scahill, L., Gadow, K. D., Arnold, L. E., Aman, M. G., McDougle, C. J., et al. (2008). Parent-rated anxiety symptoms in children with pervasive developmental disorders: Frequency and association with core autism symptoms and cognitive functioning. *Journal of Abnormal Child Psychology, 36,* 117–128. doi:10.1007/s10802-007-9165-9.

Thede, L. L., & Coolidge, F. L. (2007). Psychological and neurobehavioral comparisonsof children with Asperger's disorder versus high-functioning autism. *Journal of Autismand Developmental Disorders, 37,* 847–854.

Tonge, B. J., Brereton, A. V., Gray, K. M., & Einfeld, S. L. (1999). Behavioural and emotional disturbance in high-functioning autism and Asperger syndrome. *Autism, 3*(2), 117–130.

Ung, D., Arnold, E. B., Lewin, A. B., Nadeau, J. M., Jones, A. M., De Nadai, A. S.,Storch, E. A., & Murphy, T. K. (2013). The effect of cognitive-behavioral therapy versus treatment as usual for anxiety in children with autism spectrum disorders: a randomized, controlled trial. *Journal of the American Academy of Child & Adolescent Psychiatry, 52,* 132–142.

van Steensel, F. J., Bogels, S. M., & Perrin, S. (2011). Anxiety disorders in children and adolescents with autistic spectrum disorders: A meta-analysis. *Clinical Child and Family Psychology Review, 14,* 302–317. doi:10.1007/s10567-011-0097-0.

Weisbrot, D. M., Gadow, K. D., DeVincent, C. J., & Pomeroy, J. (2005). The presentation of anxiety in children with pervasive developmental disorders. *Journal of Child & Adolescent Psychopharmacology, 15,* 477–496. doi:10.1089/cap.2005.15.477.

White, S. W., Oswald, D., Ollendick, T., & Scahill, L. (2009). Anxiety in children and adolescents with autism spectrum disorders. *Clinical Psychology Review, 29,* 216–229. doi:10.1016/j.cpr.2009.01.003.

White, S. W., & Roberson-Nay, R. (2009). Anxiety, social deficits, and loneliness in youth with autism spectrum disorders. *Journal of Autism and Developmental Disorders, 39,* 1006–1013. doi:10.1007/s10803-009-0713-8.

Wood, J. J., Drahota, A., Sze, K., Har, K., Chiu, A., & Langer, D. A. (2009). Cognitive behavioral therapy for anxiety in children with autism spectrum disorders: A randomized, controlled trial. *Journal of Child Psychology and Psychiatry, 50,* 224–234.

Wood, J. J., & Gadow, K. D. (2010). Exploring the nature and function of anxiety in youth with autism spectrum disorders. *Clinical Psychology: Science and Practice, 17,* 281–292. doi:10.1111/j.1468-2850.2010.01220.x.

Worley, J. A., Matson, J. L., Sipes, M., & Koziowski, A. M. (2010). Prevalence of autism spectrum disorders in toddlers receiving early intervention services. *Research in Autism Spectrum Disorders, 5,* 920–925. doi:10.1016/j.rasd.2010.10.007.

Zandt, F., Prior, M., & Kyrios, M. (2007). Repetitive behaviour in children with high functioning autism and obsessive compulsive disorder. *Journal of Autism and Developmental Disabilities, 37,* 251–259. doi:10.1007/s10803-006-0158-2.

Carla A. Mazefsky and John D. Herrington

Although there is growing consensus that anxiety is common in autism spectrum disorder (ASD), the mechanisms that are associated with this symptom overlap are poorly understood at this time. Background on the etiological mechanisms of anxiety disorders in non-ASD populations is also provided in the introduction chapter and Chap. 3. In this chapter, we consider additional theoretical frameworks for understanding the increased risk for anxiety in ASD. The first half of the chapter is focused on cognitive and behavioral processes that may increase the risk for anxiety in ASD. This includes a discussion of core diagnostic features of ASD as well as processes that cut across disorders (e.g., transdiagnostic processes), such as emotion regulation. The second half of the chapter focuses on neurobiology. This discussion focuses on abnormalities in brain areas implementing social and emotional processes (particularly amygdala and PFC) across disorders, with a particular emphasis on how to interpret amygdala differences in ASD in light of both social deficits and anxiety.

Intersection of Core Diagnostic Features of ASD and Anxiety

Studies have found that overall autism spectrum disorder (ASD) symptom severity is significantly associated with anxiety (Kelly et al. 2008). There are many ways in which the core symptoms of ASD may increase the risk for anxiety. This relationship is likely bidirectional, such that symptoms of ASD may lead to anxiety and anxiety may exacerbate ASD symptoms. Although we will reference this bidirectionality where appropriate, our discussion below focuses on how characteristics of ASD may increase the risk for anxiety.

Social Deficits and Anxiety

Individuals with ASD have problems with social and emotional reciprocity and difficulty establishing and maintaining friendships and relationships. Wood and Gadow (2010) proposed that social confusion and the unpredictability stemming from social encounters may lead to social anxiety in ASD. Although this was a hypothetical model, there are numerous accounts of social deficits in ASD that lead to confusion and feeling overwhelmed in social encounters. One example is problems with the "theory of mind," or being able to take other's perspectives (Baron-Cohen 1997). In addition, despite some inconsistencies across studies, it is widely accepted that individuals with ASD struggle to identify other's emotions and may miss or misperceive nonverbal cues (Harms et al. 2010). Being unable to

C. A. Mazefsky (✉)
Psychiatry Department, The University of Pittsburgh School of Medicine, Webster Hall, Suite 300, 3811 O'Hara Street, Pittsburgh, PA 15213, USA
e-mail: mazefskyca@upmc.edu

J. D. Herrington
Center for Autism Research, The Children's Hospital of Philadelphia
PA, USA

T. E. Davis III et al. (eds.), *Handbook of Autism and Anxiety,* Autism and Child Psychopathology Series,
DOI 10.1007/978-3-319-06796-4_7, © Springer International Publishing Switzerland 2014

accurately interpret another person's intentions in the context of a rapidly moving social interaction could produce discomfort or anxiety.

This pathway is likely magnified among those with ASD who are socially motivated. Many individuals with ASD desire friendships and report loneliness (Bauminger and Kasari 2000). For these individuals, unsuccessful attempts at social engagement may be experienced as highly distressing, particularly if the peer's response involves teasing or an outright form of rejection. As many as 70 % of children with ASD are victims of bullying, with verbal and social forms of bullying being the most common (Cappadocia et al. 2012). Therefore, some individuals with ASD may develop a realistic expectation of negative outcomes in social situations. This expectancy may generalize to a broader negative fear of evaluation, which is a major facet of social anxiety (American Psychiatric Association 2013). Indeed, a large study found that children with ASD who were bullied at least once a week were rated by their parents as having significantly more anxiety than children with ASD who experienced less frequent or no victimization (Cappadocia et al. 2012). Social anxiety may be the most common outcome but these same patterns of symptoms and experiences may produce other types of anxiety as well.

Repetitive Behaviors and Anxiety

Guttmann-Steinmetz et al. (2010) found that the perseverative symptoms of ASD were even more strongly correlated with anxiety symptoms than social or communication symptoms. Although this pattern was true for both parent and teacher report, the direction of the effect cannot be determined because the study was cross-sectional. Thus, it is possible that the stronger relationship between anxiety and perseverative behaviors arose because the presence of anxiety leads to an increase in repetitive behaviors rather than vice versa. It has been argued that repetitive behaviors may both increase as a sign of distress and serve as a coping mechanism (Mazefsky et al. 2013). Similar to the reciprocal relationship between social deficits and social anxiety, it is perhaps

most likely that the relationship between repetitive behaviors and anxiety is bidirectional. There are several potential mechanisms by which the restricted and repetitive behaviors of ASD may directly contribute to an increased risk of anxiety. Below we focus on how difficulty adjusting to change and sensory problems in particular may lead to the development or exacerbation of anxiety.

Resistance to Change

Difficulty adjusting to change and transitions is a commonly reported concern in ASD. The *Autism Comorbidity Interview* (ACI) includes a "transition-related anxiety" section given how frequently this anxiety trigger is observed clinically (Lainhart et al. 2003). A study that included 31 high-functioning adolescents with ASD found that one-third of the sample satisfied ACI criteria for clinically significant transition-related anxiety, which included similar requirements for impairment and severity as traditional DSM-defined anxiety disorders (Mazefsky et al. 2010). Although this was a small sample, it does suggest that severe anxiety related to transitions is common in ASD, raising the possibility that resistance to change may impose risk for anxiety.

Longitudinal research from the temperament literature in typically developing populations lends credence to the notion that resistance to change could lead to anxiety. Children who are classified as behaviorally inhibited, which includes being shy and having difficulty adjusting to novel situations and stimuli, are more likely to develop anxiety disorders (Muris and Ollendick 2005). There have not been any longitudinal studies testing the association between resistance to change and anxiety in ASD, but a recent study supports a correlation between the two constructs. Specifically, Rodgers et al. (2012) compared adolescents with ASD with and without anxiety and found that greater resistance to change was associated with more anxiety in the anxiety sample. Interestingly, resistance to change was not correlated with anxiety in the low-anxiety group. This is consistent with findings in non-ASD populations that intolerance of uncertainty is able to distinguish clinically anxious individuals from those without clinical anxiety (Dugas 1998). However, understanding this relationship in ASD may be more complex, given that resistance to change is quite common, even among those without high levels of anxiety. Thus, additional research is needed to understand why and how resistance to change is associated with (or may lead to) anxiety in some individuals with ASD.

Differences in Sensory Processing

Sensory dysfunction, which is now also considered a diagnostic indicator of repetitive behaviors in ASD (American Psychiatric Association 2013), is also speculated to play a role in anxiety in ASD. Most of the research on the relationship between sensory processing and affective or anxiety concerns in ASD has focused on the role of sensory hypersensitivity. This research stems from the notion that children respond behaviorally in accordance with their individual sensory threshold, such that a child with a high threshold for sensory information may seek high levels of sensory input while a child who has a low threshold for sensory information may avoid sensory input or find it distressing (Dunn 1997). One might imagine how having a low threshold for sensory information (hypersensitive) may lead to anxiety in situations when it is not possible to control the amount of stimulation received (e.g., a loud cafeteria, fireworks). Through classical fear conditioning, the child with ASD may then develop a phobic response to stimuli that were previously paired with an aversive sensory reaction (Green and Ben-Sasson 2010). This could explain why children with ASD have been found to have high rates of phobias that are uncommon in the general population, such as "noise phobias" (Leyfer et al. 2006).

However, the existing research probing the link between sensory over-responsivity and anxiety in ASD has been inconsistent with regard to the degree of association with anxiety, and it is generally difficult to establish this link with certainty due to methodological flaws in these studies (Kerns and Kendall 2012). One explanation for the inconsistent findings is that there may be an even more complex mechanism underlying the anxiety–sensory relationship in ASD than the over-sensitivity hypothesis suggests. A recent neuroimaging study found that the processing of elementary sensory information was highly variable within individuals with ASD, such that the same stimulus evoked a different neurobiological response across time (Dinstein et al. 2012). Thus, rather than neatly fitting into a category of hyper- or hyposensitive, the same type and magnitude of sensory information may be perceived differently at different times by the same individual. Unpredictable responses to sensory stimuli, combined with a common preference for consistency and structure in ASD, could lead to increased anxiety, even if global categorizations of sensory style as hyper- or hyposensitive may miss the association (or find it inconsistently).

Transdiagnostic Behavioral Processes

In addition to the diagnostic features of ASD, there are other common cognitive and behavioral characteristics in this population that may underlie their experience of anxiety. Some of these disrupted processes may be shared with other populations. Transdiagnostic models focus on etiologic mechanisms that are present across disorders and help to explain overlap in behavioral presentation. This focus on fundamental dysfunctional processes helps to illuminate the understanding of psychopathology as well as comorbidity between disorders (Nolen-Hoeksema and Watkins 2011). Thus, transdiagnostic processes may be informative in understanding the etiology of anxiety in ASD well.

Perseveration or Rumination and Anxiety

Although the terminology used in other populations may differ, perseveration is a transdiagnostic concept that may have relevance to anxiety in ASD. Research on perseveration in ASD has predominantly investigated the tendency to get stuck on things that the individual enjoys (e.g., circumscribed interests). Although perseveration can be construed primarily as a cognitive or sensory process, there is likely an emotional component to perseveration as well. Individuals with ASD may experience difficulty shifting thoughts away from unpleasant and distressing ideas, which could in turn lead to anxiety or other emotional concerns (Mazefsky et al. 2012). Such emotionally laden perseveration is similar to rumination, which is defined as the tendency to persistently think about emotional topics. Rumination is a primary component of models of depression, anxiety, and other disorders (Siegle 2008). There is strong support for the role of rumination in predicting the onset of depression, and more mixed evidence for its role in anxiety (Aldao et al. 2010). Unfortunately, there are no published studies of rumination, or the emotional aspects of perseveration, in ASD. However, a study of college students provides support for a positive association between anger-focused rumination and ASD traits (Pugliese et al. submitted), suggesting that further research in this area is warranted.

Emotion Regulation

A broader construct that has played a major role in understanding the development of psychopathology is emotion regulation. Emotion regulation involves both conscious and unconscious processes related to modifying the temporal features, valence, or intensity of emotional reactions (Thompson 1994). The term emotion regulation generally infers an effort to control emotional reactions in order to promote adaptive or goal-directed behavior (Cole et al. 2004). The field of emotion regulation research has grown exponentially in the past decades, moving from questions about the construct definition itself to considerations of processes that facilitate successful emotion regulation and how abnormalities in these processes can lead to psychopathology (Tamir 2011). Maladaptive emotion regulation is apparent across psychiatric disorders (Gross 2007), though the way that emotion regulation is disrupted and the underlying mechanisms may be disorder specific (Aldao et al. 2010).

Many have posited that problems with emotion regulation play a central role in the development of anxiety disorders (e.g., Cisler et al. 2010; Hannesdottir and Ollendick 2007; Suveg and Zeman 2004). Mennin et al. (2006) proposed

a two-pronged model of emotion regulation in anxiety. Specifically, they suggested that anxiety involves both aberrant regulation of the expression and experience of emotion and overreliance on attempts to suppress emotion. This theory has been empirically supported by studies finding greater use of suppression and reduced or less effective use of cognitive reappraisal emotion regulation strategies in anxiety samples (e.g., Amstadter 2008). Interestingly, a recent study of adults with ASD also found more self-reported use of suppression and less cognitive appraisal than typically developing adults (Samson et al. 2012).

Aside from this single adult study, and two studies using observational frustration-oriented tasks with young children with ASD (Jahromi et al. 2012; Konstantareas and Stewart 2006), there has been very little ASD research focused explicitly on emotion regulation processes. However, two recent review papers highlight the ways in which emotion regulation may be disrupted in ASD (Mazefsky et al. 2013; Mazefsky and White in press). These reviews emphasize that the disruption of emotion regulation in ASD is quite likely a multifaceted and complex process, involving both factors that are inherent in having ASD and those shared with other disorders.

In terms of ASD-related characteristics, the diagnostic features of ASD discussed earlier may impact anxiety through their negative impact on emotion regulation (e.g., mediation). For example, effective emotion regulation is typically context-dependent and applied selectively to fit situational demands and goals (Sheppes and Gross 2011). The social impairments in ASD, such as a poor theory of mind and problems accurately identifying social cues, may interfere with the timing of emotion regulation as well as the ability to identify critical aspects of the situation (Mazefsky et al. 2013). Similarly, problems with change and rigidity may interfere with the flexible use of emotion regulation strategies. In addition, the drive to meet sensory needs may take precedence over emotion regulation and lead to failure in applying regulation strategies as needed (Mazefsky et al. 2013). Other common characteristics of ASD not previously discussed may also interfere with emotion regulation. For example, difficulty identifying and describing emotional experiences is common in ASD (Ciarrochi et al. 2008) and may make it difficult to communicate with others about emotional experiences and engage in joint problem solving (Mazefsky and White in press).

Emotion regulation disruption in ASD may begin at the earliest stages of the emotional experience as well. Clinical observations suggest that those with ASD may react to emotional stimuli with great intensity (Mazefsky et al. 2013) and greater baseline levels of distress and irritability have been observed as early as infancy (Rogers 2009). In line with models of anxiety proposed by Cisler et al. (2010), this greater intensity of negative affective responding (e.g., fear) may increase the likelihood of maladaptive emotion regulation strategies (avoidance, suppression) as well as serve to strengthen the anxiety response upon additional encounters with the fear-provoking stimulus. This process may derive in part from physiological hyperarousal, which has played a central role in long-standing theories of anxiety (Watson et al. 1991). Although evidence for physiological hyperarousal in ASD is comparatively more limited and mixed, the possibility warrants further attention (Mazefsky et al. 2013).

Core Diagnostic Features and Transdiagnostic Processes: Concluding Remarks

Unfortunately, our understanding of the cognitive and behavioral processes that may produce or increase risk for high levels of anxiety in ASD is limited. Further, there has been little longitudinal research, which is important in establishing causal connections. Nonetheless, several review papers have recently been published that describe plausible cognitive and behavioral pathways to anxiety in ASD that dovetail nicely with the anxiety disorders literature (Kerns and Kendall 2012; Mazefsky et al. 2013; Mazefsky and White in press; Wood and Gadow 2010).

One prominent theme is that symptoms of ASD themselves may confer increased risk for anxiety. Widely documented impairments in ASD, as well as core diagnostic features, may

intersect with demanding social situations and daily stressors to create a situation ripe for anxiety. ASD research might benefit from a deeper consideration of anxiety models from typically developing populations, especially models related to emotion regulation. Given how intertwined emotional deficits and differences are with the diagnostic features of ASD, as well as how common anxiety and other manifestations of emotion dysregulation are in ASD, it is possible that emotion dysregulation itself should be considered intrinsic to ASD (Mazefsky et al. 2013). Identifying some of the core mechanisms that underlie anxiety and other manifestations of poor emotional control in ASD (e.g., emotion regulation) and targeting them in treatment could produce improvements in functioning whether or not an official comorbid anxiety diagnosis is present.

However, in addition to the need for longitudinal studies and empirical evidence to support the conceptual models, there remain critical questions about heterogeneity in emotional functioning, and anxiety, in ASD. Not all individuals with ASD experience anxiety; some display other serious emotional concerns, and others are seemingly not impaired in any of these areas. Although we need to consider how individual differences in behavioral and cognitive processes may play a role, it is also becoming increasingly clear that the neurobiology underlying ASD is just as heterogeneous and complex as the clinical manifestations. Thus, now we turn to the consideration of the role of neurobiology in anxiety in ASD.

Common Neurobiological Etiologies of Anxiety and ASD

Existing transdiagnostic research on the neurobiology of emotional processes is an important part of the narrative on the co-occurrence of anxiety in ASD. There is a wealth of data from psychophysiology and cognitive neuroscience associating anxiety and ASD with specific patterns of nervous system function and dysfunction. This research is undergoing a shift from modular (i.e., structure-based) to connectionist (i.e., network-based) models of brain function. Yet, the amygdala and portions of the prefrontal cortex (PFC) remain among the most widely implicated structures in these literatures and are therefore the primary focus of this chapter. Abnormalities in amygdala and PFC function and connectivity are likely related to abnormal emotion processes across psychological disorders.

The majority of the existing literature on the amygdala in ASD holds that the primary consequence of abnormal amygdala function is social withdrawal and deficits in social information processing (Baron-Cohen et al. 1999, 2000; Schultz 2005). This putatively causal relationship fits well with our understanding of the social functions of the amygdala, as well as the clinical picture of ASD where social disinterest is often prominent. However, there is a growing consensus that this relationship is also an oversimplification of a complicated clinical and neurobiological phenomenon—one where social disinterest may coincide with, or be superseded by, symptoms of anxiety that uniquely contribute to deficits in social function (Kleinhans et al. 2009; Schumann et al. 2011). Although the neurobiological systems involved in the experience of negative affect are inherently transdiagnostic (as suggested by the Negative Affect System proposed by the National Institute of Mental Health's Research Domain Criteria Project), these systems have been strongly implicated in ASD in particular. In the sections that follow, we briefly review the literatures on amygdala and PFC function in ASD and anxiety disorders, emphasizing commonalities and unexplored synergies between these literatures.

Prevailing Models of Amygdala Function and Dysfunction in ASD

There have been numerous reviews of the role of amygdala dysfunction in ASD (e.g., Baron-Cohen et al. 2000; Dziobek et al. 2010; Schultz 2005). The majority of these reviews (and the articles they reference) attribute deficits to diminished social engagement and social perception in ASD. This social-intelligence-oriented perspective on amygdala function in ASD has clearly been inherited from long-standing preclinical research on samples with amygdala lesions, where social deficits have generally been more salient than affective ones (assays of affective states are of course limited in preclinical samples). For example, the most widely cited influence on the amygdala/ASD connection is arguably that of Kluver and Bucy (1937), who invoke "psychic blindness" as the main outcome—a construct that bears more similarity to social perception and Theory of Mind than affect per se. This construal dovetails with a second reason that social intelligence accounts of amygdala dysfunction in ASD predominate—the emphasis on behavioral manifestations of a disorder where access to internal affective states is even more limited than among typically developing children (often due to communication deficits).

Overall, formal considerations of amygdala dysfunction in ASD emphasize social perception deficits and, to a lesser extent, emotion perception deficits; the amygdala's relationship to the experience of affect is rarely considered. In an influential review of the neurobiology of ASD (Schultz 2005), the words anxiety, affect, and emotion do not appear anywhere in reference to the amygdala. In a recent review, Neuhaus et al. (2010; p. 736) stated that "studies of amygdala functioning point to its involvement in face processing, identification of emotion, perspective taking, social judgments, empathy, and threat detection." In another review, Monk (2008) discusses how amygdala dysfunction relates separately to ASD, anxiety disorders, and depression, but acknowledges that the interrelationships between these disorders and amygdala function are presently unclear. Monk (2008) concludes that "further work must be done to clarify whether [amygdala] disturbances relate to social functioning, emotion processing or both in ASD" (p. 1241).

Amygdala Activity, Anxiety, and ASD

Given the emphasis on the social functions of the amygdala, it is not surprising that findings of amygdala *hypoactivity* have been prominent in neuroimaging studies of ASD. In one of the earliest functional magnetic resonance imaging (fMRI) studies on the amygdala in those with ASD, Baron-Cohen et al. (1999) scanned six individuals as they performed an emotion recognition task on facial stimuli cropped around the eyes. The authors reported decreased amygdala activation during this task, arguing that their data supported the "amygdala theory of autism" (p. 1891; see Baron-Cohen et al. 2000, for a discussion of this theory).

Other studies reporting hypoactivation of the amygdala in those with ASD make more specific reference to emotion processes, though generally from the perspective of emotion perception rather than the affective states of the individuals being scanned. The paper by Critchley et al. (2000) on facial emotion perception in ASD considers their finding of amygdala hypoactivation in terms of emotion perception as well as Theory of Mind deficits. Corbett et al. (2009) also reported amygdala hypoactivation during an emotion matching task. They interpreted their results in terms of the diminished emotional salience of these faces for individuals with ASD. Lastly, Pelphrey et al. (2007) reported decreased activation of the amygdala, fusiform gyrus, and superior temporal sulcus during the perception of dynamic facial expressions, but not for static facial expressions. Interestingly, although the authors offer interpretations of their findings that reference emotion *perception*, they also discuss the possibility that the observed amygdala hypoactivation may be related to the blunted *experience* of affect in the ASD sample. Specifically, they interpret the absence of amygdala hypoactivation for static faces as related to the relatively limited "emotional impact" these faces afforded (relative to dynamic faces; p. 417).

Each of these studies dovetails nicely with accounts of abnormal social intelligence and emotion perception in ASD. However, there are a growing number of studies that show *hyperactivity* of the amygdala in those with an ASD. In an influential study by Dalton et al. (2005), the ASD group showed significantly increased activity in the left amygdala and the ventral PFC (orbitofrontal cortex) relative to controls during a facial emotion discrimination task. The authors

also reported that amygdala activity was strongly correlated with the amount of time individuals with ASD spent looking at the eyes of the presented stimuli. This same correlation was nonsignificant in the control group. In interpreting these findings, the authors offered the first account of amygdala activity in ASD focused squarely on the experience of affect: "within the autistic group, eye fixation is associated with negatively valenced overarousal mediated by activation in limbic regions such as the amygdala" (p. 524).

When interpreting the findings of Dalton et al. (2005), it is important to consider that research on affective neuroscience draws clear associations between amygdala function and the processing and experience of emotion. Decades of research on mood and anxiety disorders have implicated abnormal amygdala function (see Blackford and Pine 2012). These studies strongly support amygdala hyperactivity in anxiety. These studies elicit amygdala activity using a wide array of state and trait manipulations, though the perception of emotional faces is generally the most common and likely the most robust (Blackford and Pine 2012; Sergerie et al. 2008). The presence of hyperactivity during the perception of negative emotional faces is consistent with the role of the amygdala in the stimulus-reinforcement learning of fear, as well as the production of fear (Davis 1992; Kalin et al. 2007; Sergerie et al. 2008). The amygdala also plays a critical role in the encoding of emotional information (i.e., memory; for example, see Shaw et al. 2005). Each of these processes is enhanced in anxiety—consistent with a pattern of amygdala hyperactivity. When considering elevated rates of co-occurring anxiety in ASD, it should not come as a surprise that some ASD samples present with amygdala hyperactivation rather than hypoactivation. Just as with the role of emotion regulation in anxiety noted above, it is likely that amygdala hyperactivation is a transdiagnostic process present in anxious samples both with and without ASD.

Findings of increased amygdala activation in ASD have been reported in at least four other studies since Dalton et al. (2005). Using an attentional bias task that is widely deployed in anxiety disorder samples (see Roy et al. 2008), Monk et al. (2010) showed increased amygdala activation in ASD during the perception of emotional faces. Monk later replicated this finding using a task where participants were asked to identify the gender of a series of emotional faces (Weng et al. 2011). In the Weng et al. study, two possible interpretations of the finding of amygdala hyperactivation are presented. The first is that the emotional expressions are inherently more ambiguous to individuals with ASD. This interpretation is consistent with evidence that the amygdala is responsive to the perception of ambiguous emotional information (for review, see Whalen 2007). The second interpretation is that individuals in the ASD group had a stronger affective response to the faces.

The Dalton et al. (2005) and Monk et al. (2010) studies were similar to the majority of fMRI studies in ASD, in that affective symptoms were not formally assessed. It is therefore difficult to infer from these studies whether amygdala hyperactivity was observed for the same reasons that it is frequently observed in affective neuroscience—the presence of elevated anxiety. However, anxiety was measured in the Weng et al. (2011) study—groups were matched for anxiety symptoms using the Spence Child Anxiety Scale (though, as the authors acknowledged, there may have been differences in affective state between the groups that was not reflected in this scale). Theirs is one of the only existing studies that presents counterevidence to affective accounts of amygdala dysfunction in ASD.

On the other hand, data in favor of affective accounts continue to accumulate. The strongest published evidence to date associating amygdala hyperactivity with anxiety symptoms in ASD comes from Kleinhans et al. (2010). Using a facial affect matching task, the authors found increased activation in the amygdala compared to controls. Furthermore, the magnitude of amygdala activation was significantly correlated with responses on measure of social anxiety. Their chapter argues persuasively that considerations of anxiety symptoms in ASD are needed if we are to better understand the amygdala in those with ASD.

It is important to note that a positive association between anxiety symptoms and amygdala activity in ASD does not contradict the relationship between amygdala and social functions, nor does it require that findings of amygdala hypoactivation in ASD be considered suspect. Instead, the association requires a more sophisticated and nuanced perspective on the social and emotional functions of the amygdala and on the relevance of these functions to individual differences in ASD. Despite the large literature on amygdala function and anxiety disorders, there have been almost no systematic investigations to date into whether individual differences in anxiety can predict patterns of amygdala hypo- or hyperactivation in ASD. More detailed considerations of mood and anxiety disorder status are clearly needed if we are to further our understanding of amygdala function in ASD.

PFC Function, Anxiety, and ASD

This chapter has focused primarily on amygdala function, as the research on this structure best illustrates the neurobiological overlap between anxiety and ASD. However, a similar narrative can be constructed around research on PFC function in ASD and anxiety disorders. Theories on the social and emotional functions of the PFC tend to divide this area along dorsal/ventral and medial/lateral axes. Deficits in social intelligence and perspective taking in ASD have frequently been associated with hypoactivation of the dorsomedial aspects of the PFC (for example, the medial aspects of Brodmann Areas 9 and 10; see Shalom 2009). However, studies also associated social intelligence deficits to hypoactivation of the ventral regions of the PFC (Swartz et al. 2013; Watanabe et al. 2012).

The observation of diminished ventral PFC activation in ASD is noteworthy, as abnormal ventral PFC function has long been implicated in anxiety disorders (Blackford and Pine 2012). In addition to a primary role in the experience of affect, the ventral PFC (vPFC) is thought to influence emotion processes via modulation of amygdala activity. The preclinical literature on vPFC/amygdala connectivity indicates that this relationship is primarily inhibitory (via GABAergic neuronal projections; Amano et al. 2010). Furthermore, there are now numerous studies implicating abnormal connectivity between the vPFC and the amygdala (for review, see Kim et al. 2011; though see Pfeifer and Allen 2012, for a counter-perspective on these articles).

As with the amygdala, the ASD literature on abnormal PFC function has seldom drawn from this anxiety disorder literature. The failure to integrate these literatures is particularly surprising when considering findings of abnormal white matter development in those with ASD (for review, see Herrington and Schultz 2010)—abnormalities that may affect the same tissue connecting the vPFC to the amgydala (Baur et al. 2013; Modi et al. 2013). It is intriguing to hypothesize that those individuals with ASD who have co-occurring anxiety are those individuals who have white matter abnormalities that differentially affect vPFC/amygdala connectivity. To our knowledge, this hypothesis has yet to be formally tested.

Anxiety, ASD, and Amygdala/PFC: Concluding Remarks

The most salient implication of our growing awareness of the co-occurrence of transdiagnostic anxiety processes within ASD is that long-standing models of brain function in ASD are likely to warrant revision. Specifically, a more nuanced model of amygdala function will need to be developed to understand what role it has (or does not have) in the clinical manifestations of ASD. Specifically, models of the amygdala in those with ASD will likely need to consider a "hybrid signal" framework whereby the amygdala supports both approach (pro-social) and avoidance (fear) tendencies. Given how extensively the amygdala has been studied in those with ASD, and its well-established role in the anxiety disorders, it is somewhat surprising that accounts of how it can serve both approach and avoidance functions do not seem more readily available. One example of a possible framework for understanding the hybrid approach/avoidance functions of the amygdala is afforded by the circumplex model of

emotion—i.e., the notion that emotions consist of valence (pleasant vs. unpleasant) and arousal (high vs. low) dimensions (i.e., Russell 1980). If the amygdala functions as an arousal regulation mechanism that operates irrespective of valence, it could facilitate both pro-social and fear-oriented functions (i.e., optimizing biological readiness to either approach or avoid stimuli and events). There is some evidence that the functions of the amygdala can be encompassed by a general arousal construct, though the evidence is mixed; numerous studies show amygdala activity during pleasant as well as unpleasant affect manipulations (for an early but prototypical example, see Garavan et al. 2001). However, the preponderance of evidence continues to point to a specific relationship between the amygdala and negative affect (which may be superimposed on a more global arousal mechanism). Another unique but overlapping model of amygdala function is that it coordinates responses to ambiguous information in the environment—particularly information associated with affect. The influential work of Adolphs (2003), Phelps and LeDoux (2005), Whalen (2007), and numerous other scientists generally support this perspective. And yet, this perspective does not seem to adequately explain why some individuals with ASD are disinterested and/or confused by their social world and others are fearful of it (though all hypothetically have deficits in amygdala function). The presence of social anhedonia versus elevated fear and aversion responses within the same disorder (ASD) requires an organizing principle beyond arousal or socio-emotional salience accounts of amygdala function. Ultimately, one of the many reasons why the study of anxiety in ASD is so important is that it may shed light on these fundamental questions about the "social" and "emotional" brain.

Ultimately, the amygdala and the PFC may have untapped potential as biomarkers of anxiety in general, and social aversion in particular, among individuals with ASD. It has long been held that many individuals with ASD have an aversive response to social contact (whereas others present with social disinterest only) that is likely related to the experience of anxiety. However, it has proven challenging to gather formal empirical evidence for this perspective, as avoidance and disinterest of social contact with other people can lead to identical behaviors (i.e., diminished social interaction). Recent work by Kliemann et al. (2010, 2012) has been among the most promising to date in identifying patterns of anxiety-mediated social aversion in ASD, tying this aversion to hyperactivation of the amygdala. Notwithstanding the need for a theory of amygdala function that encompasses both pro-social and fear responses, it is possible that the direction of activation within the amygdala and the PFC may help identify individuals who have an aversive (hyperactivity) or an indifferent (hypoactivity) response to social and affective information from others. Given that these two groups of individuals are likely to benefit from distinct forms of intervention, the identification of biomarkers of these groups could resonate through many areas of ASD research and treatment.

As we develop more sophisticated models of amygdala/PFC function in anxiety and ASD, we will also need to consider that anxiety disorders are themselves a spectrum. Most of this chapter has treated anxiety in ASD as if it were a monolithic construct. There are strong reasons to suppose that many manifestations of anxiety stem from the same diathesis (e.g., transdiagnostic in origin)—this is especially true for generalized anxiety, separation anxiety, and social phobia, which are highly comorbid with one another (Brady and Kendall 1992). But there is variance among anxiety disorders that may ultimately be associated with distinct neurobiological profiles. One example of this variance is the arousal construct itself, which ranges from relatively low (generalized anxiety) to relatively high (panic). It remains to be seen which dimension of anxiety is likely to capture the most variance in amygdala/PFC function among individuals with ASD.

Conclusions

The etiology of anxiety in those with ASD is clearly complex and multifaceted. As with all psychopathology, manifestations of anxiety likely stem from an interaction of underlying neurobiology, cognitive and behavioral characteristics, and life experiences. However, understanding the development of anxiety in those with ASD is perhaps even more complicated, given the need to conceptualize the anxiety within the framework of ASD-related impairments and ASD's underlying neural circuitry. We have argued for the importance of a transdiagnostic approach, and it is quite clear that some of the same factors at work in anxiety in non-ASD populations are likely influential in an ASD population as well (e.g., emotion regulation, differences in amygdala/PFC function). Yet it is clear that the interpretation and exploration of these models within ASD will require careful consideration of how having ASD may alter conclusions. Within the behavioral realm, we described ways in which ASD-related characteristics may themselves produce risk for anxiety, perhaps through their impact on emotion regulation. Thus, when considering emotion regulation in ASD, it will be important to consider both well-established factors from models in other populations and how these models differ or what else may be influencing them in ASD. For neurobiological approaches, we argue that the interpretation of amygdala dysfunction may be highly dependent on the anxiety level of the sample and will require careful concurrent consideration of the roles of both social and anxiety concerns.

References

Adolphs, R. (2003). Cognitive neuroscience of human social behaviour. *Nature Reviews: Neuroscience, 4*, 165–178. doi:10.1038/nrn1056.

Aldao, A., Nolen-Hoeksema, S., & Schweizer, S. (2010). Emotion-regulation strategies across psychopathology: A meta-analytic review. *Clinical Psychology Review, 30*, 217–237. doi:10.1016/j.cpr.2009.11.004.

Amano, T., Unal, C. T., & Paré, D. (2010). Synaptic correlates of fear extinction in the amygdala. *Nature Neuroscience, 13*, 489–494. doi:10.1038/nn.2499.

American Psychiatric Association. (2013). Diagnostic and statistical manual of mental disorders, (5th ed., DSM-5). Washington, D.C.: American Psychiatric Association.

Amstadter, A. (2008). Emotion regulation and anxiety disorders. *Journal of Anxiety Disorders, 22*, 211–221. doi:10.1016/j.janxdis.2007.02.004.

Baron-Cohen, S. (1997). Mindblindness: An essay on autism and theory of mind. Palatino: MIT Press.

Baron-Cohen, S., Ring, H. A., Wheelwright, S., Bullmore, E. T., Brammer, M. J., Simmons, A., & Williams, S. C. (1999). Social intelligence in the normal and autistic brain: An fMRI study. *The European Journal of Neuroscience, 11,* 1891–1898. doi:10.1046/j.1460-9568.1999.00621.x.

Baron-Cohen, S., Ring, H., Bullmore, E., Wheelwright, S., Ashwin, C., & Williams, S. (2000). The amygdala theory of autism. *Neuroscience & Biobehavioral Reviews, 24,* 355–364. doi:10.1016/S0149-7634(00)00011-7.

Bauminger, N., & Kasari, C. (2000). Loneliness and friendship in high-functioning children with autism. *Child Development, 71,* 447–456. doi:10.1111/1467-8624.00156.

Baur, V., Hänggi, J., & Jäncke, L. (2013). Volumetric associations between uncinate fasciculus, amygdala, and trait anxiety. *BMC Neuroscience, 13,* 437–446. doi:10.1186/1471-2202-13-4.

Blackford, J. U., & Pine, D. S. (2012). Neural substrates of childhood anxiety disorders: A review of neuroimaging findings. *Child and Adolescent Psychiatric Clinics of North America, 21,* 501–525. doi:10.1016/j.chc.2012.05.002.

Brady, E. U., & Kendall, P. C. (1992). Comorbidity of anxiety and depression in children and adolescents. *Psychological Bulletin, 111,* 244–255. doi:10.1037/0033-2909.111.2.244.

Cappadocia, M. C., Weiss, J. A., & Pepler, D. (2012). Bullying experiences among children and youth with autism spectrum disorders. *Journal of Autism and Developmental Disorders, 42,* 266–277. doi:10.1007/s10803-011-1241-x.

Ciarrochi, J., Heaven, P. C. L., & Supavadeeprasit, S. (2008). The link between emotion identification skills and socio-emotional functioning in early adolescence: A 1-year longitudinal study. *Journal of Adolescence, 31,* 565–582. doi:10.1016/j.adolescence.2007.10.004.

Cisler, J. M., Olatunji, B. O., Feldner, M. T., & Forsyth, J. P. (2010). Emotion regulation and the anxiety disorders: An integrative review. *Journal of Psychopathology and Behavioral Assessment, 32,* 68–82. doi:10.1007/s10862-009-9161-1.

Cole, P. M., Martin, S. E., & Dennis, T. A. (2004). Emotion regulation as a scientific construct: Methodological challenges and directions for child development research. *Child Development, 75*(2), 317–333. doi:10.1111/j.1467-8624.2004.00673.x.

Corbett, B. A., Carmean, V., Ravizza, S., Wendelken, C., Henry, M. L., Carter, C., & Rivera, S. M. (2009). A functional and structural study of emotion and face processing in children with autism. *Psychiatry Research, 173,* 196–205. doi:10.1016/j.pscychresns.2008.08.005.

Critchley, H., Daly, E., Bullmore, E., Williams, S., van Amelsvoort, T., Robertson, D., & Murphy, D. (2000). The functional neuroanatomy of social behaviour: Changes in cerebral blood flow when people with autistic disorder process facial expressions. *Brain: a journal of neurology, 123,* 2203–2212. doi:10.1093/brain/123.11.2203.

Dalton, K. M., Nacewicz, B. M., Johnstone, T., Schaefer, H. S., Gernsbacher, M. A., Goldsmith, H. H., et al. (2005). Gaze fixation and the neural circuitry of face processing in autism. *Nature Neuroscience, 8,* 519–526. doi:10.1038/nn1421.

Davis, M. (1992). The role of the amygdala in fear and anxiety. *Annual Review of Neuroscience, 15,* 353–375. doi:10.1146/annurev.ne.15.030192.002033.

Dinstein, I., Heeger, D. J., Lorenzi, L., Minshew, N. J., Malach, R., & Behrmann, M. (2012). Unreliable evoked responses in autism. *Neuron, 75,* 981–991. doi:10.1016/j.neuron.2012.07.026.

Dugas, M. (1998). Generalized anxiety disorder: A preliminary test of a conceptual model. *Behaviour Research and Therapy, 36,* 215–226. doi:10.1016/S0005-7967(97)00070-3.

Dunn, W. (1997). The impact of sensory processing abilities on the daily lives of young children and their families: A conceptual model. *Infants and Young Children, 9*(4), 24–35.

Dziobek, I., Bahnemann, M., Convit, A., & Heekeren, H. (2010). The role of the fusiform-amygdala system in the pathophysiology of autism. *Archives of General Psychiatry, 67,* 397–405. doi:10.1001/archgenpsychiatry.2010.31.

Garavan, H., Pendergrass, J., Ross, T., Stein, E., & Risinger, R. (2001). Amygdala response to both positively and negatively valenced stimuli. *Neuroreport, 12*(12), 2779–2783.

Green, S. A., & Ben-Sasson, A. (2010). Anxiety disorders and sensory over-responsivity in children with autism spectrum disorders: Is there a causal relationship? *Journal of Autism and Developmental Disorders, 40,* 1495–1504. doi:10.1007/s10803-010-1007-x.

Gross, J. J. (2007). *Emotion regulation: Conceptual foundations. Handbook of emotion regulation* (pp. 3–24). New York: Guilford Press/Guilford Publications, Inc.

Guttmann-Steinmetz, S., Gadow, K. D., DeVincent, C. J., & Crowell, J. (2010). Anxiety symptoms in boys with autism spectrum disorder, attention-deficit hyperactivity disorder, or chronic multiple tic disorder and community controls. *Journal of Autism and Developmental Disorders, 40,* 1006–1016. doi:10.1007/s10803-010-0950-x.

Harms, M. B., Martin, A., & Wallace, G. L. (2010). Facial emotion recognition in autism spectrum disorders: A review of behavioral and neuroimaging studies. *Neuropsychology Review, 20,* 290–322. doi:10.1007/s11065-010-9138-6.

Hannesdottir, D. K., & Ollendick, T. H. (2007). The role of emotion regulation in the treatment of child anxiety disorders. *Clinical Child and Family Psychology Review, 10,* 275–293. doi:10.1007/s10567-007-0024-6.

Herrington, J. D., & Schultz, R. T. (2010). Neuroimaging of developmental disorders. In M. Shenton & B. I. Turetsky (Eds.), *Understanding Neuropsychiatric*

Disorders: Insights from Neuroimaging. Cambridge: Cambridge University Press.

Jahromi, L. B., Meek, S. E., & Ober-Reynolds, S. (2012). Emotion regulation in the context of frustration in children with high functioning autism and their typical peers. *Journal of Child Psychology and Psychiatry, and Allied Disciplines, 53,* 1250–1258. doi:10.1111/j.1469-7610.2012.02560.x.

Kalin, N. H., Shelton, S. E., & Davidson, R. J. (2007). Role of the primate orbitofrontal cortex in mediating anxious temperament. *Biological Psychiatry, 62*(10), 1134–1139. doi:10.1016/j.biopsych.2007.04.004.

Kelly, A. B., Garnett, M. S., Attwood, T., & Peterson, C. (2008). Autism spectrum symptomatology in children: The impact of family and peer relationships. *Journal of Abnormal Child Psychology, 36,* 1069–1081. doi:10.1007/s10802-008-9234-8.

Kerns, C. M., & Kendall, P. C. (2012). The presentation and classification of anxiety in autism spectrum disorder. *Clinical Psychology: Science and Practice, 19,* 323–347. doi:10.1111/cpsp.12009.

Kim, M. J., Loucks, R. A., Palmer, A. L., Brown, A. C., Solomon, K. M., Marchante, A. N., & Whalen, P. J. (2011). The structural and functional connectivity of the amygdala: From normal emotion to pathological anxiety. *Behavioural Brain Research, 223,* 403–410. doi:10.1016/j.bbr.2011.04.025.

Kliemann, D., Dziobek, I., Hatri, A., Steimke, R., & Heekeren, H. R. (2010). Atypical reflexive gaze patterns on emotional faces in autism spectrum disorders. *The Journal of Neuroscience, 30,* 12281–12287. doi:10.1523/JNEUROSCI.0688-10.2010.

Kliemann, D., Dziobek, I., Hatri, A., Baudewig, J., & Heekeren, H. R. (2012). The role of the amygdala in atypical gaze on emotional faces in autism spectrum disorders. *The Journal of Neuroscience, 32,* 9469–9476. doi:10.1523/JNEUROSCI.5294-11.2012.

Kleinhans, N. M., Johnson, L. C., Richards, T., Mahurin, R., Greenson, J., Dawson, G., & Aylward, E. (2009). Reduced neural habituation in the amygdala and social impairments in autism spectrum disorders. *The American Journal of Psychiatry, 166,* 467–475. doi:10.1176/appi.ajp.2008.07101681.

Kleinhans, N. M., Richards, T., Weaver, K., Johnson, L. C., Greenson, J., Dawson, G., & Aylward, E. (2010). Association between amygdala response to emotional faces and social anxiety in autism spectrum disorders. *Neuropsychologia, 48,* 3665–3670. doi:10.1016/j.neuropsychologia.2010.07.022.

Kluver, H., & Bucy, P. (1937). "Psychic blindness" and other symptoms following bilateral temporal lobectomy in Rhesus monkeys. *American Journal of Physiology, 119,* 352–353.

Konstantareas, M. M., & Stewart, K. (2006). Affect regulation and temperament in children with autism spectrum disorder. *Journal of Autism and Developmental Disorders, 36,* 143–154. doi:10.1007/s10803-005-0051-4.

Lainhart, J. E., Leyfer, O. T., & Folstein, S. E. (2003). Autism comorbidity interview-Present and lifetime version (ACI-PL). Salt Lake City: University of Utah Press.

Leyfer, O. T., Folstein, S. E., Bacalman, S., Davis, N. O., Dinh, E., Morgan, J., et al. (2006). Comorbid psychiatric disorders in children with autism: Interview development and rates of disorders. *Journal of Autism and Developmental Disorders, 36,* 849–861. doi:10.1007/s10803-006-0123-0.

Mazefsky, C. A., Conner, C. M., & Oswald, D. P. (2010). Association between depression and anxiety in high-functioning children with autism spectrum disorders and maternal mood symptoms. *Autism Research, 3,* 120–127. doi:10.1002/aur.133.

Mazefsky, C. A., Pelphrey, K. A., & Dahl, R. E. (2012). The need for a broader approach to emotion regulation research in autism. *Child Development Perspectives, 6,* 92–97. doi:10.1111/j.1750-8606.2011.00229.x.

Mazefsky, C. A., Herrington, J., Siegel, M., Scarpa, A., Maddox, B. B., Scahill, L., & White, S. W. (2013). The role of emotion regulation in autism spectrum disorders. *Journal of the American Academy of Child & Adolescent Psychiatry, 52,* 679–688. doi:10.1016/j.jaac.2013.05.006.

Mazefsky, C. A., & White, S. (in press). Emotion regulation in autism spectrum disorder; concepts and practice (Special Issue: Autism and developmental disorders: Management of serious behavioral disturbance). *Child and Adolescent Psychiatric Clinics of North America.*

Mennin, D. S., Heimberg, R. G., Turk, C. L., & Fresco, D. M. (2006). Applying an emotion regulation framework to integrative approaches to generalized anxiety disorder. *Clinical Psychology: Science and Practice, 9,* 85–90. doi:10.1093/clipsy.9.1.85.

Modi, S., Trivedi, R., Singh, K., Kumar, P., Rathore, R. K. S., Tripathi, R. P., & Khushu, S. (2013). Individual differences in trait anxiety are associated with white matter tract integrity in fornix and uncinate fasciculus: Preliminary evidence from a DTI based tractography study. *Behavioural Brain Research, 238,* 188–192. doi:10.1016/j.bbr.2012.10.007.

Monk, C. S. (2008). The development of emotion-related neural circuitry in health and psychopathology. *Development and Psychopathology, 20,* 1231–1250. doi:10.1017/S095457940800059X.

Monk, C. S., Weng, S.-J., Wiggins, J. L., Kurapati, N., Louro, H. M. C., Carrasco, M., et al. (2010). Neural circuitry of emotional face processing in autism spectrum disorders. *Journal of Psychiatry & Neuroscience, 35,* 105–114. doi:10.1503/jpn.090085.

Muris, P., & Ollendick, T. H. (2005). The role of temperament in the etiology of child psychopathology. *Clinical Child and Family Psychology Review, 8,* 271–289. doi:10.1007/s10567-005-8809-y.

Neuhaus, E., Beauchaine, T. P., & Bernier, R. (2010). Neurobiological correlates of social functioning in autism. *Clinical Psychology Review, 30,* 733–748. doi:10.1016/j.cpr.2010.05.007.

Nolen-Hoeksema, S., & Watkins, E. R. (2011). A heuristic for developing transdiagnostic models of psychopathology: Explaining multifinality and divergent trajectories. *Perspectives on Psychological Science, 6,* 589–609. doi:10.1177/1745691611419672.

Pelphrey, K. A., Morris, J. P., McCarthy, G., & Labar, K. S. (2007). Perception of dynamic changes in facial affect and identity in autism. *Social Cognitive and Affective Neuroscience, 2,* 140–149. doi:10.1093/scan/nsm010.

Pfeifer, J. H., & Allen, N. B. (2012). Arrested development? Reconsidering dual-systems models of brain function in adolescence and disorders. *Trends in Cognitive Sciences, 16,* 322–329. doi:10.1016/j.tics.2012.04.011.

Phelps, E. A., & LeDoux, J. E. (2005). Contributions of the amygdala to emotion processing: From animal models to human behavior. *Neuron, 48*(2), 175–187. doi:10.1016/j.neuron.2005.09.025.

Pugliese, C., Fritz, M., & White, S. W. (submitted). Kindling the flame: ASD traits intensify the relationship between social anxiety and aggression.

Rodgers, J., Glod, M., Connolly, B., & McConachie, H. (2012). The relationship between anxiety and repetitive behaviours in autism spectrum disorder. *Journal of Autism and Developmental Disorders, 42,* 2404–1409. doi:10.1007/s10803-012-1531-y.

Rogers, S. J. (2009). What are infant siblings teaching us about autism in infancy? *Autism Research, 2,* 125–137. doi:10.1002/aur.81.

Roy, A. K., Vasa, R. A., Bruck, M., Mogg, K., Bradley, B. P., Sweeney, M., et al. (2008). Attention bias toward threat in pediatric anxiety disorders. *Journal of the American Academy of Child and Adolescent Psychiatry, 47,* 1189–1196. doi:10.1097/CHI.0b013e3181825ace.

Russell, J. (1980). A circumplex model of affect. *Journal of Personality & Social Psychology, 39,* 1161–1178.

Samson, A. C., Huber, O., & Gross, J. J. (2012). Emotion regulation in Asperger's syndrome and high-functioning autism. *Emotion (Washington, D. C.), 12,* 659–665. doi:10.1037/a0027975.

Schultz, R. T. (2005). Developmental deficits in social perception in autism: The role of the amygdala and fusiform face area. *International Journal of Developmental Neuroscience, 23,* 125–141. doi:10.1016/j.ijdevneu.2004.12.012.

Schumann, C. M., Bauman, M. D., & Amaral, D. G. (2011). Abnormal structure or function of the amygdala is a common component of neurodevelopmental disorders. *Neuropsychologia, 49,* 745–759. doi:10.1016/j.neuropsychologia.2010.09.028.

Sergerie, K., Chochol, C., & Armony, J. L. (2008). The role of the amygdala in emotional processing: A quantitative meta-analysis of functional neuroimaging studies. *Neuroscience and Biobehavioral Reviews, 32,* 811–830. doi:10.1016/j.neubiorev.2007.12.002.

Shalom, D. B. (2009). The medial prefrontal cortex and integration in autism. *The Neuroscientist, 15,* 589–598. doi:10.1177/1073858409336371.

Shaw, P., Brierley, B., & David, A. S. (2005). A critical period for the impact of amygdala damage on the emotional enhancement of memory? *Neurology, 65,* 326–328. doi:10.1212/01.wnl.0000168867.40688.9b.

Sheppes, G., & Gross, J. J. (2011). Is timing everything? Temporal considerations in emotion regulation. *Personality and Social Psychology Review, 15,* 319–331. doi:10.1177/1088868310395778..

Siegle, G. (2008). Introduction to special issue on rumination: From mechanisms to treatment. *Cognitive Therapy and Research, 32,* 471–473. doi:10.1007/s10608-008-9207-9.

Suveg, C., & Zeman, J. (2004). Emotion regulation in children with anxiety disorders. *Journal of Clinical Child and Adolescent Psychology, 33*(4), 750–759.

Swartz, J. R., Wiggins, J. L., Carrasco, M., Lord, C., & Monk, C. S. (2013). Amygdala habituation and prefrontal functional connectivity in youth with autism spectrum disorders. *Journal of the American Academy of Child and Adolescent Psychiatry, 52,* 84–93. doi:10.1016/j.jaac.2012.10.012.

Tamir, M. (2011). The maturing field of emotion regulation. *Emotion Review, 3,* 3–7. doi:10.1177/1754073910388685.

Thompson, R. A. (1994). *Emotion regulation: A theme in search of definition. Monographs of the society for research in child development* (pp. 25–52). Chicago: University of Chicago Press.

Watanabe, T., Yahata, N., Abe, O., Kuwabara, H., Inoue, H., Takano, Y, et al. (2012). Diminished medial prefrontal activity behind autistic social judgments of incongruent information. *PloS One, 7,* e39561. doi:10.1371/journal.pone.0039561.

Watson, D., Clark, L. A., & Weber, K. (1991). Tripartite model of anxiety and depression: Psychometric evidence and taxonomic implications. *Journal of Abnormal Psychology, 100*(3), 316–336.

Weng, S.-J., Carrasco, M., Swartz, J. R., Wiggins, J. L., Kurapati, N., Liberzon, I., & Monk, C. S. (2011). Neural activation to emotional faces in adolescents with autism spectrum disorders. *Journal of Child Psychology and Psychiatry, and Allied Disciplines, 52,* 296–305. doi:10.1111/j.1469-7610.2010.02317.x.

Whalen, P. (2007). The uncertainty of it all. *Trends in Cognitive Sciences, 11,* 499–500. doi:10.1016/j.tics.2007.08.016.

Wood, J. J., & Gadow, K. D. (2010). Exploring the nature and function of anxiety in youth with autism spectrum disorders. *Clinical Psychology: Science and Practice, 17,* 281–292. doi:10.1111/j.1468-2850.2010.01220.x.

Part II

Autism Spectrum Disorder and Specific Anxiety Disorders

Obsessions, Compulsions, and Repetitive Behavior: Autism and/or OCD

Monica S. Wu, Brittany M. Rudy and Eric A. Storch

Clinical Presentations of Obsessive–Compulsive Disorder and Autism Spectrum Disorder

Obsessive–compulsive disorder (OCD) has a variable presentation, but is characterized by the presence of recurrent obsessions and/or compulsions that take more than 1 hour a day (American Psychiatric Association 2013). OCD affects an estimated 1–2 % of the pediatric population and 1 % of the typically developing adult population (Kessler et al. 2005; Geller 2006). OCD is associated with significant impairment in various domains of life, including social relationships, occupational requirements, and family life (Piacentini et al. 2003; Mancebo et al. 2008).

Obsessions are intrusive thoughts, images, urges, or sounds that repeatedly enter an affected individual's mind and often cause distress (Rahman et al. 2011). Common examples of obsessions include experiencing excessive fears of being contaminated, being responsible for something terrible happening, having excessive concerns about certain numbers or words, and having intrusive religious/scrupulous concerns (e.g., being overly concerned with what is right/wrong or offending religious objects) or sexual obsessions (e.g., distressing images of sexual acts; Moore et al. 2007). Compulsions are

behaviors that an individual performs typically to mitigate anxiety or distress resulting from obsessions (Rahman et al. 2011). Compulsions can take the form of overt, observable behaviors or covert mental rituals. Common manifestations of compulsions can present as repetitive checking, counting, ordering, or cleaning behaviors (Swedo et al. 1989; Masi et al. 2005). Compulsions can involve other people as well, such as seeking reassurance to assuage the fear that something catastrophic will happen, or they may manifest as mental rituals, where the individual must complete acts repeatedly in their mind (e.g., silently praying to self).

Autism spectrum disorder (ASD) affects approximately 1 in 88 youth and about 1 % of adults (Brugha et al. 2011; Centers for Disease Control and Prevention 2012) and is characterized by marked impairment in various developmental areas. Individuals with ASD often have difficulties in social interactions, communication, and/or restrictive and stereotyped behaviors, activities, or interests (American Psychiatric Association 2013). Within social interactions, individuals with ASD often have difficulty creating and maintaining peer relationships and lack reciprocal social interaction skills. Regarding communication, these individuals are frequently delayed in language development and may display problems in maintaining conversations with others. See Chaps. 1, 2, and 7 for a full description of the diagnostic criteria, etiology, and phenotypic variability in the clinical features of ASD.

E. A. Storch (✉) · M. S. Wu · B. M. Rudy
University of South Florida, 880 6th Street South, Suite 460, Box 7523, St. Petersburg, FL 33701, USA
e-mail: estorch@health.usf.edu

Within the context of ASD, restricted and repetitive behaviors and interests (RRBI) are often observed, characterized by stereotyped motor movements, restricted interests, fixations on certain objects, and rigid routines. The frequency and the familial distress associated with the repetitive behaviors have been linked to increased functional impairment (South et al. 2005). Self-stimulatory behaviors and motor stereotypies can present in various ways, such as hand flapping or body rocking. Individuals with ASD may also possess restricted interests or fixations with certain objects and often have difficulty diverging from their fixated interest in conversations with others. For instance, a youth with ASD may harbor a particular, intense interest in sports statistics, spending excessive time researching figures and constantly talking about them. These individuals may also display rigidity with certain schedules and can be inflexible to any changes in routine (Militerni et al. 2002). As an example, an individual with ASD may feel the need to go through the same idiosyncratic order of events each day because it is the daily routine. Disruptions in the daily routine commonly cause great distress, due to rigidity and inflexibility with change.

Obsessions, fixated interests, compulsions, and repetitive behaviors are enigmatic of both OCD and ASD. Although the symptoms may be different when considering pure OCD or ASD caseness, their similar outward presentation can pose a challenge when trying to make an accurate diagnosis. As such, it is important to consider various factors and contextual influences when attempting to parse out the symptom overlap.

Symptom Overlap and Differential Diagnosis

Providing an accurate differential diagnosis for an individual presenting with certain repetitive thoughts/behaviors, fixations, or rituals can be complicated due to similar phenotypic presentations of OCD and ASD and requires the ability to correctly discriminate between symptoms of the two disorders. For example, obsessions in OCD and fixated interests in ASD both involve continuous repetitive thoughts. Compulsions within the

context of OCD and stereotyped behaviors within the framework of ASD both involve symptoms that exhibit as repetitive behaviors that need to be carried to completion, otherwise causing distress. As such, there is a need for strategies that help clinicians to accurately parse the symptoms apart.

Obsessions consistent with OCD caseness are typically regarded as ego-dystonic, or contrary to the individual's self-concept and belief system (American Psychiatric Association 2013). As such, obsessions often cause distress, are regarded as intrusive, and they do not provide pleasure or gratification. The individual typically does not want to engage in such repeated thoughts, resulting in considerable distress. On the contrary, individuals with ASD with fixated interests often enjoy the content of the repetitive thoughts and may possess an intense investment in a particular topic (Turner-Brown et al. 2011). Individuals may repeatedly focus on these thoughts and they may occupy a considerable amount of time; furthermore, the thoughts are not usually regarded as distressing, but the act of stopping the thoughts may trigger distress (Turner-Brown et al. 2011).

In some cases, repetitive thoughts in OCD and ASD may phenotypically display more similarly and require more nuanced distinctions. In these instances, uncovering the context of the thoughts and source of distress can be valuable in correctly establishing a differential diagnosis. Obsessions consistent with OCD caseness are typically more persistent, in the sense that these intrusive thoughts are frequently in the forefront. On the contrary, the same symptoms within an ASD framework may only be triggered upon observing a behavior that violates their rigid, perceived set of rules. For instance, a child may have a repeated thought about consistently following rules and making sure everything is done in the "right" manner. This symptom could be consistent with OCD caseness, whereby the intrusive thought is frequently present and disabling. Specifically, this child may be experiencing distress in trying to do things "morally," such as taking excessive care to ensure that he never says a bad word or hurts anybody, for fear of being a "horrible" person (Amir et al. 2001). Alternatively, this same behavior could also manifest as a symptom of

ASD when, for instance, the child is experiencing the same intrusive thoughts about rigidly adhering to rules. While these thoughts can apply consistently across situations, in an individual with ASD, clinical experience dictates that the thoughts typically are not triggered until witnessing someone "breaking the rules," such as cutting in line or saying a bad word. Oftentimes, these thoughts are viewed from the perspective that certain rules must be followed inflexibly, akin to following a daily routine. Here, the intrusive thought lacks the fear about the actions' implications on character or bad outcomes and displays more of an influence driven by rigidity.

Repetitive behaviors within the context of OCD are typically intended to reduce distress or anxiety resulting from an obsessional trigger. These compulsions serve as a vehicle for distress reduction in a way that is unrealistically tied to the feared consequences and/or is excessive in nature (American Psychiatric Association 2013). On the other hand, repetitive behaviors within the ASD framework often impart alternative purposes, serving as operant (e.g., social/non-social reinforcements) or self-stimulatory behaviors (Cunningham and Schreibman 2008). Although the repetitive behaviors may increase in frequency when the individual is stressed (Groden et al. 2005) and the individual may become distressed if prevented from engaging in these behaviors (Turner-Brown et al. 2011), there is a less robust connection between the repetitive behavior and a specific anxiety-provoking obsession (Mack et al. 2010). The presence of intellectual disabilities and level of IQ may also be associated with the frequency of repetitive behaviors in individuals with ASD, though results are mixed; lower IQ has generally been linked to an increase in repetitive behaviors, but certain types of RRBI (e.g., restricted interests) and younger individuals have shown less robust relationships (Bishop et al. 2006; Matson et al. 2008).

Compulsions and repetitive behaviors in OCD and ASD can be difficult to distinguish due to their outwardly similar phenotypic presentation, so it can be helpful to investigate what purpose the behavior serves for the affected individual, as well as the context the behavior occurs in

(Joosten et al. 2009). For example, an individual may feel the need to repeatedly tap the table. If the individual has OCD, there may be a need to tap the table exactly seven times to counteract intrusive thoughts about catastrophic repercussions if failing to tap the table in a way that is "just right" (Coles et al. 2003). In this case, the repetitive tapping is intended to counteract the specific obsession and temporarily relieves distress which contributes to the maintenance of symptoms. Individuals with ASD who engage in the same behavior may be tapping their fingers as a way of self-soothing or serving as a distraction from the surroundings (Joshi et al. 2010). Overtly, the behaviors can look exactly the same; however, the latter individual is engaging in these behaviors as a calming mechanism that is not necessarily tied to a specific thought or worry, as the tapping is not intended to mitigate a feared consequence. While the repetitive behaviors may attenuate anxiety at any given moment (due to its comforting quality), these repetitive motor behaviors do not exclusively occur in anxiety-related situations (Mack et al. 2010). Specifically, identifying the reinforcement paradigms that the symptoms operate through may be helpful in distinguishing between OCD and ASD symptoms. For instance, compulsions consistent with OCD caseness typically serve as a method to mitigate or avoid the undesired stimuli, negatively reinforcing the engagement of the compulsions. Alternatively, repetitive behaviors within the context of ASD typically provide a sense of comfort or self-soothing, positively reinforcing the individual to engage in these behaviors. Furthermore, individuals with ASD may seek to engage in these behaviors with the purpose of self-stimulation due to hyposensitivity (O'Neill and Jones 1997), while those with OCD may feel distress about engaging in those same behaviors due to their disparate purpose. Ultimately, many symptoms of OCD and ASD may outwardly display similarly, but differ in terms of their purposes (Helverschou et al. 2011). However, it is possible for individuals with ASD to concurrently display bona fide OCD symptoms, particularly when the purpose of the behaviors becomes more consistent with OCD caseness.

Certain repetitive thoughts and compulsions have been reported to occur more in individuals with OCD as compared to those with ASD, such as somatic obsessions and repetitive checking behaviors (McDougle et al. 1995; Russell et al. 2005; Lewin et al. 2011). Additionally, Cath et al. (2008) found that adults with ASD generally had a lower Severity Scale score on obsessions when compared to adults with "pure" OCD, as measured by the Yale-Brown Obsessive Compulsive Scale (Y-BOCS; Goodman et al. 1989a; Goodman et al. 1989b). However, individuals with ASD may not have the ability to verbalize their obsessions due to cognitive impairment or diminished verbal expression capacities, suggesting that this inability to articulate them does not necessarily indicate they are absent (Baron-Cohen 1989; Cath et al. 2008). There are also instances when individuals may feel the need to do things until it "feels just right," which can further complicate the differential diagnosis. Specifically, some individuals with OCD simply engage in a ritual until it "feels just right" to them (instead of doing those behaviors for purposes of neutralizing a specific negative thought), which can present more similarly to individuals with ASD who experience general discomfort and distress when things are not done in a certain way (Militerni et al. 2002; Coles et al. 2003). Ultimately, the concurrent display of the symptoms and potential comorbidity of ASD and OCD make differential diagnosis more complex.

Comorbidity

With up to 37 % of youth (Leyfer et al. 2006) and 25 % of adults (Russell et al. 2005; Rydén and Bejerot 2008) with ASD having comorbid OCD, the rate at which these conditions co-occur imbues considerable, noteworthy clinical implications. A sizable subgroup of individuals with ASD also presents with subclinical obsessive–compulsive symptoms (Lewin et al. 2011; van Steensel et al. 2011). Muris et al. (1998) have reported an occurrence rate of obsessive–compulsive symptoms as high as 72 % among individuals with ASD, and some postulate that ASD and OCD

share neurobiological and genetic underpinnings (Jacob et al. 2009).

Individuals with ASD displaying obsessive–compulsive symptoms can show considerable distress related to their compounded symptoms (McDougle et al. 1995; Russell et al. 2005; Fischer-Terworth and Probst 2009). While the co-occurrence of the disorders has not been linked to an increase in obsessive–compulsive symptom severity (Lewin et al. 2011), it has been associated with increased psychosocial impairment (Mack et al. 2010). Individuals with ASD may be more prone to other comorbid psychopathology as well. Specifically, Lewin et al. (2011) found that youth with ASD and OCD diagnoses were more likely to have additional diagnoses of separation anxiety disorder, social phobia, and clinically significant inattention or hyperactive symptoms when compared to youth with only OCD.

The heightened comorbidity of OCD and ASD further complicates the clinician's ability to accurately assess and attribute symptoms to the respective disorders. Without an accurate differentiation between the respective symptoms, the ability to decide upon the appropriate treatment plan and effectively target symptoms becomes even more complex. Collectively, the high prevalence rates, compounded deleterious effects, and implications for treatment illuminate the need for valid assessment tools to parse out symptoms and make accurate diagnoses.

Assessment Recommendations

Evidence-based assessments have garnered increasing attention and are pertinent to accurate and reliable measurements of symptomology (Cohen et al. 2008). In order to be evidence based, the measures and practices must demonstrate reliability and consistency in measuring the symptoms of interest, track the symptoms in a methodical and quantitative manner, and assess symptom severity, associated impairment, and changes over the course of treatment (McGuire et al. 2012). A number of well-established measures possess good psychometric properties and the ability to assess ASD or obsessive–compulsive symptoms individually (Jacob et al. 2009).

In assessing obsessive–compulsive symptoms, the Y-BOCS (Goodman et al. 1989a; Goodman et al. 1989b) and the Children's Yale-Brown Obsessive Compulsive Scale (CY-BOCS; Scahill et al. 1997) are the most widely used measures. Each instrument assesses for the presence and severity of obsessive–compulsive symptoms, and provides a checklist and severity scores for obsessions and compulsions. Both measures are administered as semi-structured interviews and possess sound psychometric properties (Goodman et al. 1989a, b; Scahill et al. 1997; Storch et al. 2004). Additionally, various semi-structured diagnostic interviews, such as the *Anxiety Disorders Interview Schedule for DSM-IV— Child and Parent Version* (ADIS-IV-C/P; Silverman and Albano 1996), *ADIS-IV—Adult Version* (ADIS-IV; Brown et al. 1994), *ADIS-IV—Lifetime Version*(ADIS-IV-L; Brown et al. 2001), and the *Structured Clinical Interview for DSM-IV Axis I Disorders—Patient Edition* (SCID-I/P; First et al. 2002), contain modules for assessing OCD as well. While the psychometric properties of the OCD module in the ADIS are adequate (Brown et al. 2001; Brown-Jacobsen et al. 2011), these diagnostic interviews lack the level of detail that the CY-BOCS and Y-BOCS provide.

Although there are groups of measures that have been well-established in assessing obsessions and repetitive behaviors in ASD and OCD separately, there is a paucity of reliable instruments that have been validated in populations with both OCD and ASD. The *Autism Comorbidity Interview—Present and Lifetime Version* (ACI-PL) was developed as a semi-structured clinician-administered interview tailored to provide diagnoses for comorbid psychiatric disorders in children with ASD, and generally possesses good reliability and validity (Leyfer et al. 2006). Alternatively, the *ASD—Comorbid for Children* (*ASD-CC;* Matson and Wilkins 2008) and *ASD—Comorbid for Adults* (*ASD-CA;* Matson and Boisjoli 2008) were designed as self-report scales that assessed comorbid psychopathology in individuals with ASD. While the ASD-CC and ASD-CA are promising, they possess variable

reliability and cover a broad range of symptomology, precluding them from parsing out OCD and ASD symptoms. Ultimately, there is still a need for an instrument specifically designed to assess symptoms in individuals with both OCD and ASD, while having the ability to be sensitive to differential diagnosis.

The first attempt at modifying a measure to specifically assess for obsessive–compulsive symptoms in youth with pervasive developmental disorders (PDD) was conducted by Scahill et al. (2006). The *CY-BOCS—Modified for PDD* (*CY-BOCS-PDD*) is a clinician-administered measure that assesses repetitive behaviors in youth with PDD. Items assess the presence and severity of these restricted patterns of behaviors. The *CY-BOCS-PDD* possesses excellent inter-rater reliability (Intraclass Correlation, ICC = 0.97) and strong internal consistency ($\alpha = 0.85$). However, it does not allow for the opportunity to assess obsessions because of concern about the presence of obsessions and the need to infer their presence when interviewing parents.

Wu et al. (2013) examined the original *CY-BOCS* in youth with ASD and obsessive–compulsive symptoms, and found that the measure demonstrated good internal consistency, excellent inter-rater reliability, satisfactory convergent validity, and treatment sensitivity within a pediatric ASD population. The study demonstrated evidence that the *CY-BOCS* has the ability to assess for obsessions and compulsions among youth with ASD. Particularly, the *CY-BOCS* exhibited the ability to assess for obsessive–compulsive symptoms that were disparate from ASD symptoms as measured by the *Social Responsiveness Scale* (Constantino and Gruber 2005). It also demonstrated good divergent validity from anxiety, depression, and other internalizing/externalizing symptoms and the ability to assess changes in obsessive–compulsive symptoms before and after treatment for anxiety in ASD, independent of the changes in ASD symptoms. It is noted that there was some modest variability between obsessions and compulsions in inter-rater reliability between two clinicians, as there was better agreement on compulsions. This may reflect the youth's lower level of insight and difficulty articulating obsessions (Storch et al. 2012), as compared to the more observable compulsive behaviors. As such, clinicians should note that it may be more difficult to obtain a reliable endorsement of obsessions, and multiple informants may be helpful in the assessment of symptoms (Storch et al. 2012).

When assessing for OCD or ASD, it may also be helpful to examine clinical presentations of ASD outside of the symptom overlap to further inform the differential diagnosis. For example, assessing the individual's social patterns and behaviors may help with distinguishing between the disorders, as an individual who lacks emotional reciprocity or consistently engages in parallel play may be better suited under the ASD diagnosis. Descriptions of functional communication may also be helpful, as speech patterns and examinations of verbal abilities can also aid in distinguishing between neurotypical individuals and those with ASD. However, it is important to note that obsessive–compulsive symptoms may impact social functioning as well (Piacentini et al. 2007b), such as avoidance of others to prevent the triggering of certain obsessive–compulsive symptoms. As such, it is essential for clinicians to continue to assess for the purpose and motivation behind the behaviors.

In sum, clinicians should be cognizant of several things when assessing obsessions, compulsions, and/or repetitive behavior in individuals with ASD when OCD is suspected or in question. First, they should be aware of common difficulties when assessing the overlap in repetitive thoughts and behaviors. For example, individuals with ASD and/or OCD often lack insight into their symptoms, making it more difficult to assess the presence of certain symptomology, as well as the motivation behind the behaviors (Cath et al. 2008; Jakubovski et al. 2011). Moreover, distress caused by the behaviors can be challenging to assess in individuals with ASD, as ability for self-reflection is variable among this population (Cath et al. 2008). That said, distress experienced due to the obsessive–compulsive symptoms specifically can be the difference between receiving a diagnosis of OCD or not, if all other criteria are met (Muris et al. 1998). Second, clinicians should

carefully probe for the purpose of the behaviors and/or in which contexts the behaviors appear in, allowing the clinicians to appropriately attribute symptoms to the respective disorders. Additionally, assessing for ASD behaviors outside of the symptom overlap between OCD and ASD may help illuminate unique information that can aid in successful differential diagnosis. Lastly, recommendations for future directions include validation of existing measures for examining OCD symptoms in the ASD population, and/or modifying current measures to become more nuanced (e.g., providing detailed item-level anchors and examples that help differentiate between symptoms of OCD and ASD). The creation and validation of new measures possessing sound psychometric properties for use in populations with concurrent OCD and ASD diagnoses would be helpful as well. Accurately ascribing the symptoms to the respective disorders will allow for effective treatment planning and targeting of problematic behaviors.

Treatment Overview

Cognitive behavioral therapy (CBT) with exposure and response prevention (ERP) is the well-established treatment of choice for OCD for typically developing youth and adults (AACAP 2012; Lewin and Piacentini 2009) and is provided in weekly and intensive formats (Storch et al. 2007a; Storch et al. 2010). ERP involves exposing an individual to situations which trigger obsessional distress, and having the individual refrain from engaging in compulsions (March and Mulle 1998; Piacentini et al. 2007a; Storch et al. 2007b). Psychoeducational and cognitive strategies aimed at testing the reality of the obsessional worries (Barrett et al. 2004; Storch et al. 2007b) are generally incorporated in an adjunctive manner along with CBT programs. CBT with ERP has demonstrated superiority to relaxation (Freeman et al. 2008; Piacentini et al. 2011), wait-list control conditions (Storch et al. 2011a), as well as equivalence or superiority to selective serotonin reuptake inhibitors (SSRIs; The Pediatric OCD Treatment Study (POTS)

Team 2004; Irfan et al. 2011). Pharmacological treatment, typically SSRIs (Lewin et al. 2005), has received support in the literature with meta-analyses demonstrating a moderate effect relative to placebo controls (e.g., Geller et al. 2001, 2003; Vitiello and Waslick 2010). However, CBT alone is recommended for mild-to-moderate cases of OCD, while a combination of CBT and pharmacotherapy is suggested for more severe presentations POTS Team 2004; AACAP 2012).

Among youth with ASD, less treatment research is available, but some efficacy has been demonstrated for the treatment of comorbid OCD and ASD using cognitive-behavioral interventions. While habit reversal training or other intervention techniques may be more appropriate to treat repetitive behaviors that serve nonanxiety-related purposes (e.g., non-social, attention), personalized CBT represents the current best practice for treating overlapping OCD and ASD repetitive or ritualized (i.e., compulsive) behaviors that serve an anxiety alleviating purpose (Wood and Drahota 2005; White et al. 2010). Personalized CBT utilizes in vivo exposure (e.g., ERP for compulsions within the context of OCD) with ASD-specific modifications such as more concrete, simplified cognitive techniques, visual aids, social stories, greater inclusion of parent and teachers for generalization, and inclusion of behavioral rewards programs throughout treatment (see Chaps. 11, 12, 13, and 14 for a more thorough review of psychosocial treatments for anxiety and ASD as well as modification trends). Two case studies examining CBT protocols for treatment of OCD in a child (7 years old) with Asperger's syndrome (Reaven and Hepburn 2003) and a child (12 years old) with high-functioning autism (Lehmkuhl et al. 2008) yielded a 65% and an 83.3% decrease in obsessive–compulsive symptoms, respectively, with each child no longer meeting criteria for OCD. Additionally, several recent randomized controlled trials (RCTs) examining treatment of youth with comorbid anxiety (OCD inclusive) and ASD have demonstrated efficacy for personalized CBT protocols (Storch et al. 2013; Wood et al. 2009), with large effect sizes. In adolescents and adults (m age=26.9) with ASD, one RCT (n=46)

comparing two active treatments CBT and anxiety management for treatment of OCD symptoms found that both active treatments yielded significant symptom reduction (>25% reduction in OCD severity scores) but did not differ from one another (Russell et al. 2013). Clinical trials specifically examining CBT alone and/or combination (CBT + pharmacotherapy) treatments for comorbid *pediatric* OCD and ASD have yet to be conducted, and intensive treatment options have not been explored.

Further, pharmacological treatment alone, though frequently utilized (Coury et al. 2012), may not be as viable an option for youth with ASD. A recent controlled trial by King et al. (2009) recently conducted a controlled trial that compared the use of citalopram versus placebo in treating children with repetitive behaviors (as measured by the CYBOCS-PDD; Scahill et al. 2006) and ASD demonstrated no significant decreases in anxiety or repetitive behaviors and no between group treatment effects over 12 weeks. No other repetitive behavior or OCD-specific studies have examined pharmacotherapy for youth with ASD. At this time, additional clinical trials are necessary to examine the efficacy of pharmacotherapy alone or in combination with psychosocial interventions for treating OCD among the pediatric and adult ASD population.

DSM-5: Implications and Thoughts on Changes to ASD and OCD Diagnoses

The *Diagnostic and Statistical Manual of Mental Disorders—Fifth Edition* (*DSM-5*; American Psychiatric Association 2013) changes include the removal of OCD from classification as an anxiety disorder and reclassification under Obsessive–Compulsive and Related Disorders (OCRD), with rationale that characteristics of OCD may be more highly associated, and share neurological correlates, with other OCRD (e.g., trichotillomania, body dysmorphic disorder) than the anxiety disorders (Bartz and Hollander 2006; Leckman et al. 2010), and may, therefore, be better classified separately (see Storch et al. 2008 for a diverging perspective). Additionally, symptoms of OCD are arguably heterogeneous (e.g., traditional/neutralizing, cognitive, motoric, sensory related, rule/rigidity related) and do not always produce or follow the characteristic "anxiety" and "alleviation" response (Bartz and Hollander 2006; Matsunaga 2012), further differentiating OCD from other known anxiety disorders. Definitions of obsessions and compulsions have also been revised and simplified for clarity. Word changes such as replacing "inappropriate" with "unwanted" and "impulse" with "urge," as well as exclusion of "excessive" or "unreasonable" aim to make the definitions more distinguishable from other disorders and exclude criteria that cannot be easily operationalized (Leckman et al. 2010). Insight specifiers have been expanded to include "good or fair insight," "poor insight," and "absent insight" and an additional specifier "tic-related OCD" has been added. Further, hoarding behaviors will be classified as a separate disorder, and the Axis I exclusionary criterion has been expanded to include additional diagnoses that should be distinguished from OCD (e.g., stereotypies in stereotypic movement disorder, preoccupation with objects in hoarding disorder, repetitive patterns in ASD). These changes attempt to make diagnosis of OCD more empirical and objective; however, the full implications of these changes on diagnosis and comorbidity have yet to be determined.

Changes within *DSM-5* also aim to significantly revise diagnostic criteria for ASD. Autistic disorder, Asperger's syndrome, and PDD-not otherwise specified (PDD-NOS) are to be reclassified into a single diagnosis, "ASD." Individuals must demonstrate symptoms from two domains (in place of the three current domains for autistic disorder): (1) social/communication and (2) fixed interests and repetitive behaviors. As part of the domain restructuring, social and communication criteria are to be merged while excluding language delays as a criterion, and sensory difficulties are to be added as a restricted-repetitive criterion. Three social/communication criteria must be met, and two fixed interests and repetitive behaviors criteria must be met, with severity specified using levels (1–3) based upon impair-

ment. These changes will likely impact diagnosis, prevalence, and comorbidity, particularly when considering changes to OCRD. See Chaps. 15, 16, and 17 for further discussion of *DSM-5* changes to the diagnostic criteria for ASD and potential implications of those changes.

Given symptom overlap (e.g., repetitive or compulsive behaviors, rituals, fixations, rigidity with routine) and current comorbidity (Leyfer et al. 2006; Rudy et al. 2013), as stated above, the changes in *DSM-5* will likely influence differential diagnosis and comorbidity for ASD and OCD. The new *DSM-5* criteria may exclude some children who currently qualify for an ASD diagnosis from meeting criteria for ASD (Worley and Matson 2012; Mayes et al. 2013). Specifically, the increased requirement for repetitive and restricted behaviors, needing to exhibit two of the four symptoms, may preclude some youth from obtaining an ASD diagnosis (Frazier et al. 2012). This exclusion of some children raises many questions about what will happen to children who no longer meet diagnostic criteria for ASD.

The inclusion of additional insight specifiers may allow for a greater number of individuals to receive an OCD diagnosis. The majority of youth with ASD will likely fall into the "absent" insight specifier regarding the nature and purpose of their repetitive behaviors (Storch et al. 2012). Children who exhibit repetitive behaviors that are parallel with rituals or compulsions, but meet only one criterion for ASD repetitive domain, may no longer qualify for ASD. Instead, these children may qualify for OCD with "absent insight," leading to decreased prevalence of ASD diagnoses but an increase in the amount of OCD diagnoses given (i.e., children who may have previously had comorbid ASD and OCD diagnoses may only qualify for OCD *and* children who previously were only diagnosed with ASD may be classified as having OCD with "absent insight" instead). It may also be more difficult to distinguish whether or not children who meet full criteria for ASD (i.e., two or more criteria on the repetitive domain, with one criterion being repetitive or compulsive behavior) meet criteria for OCD with "absent insight" as well, potentially increasing the incidence of comorbidity among the two disorders and further blurring the lines of differential diagnosis. However, given that "poor insight" is an option for *DSM-IV-TR,* the extent of the implication of the addition of the "absent insight" specifier is yet to be determined.

Additionally, while it is possible the ASD and OCD comorbidity will increase, overall ASD and anxiety comorbidity prevalence may decrease when using the new *DSM-5* criteria, given that OCD is, by some reports, among the most commonly comorbid anxiety diagnosis (Leyfer et al. 2006; van Steensel et al. 2011; Rudy et al. 2013) and will no longer be classified as an anxiety disorder. Prevalence and comorbidity may also be affected by the reclassification of hoarding behaviors into a separate disorder. Hoarding symptoms often occur in individuals with ASD, but the estimated prevalence varies across studies (Bejerot 2007); some suggest that individuals with ASD have higher rates of hoarding than individuals with OCD and healthy control groups (McDougle et al. 1995; Pertusa et al. 2012), while others have found no significant differences (Storch et al. 2011b). Hoarding may be less associated with ASD traits and vice versa than other OCD behaviors and symptoms (Anholt et al. 2010; Pertusa et al. 2012). That said, children who currently meet criteria for OCD due to their propensity to save or hoard items must now be considered for hoarding disorder, adding an additional challenge to differentiating between saving items as a component of a restricted interest or due to an additional psychological concern and further increasing the possibility for diagnostic comorbidity. Furthermore, tic disorders are more common among children with OCD within the pediatric ASD population than typically developing children with OCD (Ivarsson and Melin 2008), making it likely that children with ASD who receive a comorbid diagnosis of OCD will often receive the new "tic-related" specifier; however, this change is likely to be less impactful than other, previously mentioned, proposed changes.

It is likely that *DSM-5* diagnostic reclassifications and criteria changes will have an impact on diagnosis, prevalence, and comorbidity of ASD and OCD clinically and with regard to research; yet the extent of the implications cannot be determined without empirical analyses. Assessment methods and measures, already lacking in quantity and quality, may need to be altered and/or revalidated to account for these additional nuances of differential diagnosis, while maintaining diagnostic integrity (e.g., sensitivity, specificity, accurate comorbidity classification). The suggestions put forth here are speculative, and now that *DSM-5* has been released, efforts will be needed to examine the impact of the proposed changes in an empirical fashion.

Conclusions

Obsessions, compulsions, and/or repetitive behaviors are core features that commonly present in individuals with ASD and OCD. Completing an accurate differential diagnosis can prove difficult due to the similar phenotypic expressions of the symptoms. Specifically, obsessions in OCD and ASD both present with repetitive thoughts that occupy a considerable amount of time, and compulsions exhibit as repetitive behaviors within both disorders. In such cases, assessing the motivation and cognitions behind the behaviors, the purpose that they serve, and the contexts in which they manifest are valuable pieces of information that can aid in correctly attributing symptoms to their respective disorder.

Symptoms of OCD concurrently occur in up to 72 % of individuals with ASD (Muris et al. 1998), further complicating the clinical picture. Changes to the *DSM-5* can possibly result in the recategorization of individuals into different diagnoses and may change the prevalence of comorbidity between the disorders. The co-occurrence of the disorders has been associated with deleterious effects, such as increased psychosocial impairment and other psychopathology. Fortunately, emerging research indicates that OCD symptoms can be effectively treated in people with ASD. As such, the importance of accurate assessment and differential diagnosis is highlighted. While there are well-established measures for assessing OCD and ASD symptoms individually, there is a lack of instruments that have been validated for use in both populations. As such, clinicians must be conscientious of the contexts and details of phenotypically similar symptoms while utilizing the existing assessment tools. Accurate differential diagnoses are the initial steps into effective treatment planning, eventually leading to appropriately targeted interventions for the problem behaviors. Ultimately, employing prudent methods to differentiate between the disorders is essential.

References

AACAP (2012). Practice parameters for the assessment and treatment of children and adolescents with obsessive-compulsive disorder. *Journal of the American Academy of Child & Adolescent Psychiatry, 51*(1), 98–113.

American Psychiatric Association. (2013). *Diagnostic and statistical manual of mental disorders* (5th ed.). Arlington: American Psychiatric Publishing.

Amir, N., Freshman, M., Ramsey, B., Neary, E., & Brigidi, B. (2001). Thought-action fusion in individuals with OCD symptoms. *Behaviour Research and Therapy, 39*(7), 765–776.

Anholt, G. E., Cath, D. C., van Oppen, P., Eikelenboom, M., Smit, J. H., van Megen, H., & van Balkom, A. J. (2010). Autism and ADHD symptoms in patients with OCD: Are they associated with specific OC symptom dimensions or OC symptom severity? *Journal of Autism and Developmental Disorders, 40*(5), 580–589. doi:10.1007/s10803-009-0922-1.

Baron-Cohen, S. (1989). Do autistic children have obsessions and compulsions? *The British Journal of Clinical Psychology, 28*(3), 193–200.

Barrett, P. M., Healy-Farrell, L., Piacentini, J., & March, J. S. (2004). Obsessive-compulsive disorder in childhood and adolescence: Description and treatment. In P. M. Barrett & T. H. Ollendick (Eds.), *Handbook of interventions that work with children and adolescents: Prevention and treatment* (pp. 187–216). Hoboken: Wiley.

Bartz, J. A., & Hollander, E. (2006). Is obsessive-compulsive disorder an anxiety disorder? *Progress in Neuro-Psychopharmacology & Biological Psychiatry, 30,* 338–352.

Bejerot, S. (2007). An autistic dimension: A proposed subtype of obsessive-compulsive disorder. *Autism, 11*(2), 101–110. doi: 10.1177/1362361307075699.

Bishop, S. L., Richler, J., & Lord, C. (2006). Association between restricted and repetitive behaviors and nonverbal IQ in children with autism spectrum disorders. *Child Neuropsychology, 12*(4–5), 247–267. doi:10.1080/09297040600630288.

Brown-Jacobsen, A. M., Wallace, D. P., & Whiteside, S. P. (2011). Multimethod, multi-informant agreement, and positive predictive value in the identification of child anxiety disorders using the SCAS and ADIS-C. *Assessment, 18*(3), 382–392. doi:10.1177/1073191110375792.

Brown, T. A., DiNardo, P. A., & Barlow, D. H. (1994). *Anxiety disorders interview schedule for DSM-IV—Adult version.* New York: Oxford University Press.

Brown, T. A., Di Nardo, P. A., Lehman, C. L., & Campbell, L. A. (2001). Reliability of DSM-IV anxiety and mood disorders: Implications for the classification of emotional disorders. *Journal of Abnormal Psychology, 110*(1), 49–58. doi:10.1037//0021-843x.110.1.49.

Brugha, T. S., McManus, S., Bankart, J., Scott, F., Purdon, S., Smith, J., et al. (2011). Epidemiology of autism spectrum disorders in adults in the community in England. *Archives of General Psychiatry, 68*(5), 459–465. doi:10.1001/archgenpsychiatry.2011.38.

Cath, D. C., Ran, N., Smit, J. H., van Balkom, A. J., & Comijs, H. C. (2008). Symptom overlap between autism spectrum disorder, generalized social anxiety disorder and obsessive-compulsive disorder in adults: A preliminary case-controlled study. *Psychopathology, 41*(2), 101–110. doi:10.1159/000111555.

Centers for Disease Control and Prevention. (2012, Mar 30). Prevalence of autism spectrum disorders—Autism and Developmental Disabilities Monitoring Network, 14 Sites, United States, 2008. *Morbidity and mortality weekly report, surveillance summaries, 61*(3). US Department of Health and Human Services.

Cohen, L. L., La Greca, A. M., Blount, R. L., Kazak, A. E., Holmbeck, G. N., & Lemanek, K. L. (2008). Introduction to special issue: Evidence-based assessment in pediatric psychology. *Journal of Pediatric Psychology, 33*(9), 911–915. doi:10.1093/jpepsy/jsj115.

Coles, M. E., Frost, R. O., Heimberg, R. G., & Rhéaume, J. (2003). Not just right experiences: Perfectionism, obsessive-compulsive features and general psychopathology. *Behaviour Research and Therapy, 41*(6), 681–700. doi:10.1016/s0005-7967(02)00044-x.

Constantino, J. N., & Gruber, C. P. (2005). *Social Responsiveness Scale (SRS).* Los Angeles, CA: Western Psychological Services.

Coury, D. L., Anagnostou, E., Manning-Courtney, P., Reynolds, A., McCoy, R., Witaker, A., & Perrin, J. M. (2012). Use of psychotropic medication in children and adolescents with autism spectrum disorders. *Pediatrics, 130,* 69–76.

Cunningham, A. B., & Schreibman, L. (2008). Stereotypy in autism: The importance of function. *Research in Autism Spectrum Disorders, 2*(3), 469–479. doi:10.1016/j.rasd.2007.09.006.

First, M. B., Spitzer, R. L., Gibbon, M., & Williams, J. B. W. (2002). *Structured Clinical Interview for DSM-IV-TR Axis I Disorders, Patient Edition (SCID-I/P).* New York: New York State Psychiatric Institute.

Fischer-Terworth, C., & Probst, P. (2009). Obsessive-compulsive phenomena and symptoms in Asperger's disorder and high-functioning autism: An evaluative literature review. *Life Span and Disability, 12,* 5–27.

Frazier, T. W., Youngstrom, E. A., Speer, L., Embacher, R., Law, P., Constantino, J., et al. (2012). Validation of proposed DSM-5 criteria for autism spectrum disorder.

Journal of the American Academy of Child and Adolescent Psychiatry, 51(1), 28–40.e23. doi:10.1016/j.jaac.2011.09.021.

Freeman, J. B., Garcia, A. M., Coyne, L., Ale, C., Przeworski, A., Himle, M., et al. (2008). Early childhood OCD: Preliminary findings from a family-based cognitive-behavioral approach. *Journal of the American Academy of Child and Adolescent Psychiatry, 47*(5), 593–602. doi:10.1097/CHI.0b013e31816765f9.

Geller, D. A. (2006). Obsessive-compulsive and spectrum disorders in children and adolescents. *The Psychiatric Clinics of North America, 29*(2), 353–370. doi:10.1016/j.psc.2006.02.012.

Geller, D. A., Hoog, S. L., Heiligenstein, J. H., Ricardi, R. K., Tamura, R., Kluszynski, S., et al. (2001). Fluoxetine treatment for obsessive-compulsive disorder in children and adolescents: A placebo-controlled clinical trial. *Journal of the American Academy of Child and Adolescent Psychiatry, 40*(7), 773–779.

Geller, D. A., Biederman, J., Stewart, S. E., Mullin, B., Martin, A., Spencer, T., & Faraone, S. V. (2003). Which SSRI? A meta-analysis of pharmacotherapy trials in pediatric obsessive-compulsive disorder. *American Journal of Psychiatry, 160*(11), 1919–1928.

Goodman, W. K., Price, L. H., Rasmussen, S. A., Mazure, C., Delgado, P., Heninger, G. R., & Charney, D. S. (1989a). The Yale-Brown Obsessive Compulsive Scale. II. Validity. *Archives of General Psychiatry, 46*(11), 1012–1016.

Goodman, W. K., Price, L. H., Rasmussen, S. A., Mazure, C., Fleischmann, R. L., Hill, C. L., et al. (1989b). The Yale-Brown Obsessive Compulsive Scale. I. Development, use, and reliability. *Archives of General Psychiatry, 46*(11), 1006–1011.

Groden, J., Goodwin, M. S., Baron, M. G., Groden, G., Velicer, W. F., Lipsitt, L. P., et al. (2005). Assessing cardiovascular responses to stressors in individuals with autism spectrum disorders. *Focus on Autism and Other Developmental Disabilities, 20*(4), 244–252.

Helverschou, S. B., Bakken, T. L., & Martinsen, H. (2011). Psychiatric disorders in people with autism spectrum disorders: Phenomenology and recognition. In J. L. Matson & P. Sturmey (Eds.), *International handbook of autism and pervasive developmental disorders* (pp. 53–74). New York: Springer.

Irfan, U., Khalid, S., & Waqar, S. (2011). Effectiveness of psychological and pharmacological treatments for obsessive-compulsive disorder: A qualitative review. *Pakistan Journal of Pharmacology, 28*(2), 65–74.

Ivarsson, T., & Melin, K. (2008). Autism spectrum traits in children and adolescents with obsessive-compulsive disorder (OCD). *Journal of Anxiety Disorders, 22*(6), 969–978. doi:10.1016/j.janxdis.2007.10.003.

Jacob, S., Landeros-Weisenberger, A., & Leckman, J. F. (2009). Autism spectrum and obsessive-compulsive disorders: OC behaviors, phenotypes and genetics. *Autism Research, 2*(6), 293–311. doi:10.1002/aur.108.

Jakubovski, E., Pittenger, C., Torres, A. R., Fontenelle, L. F., do Rosario, M. C., Ferrao, Y. A., et al. (2011). Dimensional correlates of poor insight in obsessive-compulsive disorder. *Progress in Neuro-Psychopharmacology & Biological Psychiatry, 35*(7), 1677–1681. doi:10.1016/j.pnpbp.2011.05.012.

Joosten, A. V., Bundy, A. C., & Einfeld, S. L. (2009). Intrinsic and extrinsic motivation for stereotypic and repetitive behavior. *Journal of Autism and Developmental Disorders, 39*(3), 521–531. doi:10.1007/s10803-008-0654-7.

Joshi, G., Petty, C., Wozniak, J., Henin, A., Fried, R., Galdo, M., et al. (2010). The heavy burden of psychiatric comorbidity in youth with autism spectrum disorders: A large comparative study of a psychiatrically referred population. *Journal of Autism and Developmental Disorders, 40*(11), 1361–1370. doi:10.1007/s10803-010-0996-9.

Kessler, R. C., Chiu, W. T., Demler, O., Merikangas, K. R., & Walters, E. E. (2005). Prevalence, severity, and comorbidity of 12-month DSM-IV disorders in the National Comorbidity Survey Replication. *Archives of General Psychiatry, 62*(6), 617–627. doi:10.1001/archpsyc.62.6.617.

King, B. H., Hollander, E., Sikich, L., McCracken, J. T., Scahill, L., Bregman, J. D., et al. (2009). Lack of efficacy of citalopram in children with autism spectrum disorders and high levels of repetitive behavior: Citalopram ineffective in children with autism. *Archives of General Psychiatry, 66*(6), 583–590. doi:10.1001/archgenpsychiatry.2009.30.

Leckman, J. F., Denys, D., Simpson, H. B., Mataix-Cols, D., Hollander, E., Saxena, S., et al. (2010). Obsessive-compulsive disorder: A review of the diagnostic criteria and possible subtypes and dimensional specifiers for DSM-V. *Depression and Anxiety, 27*(6), 507–527. doi:10.1002/da.20669.

Lehmkuhl, H. D., Storch, E. A., Bodfish, J. W., & Geffken, G. R. (2008). Brief report: Exposure and response prevention for obsessive compulsive disorder in a 12-year-old with autism. *Journal of Autism and Developmental Disorders, 38*, 977–981.

Lewin, A. B., & Piacentini, J. (2009). Obsessive-compulsive disorder in children. In B. J. Sadock, V. A. Sadock & P. Ruiz (Eds.), *Kaplan & Sadock's comprehensive textbook of psychiatry* (9th ed., Vol. 2, pp. 3671–3678). Philadelphia: Lippincott Williams & Wilkins.

Lewin, A. B., Storch, E. A., Adkins, J., Murphy, T. K., & Geffken, G. R. (2005). Current directions in pediatric obsessive-compulsive disorder. *Pediatric Annals, 34*(2), 128–134.

Lewin, A. B., Wood, J. J., Gunderson, S., Murphy, T. K., & Storch, E. A. (2011). Phenomenology of comorbid autism spectrum and obsessive-compulsive disorders among children. *Journal of Developmental and Physical Disabilities, 23*(6), 543–553. doi:10.1007/s10882-011-9247-z.

Leyfer, O. T., Folstein, S. E., Bacalman, S., Davis, N. O., Dinh, E., Morgan, J., et al. (2006). Comorbid psychiatric disorders in children with autism: Interview development and rates of disorders. *Journal of Autism and Developmental Disorders, 36*(7), 849–861. doi:10.1007/s10803-006-0123-0.

Mack, H., Fullana, M. A., Russell, A. J., Mataix-Cols, D., Nakatani, E., & Heyman, I. (2010). Obsessions and compulsions in children with Asperger's syndrome or high-functioning autism: A case-control study. *Australian and New Zealand Journal of Psychiatry, 44,* 1082–1088.

Mancebo, M. C., Greenberg, B., Grant, J. E., Pinto, A., Eisen, J. L., Dyck, I., & Rasmussen, S. A. (2008). Correlates of occupational disability in a clinical sample of obsessive-compulsive disorder. *Comprehensive Psychiatry, 49*(1), 43–50. doi:10.1016/j.comppsych.2007.05.016.

March, J. S., & Mulle, K. (1998). *OCD in children and adolescents: A cognitive-behavioral treatment manual.* New York: The Guilford Press.

Masi, G., Millepiedi, S., Mucci, M., Bertini, N., Milantoni, L., & Arcangeli, F. (2005). A naturalistic study of referred children and adolescents with obsessive-compulsive disorder. *Journal of the American Academy of Child and Adolescent Psychiatry, 44*(7), 673–681. doi:10.1097/01.chi.0000161648.82775.ee.

Matson, J. L., & Boisjoli, J. A. (2008). Autism spectrum disorders in adults with intellectual disability and comorbid psychopathology: Scale development and reliability of the ASD-CA. *Research in Autism Spectrum Disorders, 2*(2), 276–287. doi:10.1016/j.rasd.2007.07.002.

Matson, J. L., & Wilkins, J. (2008). Reliability of the Autism Spectrum Disorders-Comorbid for Children (ASD-CC). *Journal of Developmental and Physical Disabilities, 20*(4), 327–336. doi:10.1007/s10882-008-9100-1.

Matson, J. L., Dempsey, T., Lovullo, S. V., & Wilkins, J. (2008). The effects of intellectual functioning on the range of core symptoms of autism spectrum disorders. *Research in Developmental Disabilities, 29*(4), 341–350. doi:10.1016/j.ridd.2007.06.006.

Matsunaga, H. (2012). Current and emerging features of obsessive-compulsive disorder: Trends for the revision of DSM-5. *Seisbin Shinkeigaku Zasshi, 114,* 1023–1030.

Mayes, S. D., Black, A., & Tierney, C. D. (2013). DSM-5 under-identifies PDDNOS: Diagnostic agreement between the DSM-5, DSM-IV, and checklist for autism spectrum disorder. *Research in Autism Spectrum Disorders, 7,* 298–306.

McDougle, C. J., Kresch, L. E., Goodman, W. K., Naylor, S. T., Volkmar, F. R., Cohen, D. J., & Price, L. H. (1995). A case-controlled study of repetitive thoughts and behavior in adults with autistic disorder and obsessive-compulsive disorder. *American Journal of Psychiatry, 152*(5), 772–777.

McGuire, J. F., Kugler, B. B., Park, J. M., Horng, B., Lewin, A. B., Murphy, T. K., & Storch, E. A. (2012). Evidence-based assessment of compulsive skin picking, chronic tic disorders and trichotillomania in children. *Child Psychiatry and Human Development, 43*(6), 855–883. doi:10.1007/s10578-012-0300-7.

Militerni, R., Bravaccio, C., Falco, C., Fico, C., & Palermo, M. T. (2002). Repetitive behaviors in autistic disorder. *European Child & Adolescent Psychiatry, 11*(5), 210–218. doi:10.1007/s00787-002-0279-x.

Moore, P. S., Mariaskin, A., March, J., & Franklin, M. E. (2007). Obsessive-compulsive disorder in children and adolescents: Diagnosis, comorbidity, and developmental factors. In E. A. Storch, G. R. Geffkin, & T. K. Murphy (Eds.), *Handbook of child and adolescent obsessive-compulsive disorder* (pp. 17–46). Mahwah: Lawrence Erlbaum.

Muris, P., Steerneman, P., Merckelbach, H., Holdrinet, I., & Meesters, C. (1998). Comorbid anxiety symptoms in children with pervasive developmental disorders. *Journal of Anxiety Disorders, 12*(4), 387–393.

O'Neill, M., & Jones, R. S. P. (1997). Sensory-perceptual abnormalities in autism: A case for more research? *Journal of Autism and Developmental Disorders, 27*(3), 283–293.

Pertusa, A., Bejerot, S., Eriksson, J., Fernandez de la Cruz, L., Bonde, S., Russell, A., & Mataix-Cols, D. (2012). Do patients with hoarding disorder have autistic traits? *Depression and Anxiety, 29*(3), 210–218. doi:10.1002/da.20902.

Piacentini, J., Bergman, R. L., Keller, M., & McCracken, J. (2003). Functional impairment in children and adolescents with obsessive-compulsive disorder. *Journal of Child and Adolescent Psychopharmacology, 13,* S61–S69. doi:10.1089/104454603322126359.

Piacentini, J., Langley, A., & Roblek, T. (2007a). *Cognitive-behavioral treatment of childhood OCD: It's only a false alarm.* New York: Oxford University Press.

Piacentini, J., Peris, T. S., Bergman, R. L., Chang, S., & Jaffer, M. (2007b). Functional impairment in childhood OCD: Development and psychometrics properties of the Child Obsessive-Compulsive Impact Scale-Revised (COIS-R). *Journal of Clinical Child and Adolescent Psychology, 36*(4), 645–653. doi:10.1080/15374410701662790.

Piacentini, J., Bergman, R. L., Chang, S., Langley, A., Peris, T. S., Wood, J. J., et al. (2011). Controlled comparison of family cognitive behavioral therapy and psychoeducation/relaxation training for child obsessive-compulsive disorder. *Journal of the American Academy of Child & Adolescent Psychiatry, 50*(11), 1149–1161.

Rahman, O., Reid, J. M., Parks, A. M., McKay, D., & Storch, E. A. (2011). Obsessive-compulsive disorder. In D. McKay & E. A. Storch (Eds.), *Handbook of child and adolescent anxiety disorders* (pp. 323–338). New York: Springer.

Reaven, J., & Hepburn, S. (2003). Cognitive-behavioral treatment of obsessive-compulsive disorder in a child with Asperger syndrome: A case report. *Autism: The International Journal of Research and Practice, 7,* 145–164.

Rudy, B. M., Lewin, A. B., & Storch, E. A. (2013). Managing anxiety comorbidity in youth with autism spectrum disorders. *Neuropsychiatry, 3*(4), 411–421. doi:10.2217/npy.13.53.

Russell, A. J., Mataix-Cols, D., Anson, M., & Murphy, D. G. (2005). Obsessions and compulsions in Asperger syndrome and high-functioning autism. *British Journal of Psychiatry, 186*, 525–528. doi:10.1192/bjp.186.6.525.

Russell, A. J., Jassi, A., Fullana, M. A., Mack, H., Johnston, K., Heyman, I., et al. (2013). Cognitive behavior therapy for comorbid obsessive-compulsive disorder in high-functioning autism spectrum disorders: A randomized controlled trial. *Depression and Anxiety, 30*(8), 697–708. doi:10.1002/da.22053.

Rydén, E., & Bejerot, S. (2008). Autism spectrum disorders in an adult psychiatric population. A naturalistic cross-sectional controlled study. *Clinical Neuropsychiatry, 5*(1), 13–21.

Scahill, L., Riddle, M. A., McSwiggin-Hardin, M., Ort, S. I., King, R. A., Goodman, W. K., et al. (1997). Children's Yale-Brown Obsessive Compulsive Scale: Reliability and validity. *Journal of the American Academy of Child & Adolescent Psychiatry, 36*(6), 9.

Scahill, L., McDougle, C. J., Williams, S. K., Dimitropoulos, A., Aman, M. G., McCracken, J. T., et al. (2006). Children's Yale-Brown Obsessive Compulsive Scale modified for pervasive developmental disorders. *Journal of the American Academy of Child and Adolescent Psychiatry, 45*(9), 1114–1123. doi:10.1097/01.chi.0000220854.79144.e7.

Silverman, W. K., & Albano, A. M. (1996). *The anxiety disorders interview schedule for DSM-IV—Child and parent versions*. San Antonio: Graywind.

South, M., Ozonoff, S., & McMahon, W. M. (2005). Repetitive behavior profiles in Asperger syndrome and high-functioning autism. *Journal of Autism and Developmental Disorders, 35*(2), 145–158. doi:10.1007/s10803-004-1992-8.

Storch, E. A., Murphy, T. K., Geffken, G. R., Soto, O., Sajid, M., Allen, P., et al. (2004). Psychometric evaluation of the Children's Yale-Brown Obsessive-Compulsive Scale. *Psychiatry Research, 129*(1), 91–98. doi:10.1016/j.psychres.2004.06.009.

Storch, E. A., Geffken, G. R., Merlo, L. J., Jacob, M. L., Murphy, T. K., Goodman, W. K., et al. (2007a). Family accommodation in pediatric obsessive-compulsive disorder. *Journal of Clinical Child and Adolescent Psychology, 36*(2), 207–216. doi:10.1080/15374410701277929.

Storch, E. A., O'Brien, K., Adkins, J., Merlo, L. J., Murphy, T. K., & Geffken, G. R. (2007b). Cognitive-behavioral treatment of pediatric obsessive-compulsive disorder. In E. A. Storch, G. R. Geffken, & T. K. Murphy (Eds.), *Handbook of child and adolescent obsessive-compulsive disorder*. Mahwah: Lawrence Erlbaum.

Storch, E. A., Abramowitz, J., & Goodman, W. K. (2008). Where does obsessive-compulsive disorder belong in DSM-V? *Depression and Anxiety, 25*(4), 336–347. doi:10.1002/da.20488.

Storch, E. A., Lehmkuhl, H. D., Ricketts, E., Geffken, G. R., Marien, W., & Murphy, T. K. (2010). An open trial of intensive family based cognitive-behavioral therapy in youth with obsessive-compulsive disorder who

are medication partial responders or nonresponders. *Journal of Clinical Child and Adolescent Psychology, 39*(2), 260–268. doi:10.1080/15374410903532676.

Storch, E. A., Caporino, N. E., Morgan, J. R., Lewin, A. B., Rojas, A., Brauer, L., et al. (2011a). Preliminary investigation of web-camera delivered cognitive-behavioral therapy for youth with obsessive-compulsive disorder. *Psychiatry Research, 189*(3), 407–412. doi:10.1016/j.psychres.2011.05.047.

Storch, E. A., Rahman, O., Park, J. M., Reid, J., Murphy, T. K., & Lewin, A. B. (2011b). Compulsive hoarding in children. *Journal of Clinical Psychology, 67*(5), 507–516. doi:10.1002/jclp.20794.

Storch, E. A., Ehrenreich May, J., Wood, J. J., Jones, A. M., De Nadai, A. S., Lewin, A. B., et al. (2012). Multiple informant agreement on the Anxiety Disorders Interview Schedule in youth with autism spectrum disorders. *Journal of Child and Adolescent Psychopharmacology, 22*(4), 292–299. doi:10.1089/cap.2011.0114.

Storch, E. A., Arnold, E. B., Lewin, A. B., Nadeau, J. M., Jones, A. M., De Nadai, A. S., et al. (2013). The effect of cognitive-behavioral therapy versus treatment as usual for anxiety in children with autism spectrum disorders: a randomized, controlled trial. *Journal of the American Academy of Child & Adolescent Psychiatry, 52*(2), 132–142.e2. doi:10.1016/j.jaac.2012.11.007.

Swedo, S. E., Rapoport, J. L., Leonard, H., Lenane, M., & Cheslow, D. (1989). Obsessive-compulsive disorder in children and adolescents. Clinical phenomenology of 70 consecutive cases. *Archives of General Psychiatry, 46*(4), 335–341.

The Pediatric OCD Treatment Study (POTS) Team (2004). Cognitive-behavior therapy, sertraline, and their combination with children and adolescents with obsessive-compulsive disorder: The Pediatric OCD Treatment Study (POTS) randomized controlled trial. *Journal of the American Medical Association, 292*(16), 1969–1976.

Turner-Brown, L. M., Lam, K. S., Holtzclaw, T. N., Dichter, G. S., & Bodfish, J. W. (2011). Phenomenology and measurement of circumscribed interests in autism spectrum disorders. *Autism: the international journal of research and practice, 15*(4), 437–456. doi:10.1177/1362361310386507.

van Steensel, F. J., Bogels, S. M., & Perrin, S. (2011). Anxiety disorders in children and adolescents with autistic spectrum disorders: A meta-analysis. *Clinical Child and Family Psychology Review, 14*(3), 302–317. doi:10.1007/s10567-011-0097-0.

Vitiello, B., & Waslick, B. (2010). Pharmacotherapy for children and adolescents with anxiety disorders. *Psychiatric Annals, 40*(4), 185–191.

White, S. W., Albano, A. M., Johnson, C. R., Kasari, C., Ollendick, T., Klin, A., et al. (2010). Development of a cognitive-behavioral intervention program to treat anxiety and social deficits in teens with high-functioning autism. *Clinical Child and Family Psychology Review, 13*(1), 77–90. doi:10.1007/s10567-009-0062-3.

Wood, J. J., & Drahota, A. (2005). *Behavioral Interventions for Anxiety in Children with Autism (BIACA)*. Los Angeles: University of California Press.

Wood, J. J., Drahota, A., Sze, K., Har, K., Chiu, A., & Langer, D. A. (2009). Cognitive-behavioral therapy for anxiety in children with autism spectrum disorders: A randomized, controlled trial. *Journal of Clinical Psychology and Psychiatry, 50*(3), 224–234.

Worley, J. A., & Matson, J. L. (2012). Comparing symptoms of autism spectrum disorders using the current DSM-IV-TR diagnostic criteria and the proposed DSM-V diagnostic criteria. *Research in Autism Spectrum Disorders, 6,* 965–970.

Wu, M. S., McGuire, J. F., Arnold, E. B., Lewin, A. B., Murphy, T. K., & Storch, E. A. (2013). Psychometric properties of the Children's Yale-Brown Obsessive Compulsive Scale in youth with autism spectrum disorders and obsessive-compulsive symptoms. *Child Psychiatry and Human Development, 45*(2), 201–211. doi:10.1007/s10578-013-0392-8.

Social Worries and Difficulties: Autism and/or Social Anxiety Disorder?

9

Susan W. White, Amie R. Schry and Nicole L. Kreiser

Social anxiety disorder (SAD) is the third most common psychiatric disorder (Beidel and Turner 2007), with 2.8% of individuals meeting diagnostic criteria in a 12-month period (Grant et al. 2005) and lifetime prevalence estimated to be between 5.0 and 12.1% among adults (Grant et al. 2005; Kessler et al. 2005). In children, estimated prevalence of SAD is 3–4% (Beidel et al. 1999), and among adolescents, prevalence is approximately 9% (Burstein et al. 2011). While epidemiologic studies tend to find higher rates of SAD in females, the distribution of males and females in treatment-seeking samples is approximately equal (Beidel and Turner 2007).

Most individuals with SAD report onset in late childhood or adolescence. The mean age of onset is between 15.1 and 16.5 years, with a median of 12.5–14 years (Grant et al. 2005; Turner et al. 1986). Furthermore, the distribution of age of onset appears to be bimodal, with peaks at younger than 5 years of age and between the ages of 13 and 15 (Grant et al. 2005; Schneier

et al. 1992), and it appears that very few people develop SAD after the early- to the mid-20s (Grant et al. 2005). Untreated SAD runs a fairly chronic course with some waxing and waning of symptoms over time (Beidel and Turner 2007). In studies, mean duration of lifetime SAD in adults is 16.3 years (Grant et al. 2005), with the mean duration of avoidance being 15.3 years and mean duration of social distress being 20.9 years (Turner et al. 1986). The duration of symptoms is likely related to the fact that most individuals with SAD delay seeking treatment; there was an average of 12 years between mean age of onset and mean age of first treatment (Grant et al. 2005).

Diagnosis

SAD is defined by a marked fear of social situations in which one might be scrutinized by others (APA 2013). Individuals with SAD may fear a number of social situations, including, but not limited to, interacting with other people, giving speeches, maintaining conversations, and even using public restrooms (for fear of evaluation or being heard/observed by others; Beidel and Turner 2007). The anxiety can also occur when a person thinks about or anticipates feared social situations, which likely leads to avoidance behaviors (Beidel and Turner 2007). In addition to the key fear, in order to meet diagnostic criteria for SAD, the social fears need to be excessive relative to any actual threat, persistent over time, and they (or the avoidance that stems from

S. W. White (✉)
Department of Psychology, Child Study Center, Virginia Tech, Blacksburg, Virginia, USA
e-mail: sww@vt.edu

A. R. Schry
Department of Psychology, Durham Veterans Affairs Medical Center, Blacksburg, VA 24060, USA

N. L. Kreiser
Department of Neuropsychology, Kennedy Krieger Institute,
707 North Broadway, Baltimore, MD 21205, USA

T. E. Davis III et al. (eds.), *Handbook of Autism and Anxiety,* Autism and Child Psychopathology Series,
DOI 10.1007/978-3-319-06796-4_9, © Springer International Publishing Switzerland 2014

the fears) need to cause significant distress or impairment in the person's life (APA 2013). Finally, the symptoms must not be due to the effects of a substance or medical condition or be better accounted by another psychiatric disorder, such as autism spectrum disorder (ASD) or panic disorder (APA 2013).

In the recently released *Diagnostic and Statistical Manual, 5th edition* (*DSM-5*; APA 2013), there are several noteworthy changes that should be highlighted when considering the co-occurrence of, and differential diagnosis between, SAD and ASD. First, the common co-occurrence of social anxiety in ASD is, for the first time in the *DSM* nosology, explicitly underscored. ASD is listed as one of the commonly occurring comorbid disorders, along with selective mutism and major depressive disorder. The criterion that the person recognizes the irrationality of their fear was removed and replaced with the requirement that a clinician consider the fears to be excessive. Of particular importance for the diagnosis of SAD in a person with ASD, it is stated, "The fear, anxiety, or avoidance is not better explained by the symptoms of another mental disorder, such as panic disorder, body dysmorphic disorder, or autism spectrum disorder" (APA 2013, p. 203), which differs from the previous criterion that stated, "If a general medical condition or another mental disorder is present, the fear in Criterion A [i.e., the fear of scrutiny] is unrelated to it" (APA 2000, p. 456). The change in this criterion is noteworthy because it better allows for the diagnosis of SAD in ASD. While social anxiety and fear of scrutiny are not included in the diagnostic criteria for ASD, they may be related to a lack of social skills which are frequently characteristic of ASD. Therefore, the previous criterion could be seen as precluding a diagnosis of SAD in individuals with ASD, but the new criterion clearly allows for the comorbid diagnosis.

Phenomenology

Most individuals with SAD report that they fear a number of social situations. In one study, the mean number of social fears endorsed was 7.0, with 93.1 % of individuals with SAD endorsing

at least three fears and over half endorsing seven or more fears (Grant et al. 2005). Common fears in adults with SAD are public speaking, informal speaking (e.g., talking to people at a party), and eating in public (Turner et al. 1986). Among adults, SAD results in significant impairment in a number of areas, including school settings (e.g., not wanting to answer questions in class or ask questions, avoidance of participating in extracurricular activities), work environments (e.g., talking to coworkers, giving presentations, sharing opinions during meetings, which can affect likelihood of being promoted), and social relationships, including romantic relationships (Turner et al. 1986). Individuals with SAD also appear to report more chronic stress in their interpersonal relationships due to negative styles of interacting with others (Davila and Beck 2002). Specifically, individuals with SAD reported being afraid of expressing strong emotions, avoiding conflict, being less assertive, being too reliant on others, and worrying about being rejected by others (Davila and Beck 2002).

Some of the situations commonly feared by children with SAD are giving an oral report or reading out loud to others, asking their teacher a question and answering questions in class, attending parties and other social events, starting and joining conversations, speaking to new people, talking to adults, and performing in public (e.g., recitals and athletic games; Beidel et al. 1999; Rao et al. 2007). While adolescents with SAD report many of the same fears as children, they are more likely to endorse fears of attending parties and other social events, working or playing with a group, asking their teacher a question, participating in gym class, walking in hallways, inviting a friend to get together, dating, eating in front of others, writing in front of others, and talking on the telephone than children with SAD (Rao et al. 2007). Cognitively, when asked to predict how well they will do while interacting with a same-age peer, both children and adolescents with SAD expected to perform worse than peers without SAD, and when asked to rate their performance retrospectively, they believed they performed worse (Alfano et al. 2006). Behaviorally, children with SAD often have no friends or at least fewer friends than peers, and they may not join clubs or groups at school (Beidel et al. 1999). They also may not like school, and some children will refuse to go to school due to their social fears (Beidel et al. 1999). Finally, the presentation can include physiological symptoms such as stomachaches and headaches (Beidel et al. 1999).

While fear of negative evaluation is typically considered the key fear in SAD, fear of positive evaluation is also related to social anxiety (Weeks et al. 2008). In one study, men high in social anxiety who received positive feedback during a social interaction task reported worries and concerns about people expecting more of them in future interactions (Wallace and Alden 1995). Therefore, while negative feedback can be difficult for individuals with SAD to receive, positive evaluation may also be difficult because it can increase anxiety about needing to interact with those individuals or perform in front of those individuals again in the future because they have "raised the bar" for themselves.

Differential Diagnosis and Comorbidity

Formal diagnosis of SAD, like ASD, is made on the basis of observed behaviors and client (or parent, in the case of children)-reported symptoms. This taxonomic rather than functional or etiological nosology is borne of necessity, as neither diagnosis is yet tied to specific biomarkers (e.g., imaging data, genetic tests) that afford sufficient sensitivity and specificity. SAD and ASD can and do occur concurrently in the same individual, but social anxiety is not a universal epiphenomenon of ASD.

Phenotypic overlap makes it challenging at times to determine which condition best explains similar or identical observed symptoms, such as social avoidance and failing to speak in social situations (APA 2013). In a sample of children with anxiety disorder diagnoses, those "with elevated ASD symptoms were significantly more likely to list social/evaluation concerns…among their top three fears" (Settipani et al. 2012, p. 463). In a nonclinical sample of young adults, ASD traits were positively related to social anxiety (White

et al. 2011). Most of the research on prevalence and presentation of anxiety symptoms in people with ASD has used high-functioning samples (i.e., high-functioning autistic spectrum disorder, HFASD), specified in the *DSM-5* (APA 2013) as "ASD without accompanying intellectual impairment." Nearly half (49 %) of adolescents with HFASD exceeded the clinical cutoff on a measure of social anxiety (Bellini 2004). In fact, SAD is, by some reports, the most common co-occurring anxiety disorder in individuals with high-functioning ASD (Kuusikko et al. 2008), with an estimated 17–22 % of individuals with ASD meeting criteria for SAD (Lugnegård et al. 2011; van Steensel et al. 2011).

As these findings demonstrate, symptom overlap can complicate differential diagnosis. While social skill deficits are at the core of ASD, they are often also present in individuals with SAD. In fact, adults with SAD but without comorbid ASD self-reported significantly more characteristics of ASD (e.g., problems with attention switching, social skill deficits) than did nonanxious controls. Moreover, with respect to social skills, they were not significantly different from a comparison group with ASD and comorbid SAD or obsessive-compulsive disorder (OCD; Cath et al. 2008). Children with SAD have been found to be less socially skilled based on their self- (Spence et al. 1999), parent (Ginsburg et al. 1998; Spence et al. 1999), and teacher reports (Erath et al. 2007), and by raters during interaction tasks (Alfano et al. 2006; Beidel et al. 1999; Spence et al. 1999). Some specific observed deficits include shorter responses (i.e., using fewer words) during an interaction task, initiating socially with peers less often, and having longer delays before beginning to speak in an interaction task (i.e., longer speech latencies; Alfano et al. 2006; Spence et al. 1999). Wenzel et al. (2005) found that socially anxious college students displayed social skill deficits when interacting with a romantic partner. Specifically, they engaged in significantly fewer positive behaviors (e.g., using feeling statements, complimenting the partner, summarizing the partner's point) during conversations with their partner and significantly more very negative behaviors (e.g., putting down the partner, blaming the partner, summarizing their own statements) when talking about a problem with their partner. Those high in social anxiety also smiled, nodded, gestured, touched their partner, started conversation, made neutral sounds indicating listening (e.g., uh-huh, yeah), and engaged in eye contact less often than their nonanxious peers. Furthermore, they engaged in more fidgeting, they spoke softer, and they "made a less positive overall impression" (Wenzel et al. 2005, p. 515) than participants low in social anxiety.

In individuals with SAD, social skill difficulties may stem from attentional processes. For example, socially anxious persons may not be fully listening to the conversation because they are instead focusing on the other person's responses to their own behavior and planning their next response (Beidel and Turner 2007). Additionally, socially anxious people tend to lack sufficient opportunity to practice social skills due to social withdrawal (Gensler 2012) and concern about negative evaluation that results in lack of assertiveness and delayed responses, owing partially to careful consideration of the anticipated reaction. The pervasiveness and temporal course of the social skill deficits can be informative. Because individuals with SAD may interact comfortably with certain familiar people (e.g., family members), their social skill deficits may present in more context-specific ways. For instance, a child might seem quite unskilled or even disinterested when in an anxiety-provoking situation, yet communicate easily and without deficit with a parent. Since social skill deficits in SAD are conceptualized as resulting partially from social avoidance, the deficits should begin after the onset of the disorder and may develop gradually over time. In contrast, social skill deficits are a core feature of ASD and will be present from early childhood in most cases (often within the first 3 years of life; White and Schry 2011).

Avoidance of social situations is another symptom that is often present in both conditions (White et al. 2012a). In individuals with SAD, this avoidance is due to fears of evaluation, while in ASD the avoidance may be due to social skill deficits that prevent an individual from knowing when and how to initiate. Furthermore, individuals with ASD may also attempt to initiate social interactions but do so in ways that are socially inappropriate (White and Schry 2011). The same patterns may be present in social responses as well. Individuals with SAD may be less responsive and less assertive (White and Schry 2011), usually due to the fear of evaluation. In contrast, those with ASD may attempt to respond socially but do so in odd or atypical ways (White and Schry 2011). Therefore, exploration of reasons for social avoidance and assessment of inappropriate, and possibly unsuccessful, attempts can help to differentiate between the two disorders.

Given the overlap in symptoms and the high rates of SAD in ASD, it is important to consider the concepts of true and false comorbidity. False, or inaccurate, comorbidity can occur in cases where disorders are categorical conceptualizations of the same underlying dimensional problem, the diagnostic criteria overlap, one disorder is simply an early presentation of the later disorder, and one disorder is better conceptualized as part of the other, primary disorder (Caron and Rutter 1991). In contrast, true comorbidity is present when two disorders have the same or overlapping risk factors, the two disorders create another meaningful condition when they are comorbid, or one disorder serves as a risk factor for the development of the other (Caron and Rutter 1991). In a study of adolescents with ASD, Renno and Wood (2013) found that anxiety symptoms were distinct and separate from ASD symptom severity. In a factor analytic study of ASD and SAD symptoms among college undergraduates, White et al. (2012a) found statistical support for true comorbidity between the two conditions.

Social Anxiety in ASD: Prevalence and Phenomenology

There are no large-scale epidemiological studies upon which to draw firm estimates of the comorbidity between SAD and ASD. However, based on community-based samples, social anxiety (both diagnosed and subthreshold or continuously presented symptoms) is present in 10.7 (Leyfer et al. 2006) to 29.2% (Simonoff et al. 2008) of adolescents with ASD. Within clinical samples of higher-functioning individuals with ASD, upwards of half of adolescents are affected by social anxiety (Kuusikko et al. 2008). SAD is more common among adolescents with ASD than it is among neurotypical (i.e., those without ASD) teens, whose lifetime prevalence is about 9% (Burstein et al. 2011). Although we need more research on true prevalence, teens with ASD may face a threefold, or higher, elevated risk of having problems with social anxiety compared to teens without ASD.

Based on multiple lines of research (e.g., psychophysiological, neuroimaging, behavioral), it is plausible that there exists a bidirectional relationship between social impairment and social anxiety in people with ASD (e.g., White et al. 2010). For example, heightened arousal in social situations and behavioral avoidance may limit opportunities to interact appropriately with peers, augment impairments in processing and interpreting social information, and make it harder to fluidly execute learned social skills (e.g., Joseph et al. 2008; Kleinhans et al. 2010), whereas social disability (especially the awareness of such a disability) appears to contribute to emergent social anxiety for some (e.g., Bellini 2006). In addition to exacerbating the core social impairment, social anxiety has been associated with secondary problems in people with ASD such as loneliness (White and Roberson-Nay 2009), aggression (Pugliese et al. 2013), and hostility (White et al. 2012b) among adolescents and adults with ASD and features of ASD.

Cognitive ability is perhaps the primary moderator for the emergence of social anxiety in people with ASD. Individuals with HFASD are particularly likely to experience this bidirectional risk process relative to people with ASD with accompanying intellectual impairment, owing to greater social motivation, along with the awareness (insight) of their social difficulties (Kuusikko et al. 2008; Sukhodolsky et al. 2008). For instance, adolescents with HFASD have been found to place as much emphasis on the importance of approval from their peers as do non-ASD peers, while simultaneously perceiving themselves as less socially competent and less approved by their peers (Williamson et al. 2008). Age is another factor that likely affects the presence of social anxiety. Problems with social anxiety appear more likely to emerge during mid- to late adolescence, when the social milieu becomes more complex and the teen's awareness of social demands and social differences come to the forefront (Bellini 2004; Kuusikko et al. 2008; White and Roberson-Nay 2009). Social motivation, or the desire to engage with others for purely social reasons, is yet another viable moderator for the experience of social anxiety. Although some individuals with ASD lack interest in socialization (amotivation; Koegel and Mentis 1985) and do not find social stimuli in the environment important or salient (Klin et al. 2003), it is clear that many people with ASD are quite interested in having social relationships. Although interventionists have begun to explore approaches to increase social motivation in people with ASD, at this time we lack sensitive measures or precise biomarkers of social motivation and interest (Lerner et al. 2012).

Theoretical Considerations

Emergence of social anxiety among people on the autism spectrum can be thought of as representing the developmental psychopathology construct of equifinality, in which a range of processes can result in the same outcome. It is likely that multiple processes, including structural and functional neurological anomalies (e.g., Amaral et al. 2003), shared genetic vulnerabilities (e.g., Piven and Palmer 1999), and psychosocial factors (e.g., Attwood 2007), all play a role in the emergence of social anxiety in people with ASD. We do not have a single, unifying, or empirically grounded theoretical explanation for the high rate of co-occurrence. As such, we review research related to social learning, motivational, developmental, and cognitive factors that may be involved.

A host of experiential and cognitive processes may interact to produce social anxiety in young people with ASD. Especially among older children and adolescents with ASD, a history of rejection and social failures could contribute to the experience of social anxiety (Bellini 2006; Harnum et al. 2007; Shtayermman 2007; Swaim and Morgan 2001). Improved insight into one's own social impairment and differences could also play a role (Kuusikko et al. 2008). The young person recognizes, quite accurately, that attempts to engage with peers are awkward, unskilled, and seen as such by peers. Additional processes, such as a biologically based propensity to experience anxiety (i.e., evidence of greater physiological arousal and metabolic preparedness—stress responses—during social interactions) and age-related increases in motivation to interact socially with peers (Corbett et al. 2010), must also be considered.

There is evidence that social stress and anxiety become more salient during late childhood and adolescence for youth with ASD. In studies on cortisol responsivity during playground interactions with unfamiliar peers, older (though still prepubertal) children with ASD exhibited elevated cortisol levels, indicating that they found even relatively benign social situations more stressful than did peers without ASD (Corbett et al. 2010). Moreover, the older children with ASD were interacting socially more with peers, and avoiding less, compared to younger children with ASD (Corbett et al. 2010). Although neurotypical children, similar to those with ASD, exhibit increased cortisol response upon initial exposure to a social stressor, the stress response of children with ASD tends to be more prolonged (Corbett et al. 2012). Corbett et al. (2012) proposed that, with age, young people with ASD become more motivated to approach others socially, despite their felt biobehavioral stress.

Common triggers for anxiety (not just social anxiety) in children with ASD are changes in routine and social situations. Within the social domain, frequently reported situations that exacerbate anxiety include when one is the center of attention and fears ridicule (Ozsivadjian et al. 2012). Likewise, the unpredictability of the social world likely engenders a fair amount of apprehension and worry about social interactions for people on the spectrum. Similarly, deficient Theory of Mind (ToM) may contribute to social avoidance if, for instance, the young person with

ASD finds other people's behavior confusing and thereby frightening (Baron-Cohen 2008).

Deficits in ToM are commonly reported among children, adolescents, and adults with ASD (Baron-Cohen 1995). ToM deficits are typically expressed as an inability to infer others' points of view and accurately interpret the behavioral intentions of others (Baron-Cohen 1995). It is largely assumed that ToM, and some appreciation for the fact that the internal states of others may differ from one's own, is a precursor for the existence of true social anxiety given the necessity of awareness of others' perceptions for the fear of negative evaluation (as reviewed in Kerns and Kendall 2012). As such, it seems implausible that social anxiety could conceivably arise in a person with severe ToM deficits. On the other hand, it is entirely plausible that difficulty navigating and inferring others' thoughts, feelings, and intentions could engender considerable social distress. In essence, the social world becomes an unpredictable, likely frightening, place and social anxiety develops.

There is a growing scientific literature indicating the existence of atypicalities in how individuals with ASD perceive and process environmental stimuli. Most of this research has focused on social stimuli, which is understandable given that the primary deficit in social interaction defines ASD. Historically, the social disability in ASD has been presumed to be due to indifference or lack of social motivation. In ASD, decreased attending to social cues, and others' eye gaze in particular, is believed to stem from lack of appreciation for the social significance of eye gaze (e.g., Klin et al. 2003), such that social stimuli (e.g., human faces) are not highly and inherently salient, as they are for neurotypical people (e.g., Baron-Cohen 1995). In SAD, in contrast, decreased eye gaze is believed to be more intentional, an aversion to something that is highly socially meaningful albeit anxiety provoking (e.g., Garner et al. 2006).

Emerging evidence from neuroimaging, psychophysiological, and behavioral studies suggests that social disability, in at least a subset of people with ASD, is in fact associated with heightened arousal and intentional avoidance of social stimuli (Dalton et al. 2007; Joseph et al.

2008). Heightened arousal, especially in response to social-emotional information (e.g., Joseph et al. 2008), may impede accurate interpretation of social cues and appropriate responses to others. Recent studies assessing gaze patterns, neural circuitry, and autonomic arousal indicate that, for some adolescents with ASD, aversion and heightened emotional reactivity, both of which are core components of social anxiety, may contribute to the observed lack of attending to others' eye gaze and facial features (e.g., Dalton et al. 2007; Joseph et al. 2008).

On average, people with ASD exhibit a greater negative affect compared to peers without ASD (Schwartz et al. 2009). In addition, children with ASD have been found to display atypical autonomic responses to (nonsocial) anxiety-provoking situations, indicative of sympathetic overarousal and parasympathetic under-arousal, compared to peers without ASD (Kushki et al. 2013). Weaknesses in executive functioning, including inhibitory control and cognitive and behavioral flexibility, among people with ASD are also reported (e.g., D'Cruz et al. 2013). Finally, impoverished emotion regulation, or the ability to intentionally or automatically modify one's own emotional state in the service of goal-directed behavior, may be intrinsic to ASD (Mazefksy et al. 2013). It is plausible, then, that social disability, problems with fairly chronic overarousal and overstimulation, high negative affect, and difficulty managing one's emotional responses when stressed jointly explain the ontology of social anxiety among people on the spectrum. In summary, social anxiety may be conceptualized as multiply determined—a function of social motivation, severe social disability, and a tendency to experience social situations as overarousing and distressing. These theoretical mechanisms are examined through a clinical lens in the next section.

Clinical Considerations

Appreciation of the bidirectional relationship between social anxiety and ASD is imperative in the assessment and successful treatment of individuals with ASD and co-occurring SAD. Individuals with ASD who also have SAD may not always report feeling anxious in social situations (White and Schry 2011). Many individuals with SAD experience physiological symptoms of anxiety, in some cases resulting in panic attacks, when in feared situations (APA 2013). Physiological symptoms may be helpful in identifying SAD in individuals with ASD. For example, Bellini (2006) found that physical symptoms of anxiety were positively related to social anxiety in adolescents with ASD. While this finding was interpreted as suggesting physical symptoms were a risk factor of SAD in ASD, since data were cross-sectional, it could simply indicate that SAD tends to manifest physically in this population. Individuals with ASD may also show behavioral responses, such as temper tantrums, misbehaving, or engaging in more restricted, repetitive, or stereotyped behaviors, in response to social anxiety (White and Schry 2011).

Additionally, fear of negative evaluation and rejection in social situations may lead to increased repetitive, stereotyped, or rigid behaviors or behavioral problems, such as tantrums and noncompliance, for individuals with ASD (Wood and Gadow 2010). For instance, a person with ASD and social anxiety, in anxiety-provoking social situations, may begin to engage in increased self-stimulatory behavior (e.g., hand flapping) or may exhibit a heightened focus on his or her restricted interests (e.g., increased monologue speech related to interest, fixation on object of interest). Alternatively, a child or adolescent with ASD, when experiencing anxiety in a social situation, may have a "melt down" or tantrum (e.g., exhibit yelling or crying) or flee the situation in escape (e.g., run away or hide). It is important for clinicians to be aware that an increase in severity of such behaviors, often characteristic of or associated with an ASD, may be related to anxiety.

The impact of individual differences among people with ASD on the presentation and quality of social anxiety is also an important clinical consideration, given the heterogeneity inherent in ASD. It is our clinical experience that some individuals with ASD are hyperaware of the reactions from others. Due to the nature of their social and communication deficits (i.e., deficits in interpreting nonverbal cues, literal interpretation of language), they may inaccurately interpret ambiguous social information as threatening. In this case, the ASD directly increases risk of SAD. In contrast, other individuals with ASD, perhaps those with greater deficits in ToM and with less insight into others' perceptions, may exhibit a general fear of uncertainty of social situations (e.g., "I'm nervous because I don't know what to expect or what will happen when I interact with others") but without specific concerns of the evaluation of others. Still others may perceive social feedback and fear rejection in a very reality-based, almost probabilistic, way given the nature of their social deficits. They may also worry about possible consequences (e.g., bullying and victimization) but have limited insight into the reasons for others' negative evaluations of them (i.e., how their own social behaviors play a role).

Another individual difference of clinical consideration is the degree of insight into one's own emotions, thoughts, and internal states (Berthoz and Hill 2005; Lainhart and Folstein 1994). Poor insight is frequently observed in individuals with ASD. Some individuals with ASD may be unable to recognize and identify their own anxiety spontaneously or when explicitly asked, leading to clinical difficulties in understanding and teasing apart an individual's symptom presentation in understanding whether deficits or potential indicators of anxiety are accounted for by deficits inherent in ASD, more global physiological arousal and anxiety in response to environmental stimuli, or fear of negative evaluation characteristic of social anxiety. Anecdotally, some individuals with ASD might report vague "bad feelings" in social situations ("I don't like it," "I feel bad"), describe physiological arousal (e.g., heart pounding, upset stomach, headache, muscle tension), or describe patterns of avoidance of certain social situations instead of reporting symptoms indicative of the cognitive or emotional components of social anxiety.

Finally, differences in social motivation are an important consideration. In order for social anxiety to be present, it is assumed that an individual must have some level of motivation or desire to interact with others or to develop social relationships. However, by definition some individuals with ASD lack social reciprocity and lack spontaneous seeking to share enjoyment, interests, or achievement with others (APA 2013). Diagnostically, the most extreme manifestation of deficient social interaction can be thought of as complete absence of interest in peers (APA 2013). Because of the great heterogeneity in symptom presentation, it is important for clinicians to be mindful that while some individuals with ASD lack desire to interact with others, some do indeed exhibit great social motivation and a desire for friendships, and these people struggle with loneliness and isolation (e.g., Locke et al. 2010; White and Roberson-Nay 2009). Clinical observations and anecdotal evidence would also suggest that a subset of people with ASD, through repeated experiences of peer rejection, may present with denial of social interest and lack of desire to develop friendships, although such individuals may have previously exhibited social motivation (e.g., Attwood 2007).

The case of "Dan," a 15-year-old male, is illustrative of clinical considerations such as the unique manifestation of social anxiety in individuals with ASD. Dan, diagnosed with ASD several years prior, presented for treatment due to increasing problems with peer victimization and bullying, tantrums, and "meltdowns" occurring in school and increasing social withdrawal and loneliness. Although Dan experienced some bullying and peer rejection in prior grades, more recently his mother noticed that some of the children with whom he used to socialize outside of school had stopped inviting him out. His mother also reported that Dan had begun having tantrums before going to scouts meetings, crying and saying he did not want to go, and refusing to attend school activity nights, both of which he used to enjoy in prior grades. She reported that he frequently complained he was lonely and bored. Per his teacher's report, Dan rarely interacted with the other students in his class and was at times "picked on" by other kids due to some of his oddities. His teacher said that Dan frequently played with Legos during breaks and often engaged in monologues about his interest in several cartoons, leading some of his peers to laugh at him. His teacher also noted that, on several occasions, Dan became upset when interacting with other students during free time and had "meltdowns" in which he ran out of the classroom and cried. Based upon his self-report, Dan indicated that he did not like interacting with other students in his classroom because they were mean, and he said he felt bad when talking with other kids or going to boy scouts or school activity nights. He did not present obvious fears of negative evaluation or of embarrassment; but when the therapist asked him follow-up questions regarding what he did not like and what he thought might happen in social situations, he indicated he thought the other students might think he was stupid or would tease him. He indicated that he no longer wanted friends, and that the other kids in his class are "stupid."

Dan's case is illustrative of the bidirectional relationship between social deficits and social anxiety; Dan's social difficulties and immaturity presumably led to negative interactions and rejection from peers, and his awareness of such negative reactions from others exacerbated his deficits and led to increased social avoidance. Though Dan had difficulty articulating a fear of negative evaluation, he described general bad feelings and avoidance of social situations, with some concern of others making fun of him, evidencing that he has some awareness of other's perspectives. He exhibited several symptoms of anxiety in social situations, which were less typical of a traditional social anxiety presentation, including increased intensity of focus on his interests and monologue speech and, at times, acting-out behavior. Though Dan presented with some hostility to his peers, it was apparent from his history and his mother's report that he was avoiding social activities and interactions that he used to enjoy, which is perhaps evidence of avoidance due to anxiety in the presence of some social motivation.

Assessment Recommendations

Despite overlap in diagnostic criteria between social anxiety and ASD and the frequency with which social anxiety occurs in adolescents and adults with ASD, there is limited empirical guidance on how to best assess symptoms of social anxiety in people with ASD. Questionable reliability and validity of currently utilized measures to assess anxiety in individuals with ASD and the need for the development of measures that assess the unique and distinct features of anxiety as manifested in individuals with ASD (Grondhuis and Aman 2012; Ollendick and White 2012; van Steensel et al. 2011) further complicates the assessment of anxiety in this population. In this section, we review the extant research on clinical assessment of social anxiety within ASD. Because of the dearth of research in this area on adults with ASD, we focus our review on the assessment of children and adolescents.

One of the greatest challenges is distinguishing whether some symptoms (e.g., behavioral avoidance) are better accounted for by ASD or are indicative of co-occurring social anxiety. In determining how best to conceptualize a given symptom or behavior, it is important to consider the individual's social motivation, ToM capabilities, the nature of social fear, the reality-based nature of the fear, and the time course of symptoms.

Questions a clinician may ask her or himself in making this distinction include:

- Does this individual have an awareness of others' social perceptions, whether accurate or not?
- Does this individual exhibit motivation/desire to interact socially or have friends?
- Does this individual avoid social interactions due to lack of interest in social interaction or due to anxiety in social situations?
- Does this individual experience anxiety in social situations due to fear of negative evaluation or embarrassment or due to some other element toward of social situations (e.g., overarousal, environmental stimulation)?
- Is this individual's fear reality based and due to imminent threat in the environment (i.e., severe and repeated bullying)?
- Do symptoms represent a change from prior functioning or are they more reflective of chronic and pervasive social deficits related to ASD?

When there is evidence of social motivation, the avoidance seems to be due to aspects of social evaluation/social consequences, and there is evidence of a change in symptom presentation with onset of anxiety, a diagnosis of SAD should be considered. Note, however, that the young person might not be able to report accurately on mechanisms underlying social avoidance and cognitive aspects (e.g., fear of negative evaluation) involved.

A challenge inherent in the assessment of anxiety in individuals with ASD is the questionable ability of individuals with ASD to accurately self-report symptoms due to aforementioned deficits and impairments in insight, emotional awareness (alexithymia), and ability to report on their own and others' thoughts. The utilization of multi-method and multi-informant assessment with this population is strongly suggested (e.g., Kerns and Kendall 2012; Kreiser and White 2014; Mazefsky et al. 2011). Given preliminary evidence suggesting underreporting of co-occurring anxiety disorders among children with ASD (Mazefsky et al. 2011), the use of both self and parent or other report is recommended in conjunction with a semi-structured clinical interview. In our experience, the adaptation of semi-structured interviews may be necessary due to deficits inherent in ASD. Interviews such as the Anxiety Disorders Interview Schedule, Child and Parent Versions (ADIS-C/P; Silverman and Albano 1996) may be administered jointly with both parent and child together to assist with difficulties the individual with ASD may have in reporting, while still obtaining valuable information from multiple perspectives.

The most commonly utilized measures to assess social anxiety among children and adolescents with ASD are self-report questionnaires designed for typically developing child and adolescent populations. Broad multidimensional screening measures of anxiety that contain social anxiety subscales, including the Multidimensional Anxiety Scale for Children (MASC; March 1998), the Self-Report for Childhood Anxiety Related Emotional Disorders (SCARED; Birmaher et al. 1997), and the Spence Children's Anxiety Scale (SCAS; Nauta et al. 2004), and

several self-report measures of social anxiety including the Social Anxiety Scale for Adolescents (SAS-A; La Greca and Lopez 1998), Social Anxiety Scale for Children—Revised (SASC-R; La Greca and Stone 1993), and the Social Worries Questionnaire (SWQ; Spence 1995) have been frequently utilized with this population. Many studies have utilized a combination of parent- and self-report versions of these measures (Kreiser and White 2014). To date, the majority of self-report measures have been administered in their original form, with two exceptions: Kuusikko et al. (2008) removed several items deemed to have overlap with symptoms of ASD in the SAS-A and SASC-R, and there is one measure, the Social Anxiety Scale for People with ASD (SASPA), specifically designed to assess social anxiety as it presents in individuals with ASD without conflation owing to ASD symptoms (Kreiser and White 2011). Original versions of semi-structured interviews, designed for typically functioning populations, including the ADIS-C/P, have also been used to assess for social anxiety in this population, most commonly administered exclusively to parents, or with both parent and child (Kreiser and White 2014). Additionally, one interview, the Kiddie Schedule for Affective Disorders and Schizophrenia for School-Age Children—Present and Lifetime version (K-SADS-PL; Ambrosini 2000), has been modified in order to assist in distinguishing impairment associated with ASD symptoms and impairment associated with anxiety symptoms (Kimel 2009) and one semi-structured interview, the Autism Comorbidity Interview—Present and Lifetime Version (ACI-PL: Leyfer et al. 2006), has been specifically developed for use with individuals with ASD to assess for comorbid diagnoses.

Across studies, almost without exception, measures used to assess social anxiety in ASD have demonstrated acceptable-to-excellent internal consistency; however, limited data on the sensitivity and validity of such measures exist, aside from evidence of strong concordance among different measures of social anxiety, and evidence of moderate-to-strong relationships with other theoretically related constructs (e.g., social deficits, loneliness, restrictive interests, and repetitive behaviors; as reviewed in Kreiser and White 2014). Self-report measures may lack sensitivity in identifying adolescents with ASD and diagnosed SAD (Kreiser 2011). Further, given that the majority of measures utilized with this population have been designed, standardized, and validated with typically functioning populations, the degree to which the measures accurately assess social anxiety as manifested in individuals with ASD is questionable. Some of the items in existing measures may have overlap with symptoms of ASD, leading to conflation on scores, and many of the most commonly utilized measures (i.e., MASC, SCAS, SCARED) only contain items that assess cognitive and emotional components of social anxiety but do not contain items indicative of behavioral avoidance and physiological symptoms (Kreiser and White 2014). The limitations in existing measures underscore the importance of clinicians' awareness of aforementioned clinical considerations with this population and the utilization of a multi-method, multi-informant approach as the field awaits further psychometric evaluation of existing measures and the development and validation of newly designed measures.

Treatment Recommendations

Several cognitive behavioral therapy (CBT) treatments have been specifically developed and modified for children and adolescents with ASD with co-occurring anxiety with promising outcome data (e.g., Reaven et al. 2009; White et al. 2013; Wood et al. 2009); however, at present there has been no treatment-outcome research targeting social anxiety. There have been no treatments developed for social anxiety, or anxiety broadly, in adults with ASD. It is the general consensus among clinicians and researchers that modification of traditional CBT is necessary given some of the unique concerns and deficits in this population. Common CBT modifications include increased structure in session (i.e., utilization of written agenda) to avoid distress with unanticipated changes or novelty, increased fre-

quency of exposures and practice, increased parental involvement to aid in homework compliance and generalization, and increased utilization of visual aids when introducing abstract concepts (e.g., using pictures of bodies to introduce subjective feelings of anxiety; e.g., Lang et al. 2010; White et al. 2010). One goal shared by the available treatment programs is to increase awareness of anxiety, given that many individuals with ASD exhibit difficulties with insight, emotion and thought recognition, and emotion regulation. Because of such difficulties, many individuals with ASD may only recognize more extreme behavioral indicators of anxiety. Explicit instructions related to physiological, emotional, and cognitive (i.e., anxious thoughts) indicators of anxiety and the utilization of visual aids such as anxiety thermometers and cartoons may assist in this regard.

The incorporation of strategies to increase social competence and address problems with loneliness and bullying may be necessary to address in the treatment of social anxiety in adolescents, given the bidirectional and mutually exacerbating relationship between these factors and social anxiety in this population. Concurrent instruction in developmentally appropriate social skills (i.e., psychoeducation, modeling, practice, feedback) may help to reduce social anxiety and loneliness, given the reality-based nature of social fears for many adolescents and adults with ASD. Further, specific coping strategies and skills to handle bullying may be beneficial, particularly in adolescence.

Strong parental (or significant other) involvement in treatment may assist with generalization of skills to real life situations. For instance, parents are provided psychoeducation related to skills the adolescent learns in the individual therapy sessions and are expected to remind their child to use the skills between sessions in the Multimodal Anxiety and Social Skills Intervention, a treatment designed for adolescents with ASD and anxiety disorders (White et al. 2013). Additionally, parental reinforcement of anxiety and issues with overprotection may be important to discuss, as such factors can interfere with treatment compliance and response.

DSM-5: Implications and Thoughts on Changes to ASD and SAD Diagnoses

There is more scientific recognition and clinical appreciation for the possibility of co-occurrence of social anxiety in a person with diagnosed ASD. A *PsycINFO* search (July 16, 2013) using the keywords of "autism" and "social anxiety" yields only 27 peer-reviewed articles; half of these articles, however, were published in just the past 3 years. This zeitgeist is also reflected in changes to the *DSM-5*. In the text description for SAD, ASD is now listed as one of the common comorbid conditions and it is stated that anxiety is common in those with ASD diagnoses. The changes seen in *DSM-5*, notably that the criterion of recognition of the irrationality of one's social fears has been removed and that it is made explicit that people with ASD can and often do have social anxiety, will likely result in increased identification of social anxiety in people with ASD, and dual diagnosis of SAD and ASD.

As such, the importance of determining how to most sensitively assess for social anxiety in individuals (children as well as adults) with ASD cannot be overstated. There is considerable risk of "double-counting" symptoms (e.g., social avoidance, poor eye contact, few friends) to derive diagnoses of both SAD and ASD. To clarify the construct of social anxiety as it manifests in people with ASD, novel assessment approaches as well as clinical criteria should be explored. Measures of psychophysiological reactivity (e.g., heart rate and heart rate variability) or attention (e.g., reaction time tasks and eye gaze tracking), for instance, might augment more traditional indices of social anxiety such as interviews and questionnaires. Understanding the individual's ability to hypothesize about others' thoughts and feelings (theory of mind) and his or her social motivation or need for connectedness may also be useful clinically. We also need to consider intraindividual developmental factors and societal changes in evaluating social anxiety in ASD. In adolescence, for example, there is a heightened focus on social relationships and the feedback of peers. The *DSM-5* emphasizes that ASD can in-

deed be diagnosed later in life, rather than only in early childhood, and the usual age of onset of SAD is mid-adolescence. When assessing and treating adolescent clients presenting with social concerns, it is especially important to consider the history of social concerns (i.e., were deficits present prior to adolescence?) and the presence (or absence) of restricted, repetitive patterns of behavior or interests, as deficits in social communication and interaction alone are not sufficient for the ASD diagnosis. Finally, in the USA, like most other developed countries, we are simultaneously more connected to each other (via instant messaging, texting, and other forms of social media) and yet more disconnected than we have ever been. Young people meet each other and socialize electronically, perhaps more so than in person. The possible societal and clinical ramifications of these changes have yet to be empirically examined. Anecdotally, however, we have seen countless clinical examples of adolescents and young adults with extensive virtual relationships, but nonexistent human socialization.

Conclusions

In conclusion, we suggest that social anxiety is *not* simply epiphenomena associated with above and beyond core ASD symptoms; it is important that social anxiety be recognized as a separable clinical construct and treated as such and that it not be overlooked due to diagnostic overshadowing (cf. Mason and Scior 2004). It is abundantly clear that not everyone with ASD struggles with social anxiety; herein, there is both a scientific challenge and a potential opportunity to better understand the phenotypic diversity of ASD.

Clinical scientists must determine who is more susceptible to experiencing social anxiety, by exploring moderators such as age, verbal ability, and level of insight. We must also develop evidence-based tools with which to assess social anxiety in this clinical population. Social anxiety can be statistically separated from ASD symptom severity (White et al. 2012a), but ability to distinguish social anxiety, distinct from other anxiety constructs, is less clear (Renno and Wood 2013).

Additionally, within the specific anxiety disorders, social anxiety appears to be the hardest to identify clinically, and there is little agreement among raters (Renno and Wood 2013; White et al. 2012c).

Anxiety often amplifies the social impairment that is fundamental to ASD (e.g., Kleinhans et al. 2010; Wood and Gadow 2010). We propose that the presence or absence of social anxiety might be useful clinically and scientifically, as a way to parse phenotypic heterogeneity in ASD. Social anxiety must be considered in its typical form (i.e., as it manifests among people without ASD) as well as in atypical, perhaps ASD-specific, forms (e.g., fears of negative evaluation that are fairly reality-based and inability to report on specific emotions related to social fears; see Kerns and Kendall 2012, for review). Put another way, presence or absence of social anxiety, in the face of the profound social deficits that define ASD, could be both clinically informative and scientifically useful for the study of related constructs (e.g., underlying differences in cognitive processes and social motivation). There may be something both etiologically and phenomenologically unique about people with ASD and social anxiety and those with ASD without social anxiety. Moreover, its presence likely moderates treatment effects and should, therefore, be considered in treatment planning. Left untreated, social anxiety may diminish the potential benefit of interventions that target social skill deficits in isolation and contribute to the emergence of other problem behaviors (e.g., avoidance of school, poor school performance, inattention).

References

Alfano, C. A., Beidel, D. C., & Turner, S. M. (2006). Cognitive correlates of social phobia among children and adolescents. *Journal of Abnormal Child Psychology, 34*, 189–201. doi:10.1007/s10802-005-9012-9.

Amaral, D. G., Bauman, M. D., & Schumann, C. M. (2003). The amygdale and autism: Implications from non-human primate studies. *Genes, Brain, and Behavior, 2*, 295–302. doi:10.1034/j.1601-183X.2003.00043.x.

Ambrosini, P. J. (2000). Historical development and present status of the schedule for affective disorders and schizophrenia for School-Age Children (K-SADS). *Journal of the American Academy of Child and Adolescent Psychiatry, 39*, 49–58. doi:10.1097/00004583-200001000-00016.

APA (American Psychiatric Association). (2000). Diagnostic and statistical manual of mental disorders (4th ed.). (Text Revision). Washington, DC: American Psychiatric Association.

APA (American Psychiatric Association). (2013). *Diagnostic and statistical manual of mental disorders* (5th ed.). Washington, DC: American Psychiatric Association.

Attwood, T. (2007). *The complete guide to Asperger's syndrome*. London: Jessica Kingsley.

Baron-Cohen, S. (1995). Mindblindness: An essay on autism and theory of mind. In L. Gleitman, S. Carey, E. Newport, & E. Spelke (Eds.), *Learning, development, and conceptual change*. Cambridge, MA: MIT.

Baron-Cohen, S. (2008). Theories of the autistic mind. *The Psychologist, 21*(2), 112–116.

Beidel, D. C., & Turner, S. M. (2007). *Shy children, phobic adults: Nature and treatment of social anxiety disorder* (2nd ed.). Washington, DC: American Psychological Association.

Beidel, D. C., Turner, S. M., & Morris, T. L. (1999). Psychopathology of childhood social phobia. *Journal of the American Academy of Child & Adolescent Psychiatry, 38*, 643–650. doi:10.1097/00004583-199906000-00010.

Bellini, S. (2004). Social skill deficits and anxiety in high-functioning adolescents with autism spectrum disorders. *Focus on Autism and Other Developmental Disabilities, 19*(2), 78–86. doi:10.1177/10883576040190020201.

Bellini, S. (2006). The development of social anxiety in adolescents with autism spectrum disorders. *Focus on Autism and Other Developmental Disabilities, 21*(3), 138–145. doi:10.1177/10883576060210030201.

Berthoz, S., & Hill, E. L. (2005). The validity of using self-reports to assess emotion regulation abilities in adults with autism spectrum disorder. *European Psychiatry, 20*, 291–298. doi:10.1016/j.eurpsy.2004.06.013.

Birmaher, B., Khetarpal, S., Brent, D., Cully, M., Balach, L., Kaufman, J., & Neer, S. M. (1997). The Screen for Child Anxiety and Related Emotional Disorders (SCARED): Scale construction and psychometric characteristics. *Journal of the American Academy of Child and Adolescent Psychiatry, 36*, 545–553. doi:10.1097/00004583-199704000-00018.

Burstein, M., He, J.-P., Kattan, G., Albano, A. M., Avenevoli, S., & Merikangas, K. R. (2011). Social phobia and subtypes in the national comorbidity survey-adolescent supplement: Prevalence, correlates, and comorbidity. *Journal of the American Academy of Child & Adolescent Psychiatry, 50*, 870–880. doi:10.1016/j.jaac.2011.06.005.

Caron, C., & Rutter, M. (1991). Comorbidity in child psychopathology: Concepts, issues and research strategies. *Journal of Child Psychology and Psychiatry, 32*, 1063–1080. doi:10.1111/j.1469-7610.1991.tb00350.x.

Cath, D. C., Ran, N., Smit, J. H., van Balkom, A. J. L. M., & Comijs, H. C. (2008). Symptom overlap between autism spectrum disorder, generalized social anxiety disorder and obsessive-compulsive disorder in adults: A preliminary case-controlled study. *Psychophathology, 41*, 101–110. doi:10.1159/000111555.

Corbett, B. A., Schupp, C. W., Simon, D., Ryan, N., & Mendoza, S. (2010). Elevated cortisol during play is associated with age and social engagement in children with autism. *Molecular Autism, 1*(13). doi:10.1186/2040-2392-1-13.

Corbett, B. A., Schupp, C. W., & Lanni, K. E. (2012). Comparing biobehavioral profiles across two social stress paradigms in children with and without autism spectrum disorders. *Molecular Autism, 3*, 13. doi:10.1186/2040-2392-3-13.

D'Cruz, A.-M., Ragozzino, M. E., Mosconi, M. W., Shrestha, S., Cook, E. H., & Sweeney, J. A. (2013). Reduced behavioral flexibility in autism spectrum disorders. *Neuropsychology, 27*, 152–160. doi:10.1037/a0031721.

Dalton, K. M., Nacewicz, B. M., Alexander, A. L., & Davidson, R. J. (2007). Gaze-fixation, brain activation, and amygdala volume in unaffected siblings of individuals with autism. *Biological Psychiatry, 61*, 512–520. doi:10.1016/j.biopsych.2006.05.019.

Davila, J., & Beck, J. G. (2002). Is social anxiety associated with impairment in close relationships? A preliminary investigation. *Behavior Therapy, 33*, 427–446. doi:10.1016/s0005-7894(02)80037-5.

Erath, S. A., Flanagan, K. S., & Bierman, K. L. (2007). Social anxiety and peer relations in early adolescence: Behavioral and cognitive factors. *Journal of Abnormal Child Psychology, 35*, 405–416. doi:10.1007/s10802-007-9099-2.

Garner, M., Mogg, K., & Bradley, B. P. (2006). Orienting and maintenance of gaze to facial expressions in social anxiety. *Journal of Abnormal Psychology, 115*, 760–770. doi:10.1037/0021-843X.115.4.760.

Gensler, D. (2012). Autism spectrum disorder in DSM-V: Differential diagnosis and boundary conditions. *Journal of Infant, Child & Adolescent Psychotherapy, 11*(2), 86–95. doi:10.1080/15289168.2012.676339.

Ginsburg, G. S., La Greca, A. M., & Silverman, W. K. (1998). Social anxiety in children with anxiety disorders: Relation with social and emotional functioning. *Journal of Abnormal Child Psychology, 26*(3), 175–185. doi:10.1023/a:1022668101048.

Grant, B. F., Hasin, D. S., Blanco, C., Stinson, F. S., Chou, S. P., Goldstein, R. B., … Huang, B. (2005). The epidemiology of social anxiety disorder in the United States: Results from the National Epidemiologic Survey on Alcohol and Related Conditions. *Journal of Clinical Psychiatry, 66*, 1351–1361. doi:10.4088/JCP.v66n1102.

Grondhuis, S. N., & Aman, M. G. (2012). Assessment of anxiety in children and adolescents with autism spectrum disorders. *Research in Autism Spectrum Disorders, 6*, 1345–1365. doi:10.1016/j.rasd.2012.04.006.

Harnum, M., Duffy, J., & Ferguson, D. A. (2007). Adults' versus children's perceptions of a child with autism or attention deficit hyperactivity disorder. *Journal of Autism and Developmental Disorders, 37*, 1337–1343. doi:10.1007/s10803-006-0273-0.

Joseph, R. M., Ehrman, K., McNally, R., & Keehn, B. (2008). Affective response to eye contact and face recognition ability in children with ASD. *Journal of the International Neuropsychological Society, 14*, 947–955. doi:10.1017/S1355617708081344.

Kerns, C. M., & Kendall, P. C. (2012). The presentation and classification of anxiety in autism spectrum disorder. *Clinical Psychology: Science and Practice, 19*, 323–347. doi:10.1111/cpsp.12009.

Kessler, R. C., Berglund, P., Demler, O., Jin, R., Merikangas, K. R., & Walters, E. E. (2005). Lifetime prevalence and age-of-onset distributions of DSM-IV disorders in the National Comorbidity Survey Replication. *Archives of General Psychiatry, 62*(6), 593–602. doi:10.1001/archpsyc.62.6.593.

Kimel, L. K. (2009). Phenomenology of anxiety and fears in clinically anxious children with autism spectrum disorders. Unpublished doctoral dissertation. Denver: University of Denver.

Kleinhans, N. M., Richards, T., Weaver, K., Johnson, L. C., Greenson, J., Dawson, G., & Aylward, E. (2010). Association between amygdala response to emotional faces and social anxiety in autism spectrum disorders. *Neuropsychologia, 48*, 3665–3670. doi:10.1016/j.neuropsychologia.2010.07.022.

Klin, A., Jones, W., Schultz, R., & Volkmar, F. (2003). The enactive mind, or from actions to cognition: Lessons from autism. *Philosophical Transactions of The Royal Society B, 358*, 345–360. doi:10.1098/rstb.2002.1202.

Koegel, R. L., & Mentis, M. (1985). Motivation in childhood autism: Can they or won't they? *Journal of Child Psychology and Psychiatry, 26*, 185–191. doi:10.1111/j.1469-7610.1985.tb02259.x.

Kreiser, N. L. (2011). *The development of a social anxiety measure for adolescents and adults with ASD.* Unpublished master's thesis. Blacksburg: Virginia Tech.

Kreiser, N. L., & White, S. W. (2011, November). Measuring social anxiety in adolescents and adults with high functioning autism: The development of a screening instrument. In N. L. Kreiser & C. Pugliese (Co-chairs), *Co-occurring psychological and behavioral problems in adolescents and adults with features of Autism Spectrum Disorder: Assessment and characteristics.* Symposium conducted at the meeting of the Association for Behavioral and Cognitive Therapies, Toronto, Canada.

Kreiser, N. L. & White, S. W. (2014) Assessment of social anxiety in people with ASD. *Clinical Psychology: Science and Practice.*

Kushki, A., Drumm, E., Mobarak, M. P., Tanel, N., Dupuis, A., Chau, T., & Anagnostou, E. (2013). Investigating the autonomic nervous system response to anxiety in children with autism spectrum disorders. *PLoS One, 8*(4), e59730. doi:10.1371/journal.pone.0059730.

Kuusikko, S., Pollock-Wurman, R., Jussila, K., Carter, A. S., Mattila, M.-L., Ebeling, H., … Moilanen, I. (2008). Social anxiety in high-functioning children and adolescents with autism and Asperger syndrome. *Journal of*

Autism and Developmental Disorders, 38, 1697–1709. doi:10.1007/s10803-008-0555-9.

La Greca, A. M., & Lopez, N. (1998). Social anxiety among adolescents: Linkages with peer relations and friendships. *Journal of Abnormal Child Psychology, 26,* 83–94. doi:10.1023/A:1022684520514.

La Greca, A. M., & Stone, W. L. (1993). Social anxiety scale for children-revised: Factor structure and concurrent validity. *Journal of Clinical Child Psychology, 22,* 17–27. doi:10.1207/s15374424jccp2201_2.

Lainhart, J. E., & Folstein, S. E. (1994). Affective disorders in people with autism: A review of published cases. *Journal of Autism and Developmental Disorders, 24,* 587–601. doi:10.1007/BF02172140.

Lang, R., Regester, A., Lauderdale, S., Ashbaugh, K., & Haring, A. (2010). Treatment of anxiety in autism spectrum disorders suing cognitive behaviour therapy: A systematic review. *Developmental Neurorehabilitation, 13,* 53–63. doi:10.3109/17518420903236288.

Lerner, M. D., White, S. W., & McPartland, J. C. (2012). Mechanisms of change in psychosocial interventions for autism spectrum disorders. *Dialogues in Clinical Neuroscience, 14,* 307–318.

Leyfer, O. T., Folstein, S. E., Bacalman, S., Davis, N. O., Dinh, E., Morgan, J., et al. (2006). Comorbid psychiatric disorders in children with autism: Interview development and rates of disorders. *Journal of Autism Developmental Disorders, 36,* 849–861. doi:10.1007/s10803-006-0123-0.

Locke, J., Ishijima, E. H., Kasari, C., & London, N. (2010). Loneliness, friendship quality and the social networks of adolescents with high□functioning autism in an inclusive school setting. *Journal of Research in Special Educational Needs, 10*(2), 74–81. doi:10.1111/j.1471-3802.2010.01148.x.

Lugnegård, T., Hallerbäck, M. U., & Gillberg, C. (2011). Psychiatric comorbidity in young adults with a clinical diagnosis of Asperger syndrome. *Research in Developmental Disabilities, 32,* 1910–1917. doi:10.1016/j.ridd.2011.03.025.

March, J. S. (1998). *Multidimensional anxiety scale for children.* North Tonawanda: Multi-Health Systems.

Mason, J., & Scior, K. (2004). 'Diagnostic overshadowing' amongst clinicians working with people with intellectual disabilities in the UK. *Journal of Applied Research in Intellectual Disabilities, 17*(2), 85–90. doi:10.1111/j.1360-2322.2004.00184.x.

Mazefksy, C. A., Herrington, J., Siegel, M., Scarpa, A., Maddox, B. B., Scahill, L., & White, S. W. (2013). The role of emotion regulation in autism spectrum disorder. *Journal of the American Academy of Child and Adolescent Psychiatry.*

Mazefsky, C. A., Kao, J., & Oswald, D. P. (2011). Preliminary evidence suggesting caution in the use of psychiatric self-report measures with adolescents with high-functioning autism spectrum disorders. *Research in Autism Spectrum Disorders, 5,* 164–174. doi:10.1016/j.rasd.2010.03.006.

Nauta, M. H., Scholing, A., Rapee, R. M., Abbott, M., Spence, S. H., & Waters, A. (2004). A parent-report measure of children's anxiety: Psychometric properties and comparison with child-report in a clinic and normal sample. *Behaviour Research and Therapy, 42,* 813–839. doi:10.1016/S0005-7967(03)00200-6.

Ollendick, T. H., & White, S. W. (2012). The presentation and classification of anxiety in autism spectrum disorder: Where to from here? *Clinical Psychology: Science and Practice, 19,* 352–355. doi:10.1111/cpsp.12013.

Ozsivadjian, A., Knott, F., & Magiati, I. (2012). Parent and child perspectives on the nature of anxiety in children and young people with autism spectrum disorders: A focus group study. *Autism, 16*(2), 107–121. doi:10.1177/1362361311431703.

Piven, J., & Palmer, P. (1999). Psychiatric disorder and the broad autism phenotype: Evidence from a family study of multiple-incidence autism families. *The American Journal of Psychiatry, 156,* 557–563.

Pugliese, C. E., White, B. A., White, S. W., & Ollendick, T. H. (2013). Social anxiety predicts aggression in children with ASD: Clinical comparisons with socially anxious and oppositional youth. *Journal of Autism and Developmental Disorders, 43,* 1205–1213. doi:10.1007/s10803-012-1666-x.

Rao, P. A., Beidel, D. C., Turner, S. M., Ammerman, R. T., Crosby, L. E., & Sallee, F. R. (2007). Social anxiety disorder in childhood and adolescence: Descriptive psychopathology. *Behaviour Research and Therapy, 45,* 1181–1191. doi:10.1016/j.brat.2006.07.015.

Reaven, J. A., Blakeley-Smith, A., Nichols, S., Dasari, M., Flanigan, E., & Hepburn, S. (2009). Cognitive-behavioral group treatment for anxiety symptoms in children with high-functioning autism spectrum disorders: A pilot study. *Focus on Autism and Other Developmental Disabilities, 24*(1), 27–37. doi:10.1177/1088357608327666.

Renno, P., & Wood, J. J. (2013). Discriminant and convergent validity of the anxiety construct in children with autism spectrum disorders. *Journal of Autism and Developmental Disorders, 43,* 2135–2146. doi:10.1007/s10803-013-1767-1.

Schneier, F. R., Johnson, J., Hornig, C. D., Liebowitz, M. R., & Weissman, M. M. (1992). Social phobia: Comorbidity and morbidity in an epidemiologic sample. *Archives of General Psychiatry, 49*(4), 282–288.

Schwartz, C. B., Henderson, H. A., Inge, A. P., Zahka, N. E., Coman, D. C., Kojkowski, N. M., … Mundy, P. C. (2009). Temperament as a predictor of symptomotology and adaptive functioning in adolescents with high-functioning autism. *Journal of Autism and Developmental Disorders, 39,* 842–855. doi:10.1007/s10803-009-0690-y.

Settipani, C. A., Puleo, C. M., Conner, B. T., & Kendall, P. C. (2012). Characteristics and anxiety symptom presentation associated with autism spectrum traits in youth with anxiety disorders. *Journal of Anxiety Disorders, 26,* 459–467. doi:10.1016/j.janxdis.2012.01.010.

Shtayermman, O. (2007). Peer victimization in adolescents and young adults diagnosed with Asperger's syndrome: A link to depressive symptomatology, anxiety symptomatology and suicidal ideation. *Issues in Comprehensive Pediatric Nursing*, *30*(3), 87–107. doi:10.1080/01460860701525089.

Silverman, W. K., & Albano, A. M. (1996). Anxiety disorders interview schedule for DSM-IV. San Antonio, TX: The Psychological Corporation.

Simonoff, E., Pickles, A., Charman, T., Chandler, S., Loucas, T., & Baird, G. (2008). Psychiatric disorders in children with autism spectrum disorders: Prevalence, comorbidity, and associated factors in a population-derived sample. *Journal of the American Academy of Child and Adolescent Psychiatry*, *47*, 921–929. doi:10.1097/CHI.0b013e318179964f.

Spence, S. H. (1995). *Social skills training: Enhancing social competence with children and adolescents.* Windsor: Nfer-Nelson.

Spence, S. H., Donovan, C., & Brechman-Toussaint, M. (1999). Social skills, social outcomes, and cognitive features of childhood social phobia. *Journal of Abnormal Psychology*, *108*, 211–221. doi:10.1037/0021-843x.108.2.211.

Sukhodolsky, D. G., Scahill, L., Gadow, K. D., Arnold, L. E., Aman, M. G., McDougle, C. J., Vitiello, B. (2008). Parent-rated anxiety symptoms in children with pervasive developmental disorders: Frequency and association with core autism symptoms and cognitive functioning. *Journal of Abnormal Child Psychology*, *36*, 117–128. doi:10.1007/s10802-007-9165-9.

Swaim, K. F., & Morgan, S. B. (2001). Children's attitudes and behavioral intentions toward a peer with autistic behaviors: Does a brief educational intervention have an effect? *Journal of Autism and Developmental Disorders*, *31*, 195–205. doi:10.1023/A:1010703316365.

Turner, S. M., Beidel, D. C., Dancu, C. V., & Keys, D. J. (1986). Psychopathology of social phobia and comparison to avoidant personality disorder. *Journal of Abnormal Psychology*, *95*, 389–394. doi:10.1037/0021-843x.95.4.389.

van Steensel, F. J. A., Bögels, S. M., & Perrin, S. (2011). Anxiety disorders in children and adolescents with autistic spectrum disorders: A meta-analysis. *Clinical Child and Family Psychology Review*, *14*, 302–317. doi:10.1007/s10567-011-0097-0.

Wallace, S. T., & Alden, L. E. (1995). Social anxiety and standard setting following social success or failure. *Cognitive Therapy and Research*, *19*, 613–631. doi:10.1007/BF02227857.

Weeks, J. W., Heimberg, R. G., Rodebaugh, T. L., & Norton, P. J. (2008). Exploring the relationship between fear of positive evaluation and social anxiety. *Journal of Anxiety Disorders*, *22*, 386–400. doi:10.1016/j.janxdis.2007.04.009.

Wenzel, A., Graff-Dolezal, J., Macho, M., & Brendle, J. R. (2005). Communication and social skills in socially anxious and nonanxious individuals in the context of romantic relationships. *Behaviour Research and Therapy*, *43*, 505–519. doi:10.1016/j.brat.2004.03.010.

White, S. W., & Roberson-Nay, R. (2009). Anxiety, social deficits, and loneliness in youth with autism spectrum disorders. *Journal of Autism and Developmental Disorders*, *39*, 1006–1013. doi:10.1007/s10803-009-0713-8.

White, S. W., & Schry, A. R. (2011). Social anxiety in adolescents on the autism spectrum. In C. A. Alfano & D. C. Beidel (Eds.), *Social anxiety in adolescents and young adults: Translating developmental science into practice* (pp. 183–201). Washington, DC: American Psychological Association.

White, S. W., Albano, A. M., Johnson, C. R., Kasari, C., Ollendick, T., Klin, A., … Scahill, L. (2010). Development of a cognitive-behavioral intervention program to treat anxiety and social deficits in teens with high-functioning autism. *Clinical Child and Family Psychology Review*, *13*, 77–90. doi:10.1007/s10567-009-0062-3.

White, S. W., Ollendick, T. H., & Bray, B. C. (2011). College students on the autism spectrum: Prevalence and associated problems. *Autism*, *15*, 683–701. doi:10.1177/1362361310393363.

White, S. W., Bray, B. C., & Ollendick, T. H. (2012a). Examining shared and unique aspects of social anxiety disorder and autism spectrum disorder using factor analysis. *Journal of Autism and Developmental Disorders*, *42*, 874–884. doi:10.1007/s10803-011-1325-7.

White, S. W., Kreiser, N. L., Pugliese, C., & Scarpa, A. (2012b). Social anxiety mediates the effect of autism spectrum disorder characteristics on hostility in young adults. *Autism*, *16*, 453–464. doi:10.1177/1362361311431951.

White, S. W., Schry, A. R., & Maddox, B. B. (2012c). Brief report: The assessment of anxiety in high-functioning adolescents with autism spectrum disorder. *Journal of Autism and Developmental Disorders*, *42*, 1138–1145. doi:10.1007/s10803-011-1353-3.

White, S. W., Ollendick, T., Albano, A. M., Oswald, D., Johnson, C., Southam-Gerow, M. A., … Scahill, L. (2013). Randomized controlled trial: Multimodal anxiety and social skill intervention for adolescents with autism spectrum disorder. *Journal of Autism and Developmental Disorders*, *43*, 382–394. doi:10.1007/s10803-012-1577-x.

Williamson, S., Craig, J., & Slinger, R. (2008). Exploring the relationship between measures of self-esteem and psychological adjustment among adolescents with Asperger syndrome. *Autism*, *12*, 391–402. doi:10.1177/1362361308091652.

Wood, J. J., & Gadow, K. D. (2010). Exploring the nature and function of anxiety in youth with autism spectrum disorders. *Clinical Psychology: Science and Practice*, *17*, 281–292. doi:10.1111/j.1468-2850.2010.01220.x.

Wood, J. J., Drahota, A., Sze, K., Har, K., Chiu, A., & Langer, D. A. (2009). Cognitive behavioral therapy for anxiety in children with autism spectrum disorders: A randomized, controlled trial. *Journal of Child Psychology and Psychiatry*, *50*, 224–234. doi:10.1111/j.1469-7610.2008.01948.x.

Fear: Autism Spectrum Disorder and/or Specific Phobia

Thompson E. Davis III and Thomas H. Ollendick

Introduction

Autism spectrum disorder (ASD) encapsulates a variety of neurodevelopmental problems, syndromes, and disorders that are frequently comorbid with other psychopathologies (Matson and Nebel-Schwalm 2007). Among the more common comorbidities with ASD are the anxiety disorders which co-occur at rates of 11–84% (White et al. 2009). The investigation of anxiety in those with ASD has become a burgeoning area of inquiry; however, fear and specific phobias, by comparison, have been curiously neglected in this area of study (Matson and Nebel-Schwalm 2007). This oversight is particularly concerning given specific phobia has been found by some researchers to be the most common comorbid disorder in those with ASD (Leyfer et al. 2006; Muris et al. 1998; Sukhodolsky et al. 2008; Turner and Romanczyk 2012; van Steensel et al 2011). However, a great deal of difficulty lies in distinguishing ASD symptoms from fears and phobias, and judging the exact point of departure from ASD to an additional diagnosis of specific phobia can be difficult. As a result, the following chapter delves into the specific phobia and ASD diagnoses, es-pecially focusing on differential diagnosis and issues with their comorbidity. Additionally, we offer specific suggestions for assessing and treating specific phobia in those with ASD, as well as thoughts about the future of these two diagnoses as the field moves forward with the *Diagnostic and Statistical Manual of Mental Disorders, 5th edition* (*DSM-5*; American Psychiatric Association 2013).

The Phenomenology of Fear and Phobia

Fear is a multicomponent emotional response that can be construed as existing along a continuum of development and intensity (Davis et al. 2011b; Davis and Ollendick 2005; Lang 1979). The typical description has been for one end of this continuum to be the healthy, developmentally transient, or situationally appropriate expression of fear. At the other end of this spectrum, however, is specific phobia —a markedly intense fear that is excessive, unreasonable, distressing, and impairing to the person's daily functioning (*Diagnostic and Statistical Manual of Mental Disorders, 4th edition-text revision*, 2000; *DSM-IV-TR*). That said, the degree to which a fear is commonplace for a given individual at a given stage of development also needs to be considered. These considerations of intensity and developmental typicality make determining the phenomenology of specific phobia in those with ASD complex, especially given the diffi-

T. E. Davis III (✉)
Department of Psychology, Louisiana State University, Baton Rouge, Louisiana, USA
e-mail: ted@lsu.edu

T. H. Ollendick
Department of Psychology, Child Study Center, Virginia Tech, Blacksburg, Virginia, USA
e-mail: tho@vt.edu

T. E. Davis III et al. (eds.), *Handbook of Autism and Anxiety,* Autism and Child Psychopathology Series,
DOI 10.1007/978-3-319-06796-4_10, © Springer International Publishing Switzerland 2014

culties and symptoms associated with an ASD diagnosis. In addition, given the pervasiveness of ASD symptoms, the likelihood for diagnostic overshadowing (Mason and Scior 2004), or simply considering a specific phobia part of an eccentricity or symptom of the ASD or a comorbid intellectual disability (ID), is great (Matson and Sevin 1994). As a result, in this section, we start with a brief review of a neurotypical child's developmental trajectory for fear. Next, we follow this with what is known about the development of more intense or extreme fears—specific phobias in neurotypical individuals. Finally, we review the phenomenology of these intense fears in individuals with ASD, including the more unusual fears commonly comorbid with the disorder.

Fear in the Typically Developing Individual

Beginning early in life, we occasionally experience the world as a scary, fearful undertaking, as can be seen in the reflexive startle during early infancy (e.g., Moro reflex) or the fear of heights that emerges with increased depth perception and locomotive ability (i.e., the Visual Cliff; Gibson and Walk 1960). Generally, these fears are adaptive and often reflect a child's changing developmental capabilities (Davis 2009; Gullone 2000; Ollendick et al. 2004). While unpleasant, developmentally appropriate fears serve a protective function by helping mobilize an individual for action, keeping one from perceived harm, and allowing an individual to make speedy appraisals of complex emotional situations. These fears are thought to be composed of three primary components—physiological, behavioral, and cognitive—as well as an overall subjective appraisal of the emotional response (Davis et al. 2011c; Davis and Ollendick 2005; Lang 1979). When an individual is afraid, the individual's body evidences a variety of physiological responses (e.g., increased heart rate, increased cortisol), behavioral responses (e.g., freezing, running away), and cognitive responses (e.g., catastrophic thinking, perceptions of dangerousness). The totality of this experience is usually subjectively experi-

enced and interpreted by the individual as unpleasant and aversive (Barlow 2002; Davis and Ollendick 2005).

Fear generally follows a developmental path, with gains in emotional expression and more cognitively complex fears essentially piggybacking on broader cognitive-developmental gains. Specifically, fear begins in infancy (even in the first year of life) and is usually associated with concrete stimuli in the infant's immediate environment (Gullone 2000). Over the ensuing years, these fears tend to be focused increasingly on concrete stimuli associated with danger until cognitive development reaches the point at which the individual can consider more abstract fears and anxieties—usually during the ages of 6–12 (Gullone 2000); for example, with increasing gains in abstract thinking and emotional development come mounting fears of social evaluation, bodily injury, and the supernatural (Davis 2009; Davis and Ollendick 2011; Gullone 2000). More complex and cognitively abstract fears of death and dying tend to develop last (Gullone 2000). Childhood and adolescent fears of these types tend to emerge and then dissipate with disconfirmatory experiences, parental and caregiver assistance, or greater practice in the feared situation leading many to consider such fears healthy and transitional, essentially a phase children go through (Ollendick et al. 2009a). Indeed, normal and developmentally appropriate fears tend to decline as age increases, tend to occur more frequently and more intensely in girls than in boys (though this may be partially related to stereotype development and cultural experiences), and tend to occur more frequently in children from lower socioeconomic status (SES) than middle and upper SES (Gullone 2000). Normative fears are typically transient through childhood, although if they continue they may become fairly stable problems at approximately 11 years of age (Gullone 2000). Across cultures, the development of fear is generally consistent with the research in more westernized countries, showing similar changes in development, common fears, and gender differences (Gullone 2000), although some notable exceptions have been reported (King et al. 1988). Even so, some culturally specific fears may be present which are more reflective of unique cultural or environmental constructs (e.g., taijin kyofusho; see *DSM-5*, 2013).

Specific Phobia in the Typically Developing Individual

While fears are quite normal, healthy, and adaptive, in some individuals they can become problematic and reach the level of a disorder: a specific phobia. Consistent with current diagnostic criteria, Muris and Merckelbach (2012) clearly outline three key features of specific phobias: (1) the fear is circumscribed and stimulus specific, (2) exposure or confrontation with the feared stimuli evokes a strong fear response, and (3) the fear is irrational, excessive, and unreasonable to a degree that it causes significant interference for the individual. Essentially, a specific phobia can be described as the unusually intense, integrated, potentiated, and pathological fear response of a network of memories and prepotent and highly predictable responses (Davis and Ollendick 2005, 2011; Lang 1979). Similar to the experience of developmentally typical fears, phobias are composed of the same three response components: physiology, behavior, and cognition. When these responses are all activated, there is a fear response and the result is described as synchronous responding (e.g., high heart rate, running away, and thinking a dog will bite would be "fear;" Davis and Ollendick 2011; Ollendick et al. 2011). A partial, or desynchronous, response is also possible, however, with only portions of the response being activated (Hodgson and Rachman 1974; Rachman and Hodgson 1974). In these instances, avoidance behavior may occur before physiological symptoms become fully expressed (i.e., behavioral avoidance) or a catastrophic cognition may prevent exposure to the feared stimulus all together (e.g., "if I go near that field I'll see a snake and it will bite me"). These broad characteristics and considerations are also consistent with the criteria described in both the *DSM-IV-TR* and the *DSM-5* (see Table 10.1 for a side-by-side comparison of criteria).

Diagnostic Criteria   At first glance, the criteria between the two DSM editions seem remarkably similar (i.e., *DSM-IV-TR* and the *DSM-5*). In general, the criteria fall in line with the historic understanding of phobia as panic and avoidance. As well, the five different types of specific phobia have been retained in the new edition: animal type (e.g., dogs and roaches), natural environment type (e.g., storms and dark), blood-injection-injury type (e.g., seeing blood or injections), situational type (e.g., elevators and small spaces), and other type (e.g., clowns and vomit). The presentation in children is still similarly described as potentially involving freezing, clinging, crying, or tantrumming (*DSM-5*). Criteria A and B for both editions are also comparable (see Table 10.1); however, beyond those similarities, there are changes and details which require further explication.

The initial criterion for specific phobia, criterion A, in both volumes is an intense fear (*DSM-IV-TR, DSM-5*), but *DSM-5* goes on to elaborate that there can be fear *or* anxiety about a stimulus. This is a new and interesting change as the conceptual understanding of "fear" and "anxiety" has been viewed as separate and distinct for some time. Fear has generally been understood to be the ancient and evolutionary alarm–reaction to an impending threat (i.e., panic), whereas anxiety has been considered a more future-oriented worry (Barlow 2002) and "the tense anticipation of a threatening but vague event" (Rachman 1998, p. 2). This addition allows anxiety in anticipation of exposure to a circumscribed stimulus to be categorized as a phobia. Criterion B is largely consistent as well in that exposure to the feared stimulus should elicit a response; however, in *DSM-5* that response is again either fear or anxiety. *DSM-5* continues with a criterion for either an avoidance of the feared stimulus or an unpleasant endurance of symptoms if escape is not possible and one is exposed (criterion C). A change, however, is observed in criterion D as the fear or anxiety now only needs to be disproportionate to the exposure (*DSM-5*), and there is no longer a requirement that the individual recognize the excessiveness and irrationality of the fear if cognitively mature enough to do so (*DSM-IV-TR*). Similarly, a change from

Table 10.1 Specific phobia by *Diagnostic and Statistical Manual of Mental Disorders* (*DSM*) Edition

DSM-IV-TR (2000)	DSM-5 (2013)
"Marked," enduring fear that is unreasonable on in excess of what would be expected and triggered by anticipation of or the actual presence of a feared stimulus	"Marked fear or anxiety" about a stimulus
Exposure to the feared stimulus regularly evokes an immediate anxious response which may be a panic attack	The feared stimulus regularly evokes immediate anxiety or fear
Except for children, those with a phobia must recognize the fear is unreasonable or in excess of what would be expected	The feared stimulus is avoided or "endured with intense fear or anxiety"
There must be either avoidance or strong distress or anxiety if the stimulus must be endured because avoidance/escape is not possible	The "fear or anxiety" is disproportional to the risk, situation, or sociocultural context
The avoidance, anticipation, or distress while in the situation must significantly interfere with life (e.g., work, social, academic), or there must be distress about having the fear	The "fear, anxiety, or avoidance" must be enduring with a 6-month duration regardless of age. This duration, however, is not absolute
There must be a 6-month duration in children and adolescents younger than 18 years	The "fear, anxiety, or avoidance" causes significant impairment (e.g., work, social, academic) or distress
The fear is not better accounted for by another disorder	The fear cannot be better accounted for by other symptoms of a disorder
For children: The anxiety may involve "crying, tantrums, freezing, or clinging."	For children: The "fear or anxiety" may involve "crying, tantrums, freezing, or clinging"
Types: Animal, Natural Environment, Blood-Injection-Injury, Situational, and Other	Types: Animal, Natural Environment, Blood-Injection-Injury, Situational, and Other. Blood-Injection-Injury is further specified as fear of blood, injections/transfusions, other medical care, or injury per ICD-10-CM codes

See pp. 449–450 for *DSM-IV-TR*; see pp. 197–198 for *DSM-5*

DSM-IV-TR to *DSM-5* is a flexible duration requirement of 6 months that is now independent of age. Previously, a 6-month duration requirement existed only for children and adolescents to help ensure fears were actually phobias and not more transitory developmentally appropriate fear responses (*DSM-IV-TR*), and adults could essentially be diagnosed with a phobia after meeting all other criteria for any period of time. In *DSM-5*, the avoidance, anxiety, or fear must cause impairment or distress (criterion F), and the fear cannot be better conceptualized as part of another mental disorder (criterion G).

Phenomenology Little research in children and adolescents has been conducted specifically on the phenomenology of specific phobia (Davis and Ollendick 2011), even though many phobias appear beginning during early childhood and on into adolescence. Researchers have long pointed out that some fears seem more predisposed to

become phobias than others: for example, phobias of animals are more prevalent than electricity or biking (for reviews, see Mineka and Zinbarg 2006; Muris and Merckelbach 2012; Nebel-Schwalm and Davis 2013). These differences do not seem to be related to the actual danger posed by the stimulus and may be more the result of natural selection leading to an increased predisposition toward forming certain associations between stimuli and fear (see Muris and Merckelbach 2012, for a review). Overall, animal- and natural environment-type phobias are most common in children: specifically, phobias of dogs, insects, heights, the dark, and storms (Davis and Ollendick 2011; Last et al. 1992; Milne et al. 1995; Ollendick et al. 2009b, 2010a, b; Silverman et al. 1999). Generally, it seems that the presentation of specific phobias does differ by type, with natural environment phobias being more severe and impairing than animal-type phobias (Ollendick et al. 2010a, b). Compared to children and adolescents with animal phobias, children with natural environment phobias have been found to have parent ratings, suggesting that they have more social problems, are more anxious/depressed, are more withdrawn, and have more somatic complaints (Davis and Ollendick 2011; Ollendick et al. 2010a, b). In addition, Ollendick et al. (2010a, b) found that children with natural environment-type phobias had more severe and impairing self-reported symptoms too: more conviction in their catastrophic belief occurring, more somatic and anxious symptoms, more symptoms of depression, and poorer life satisfaction and quality of life. Interestingly, these two groups did not differ in the overall clinical severity of their phobias, their respective demographic or socioeconomic characteristics, or their self-reported coping ability (Ollendick et al. 2010a, b). While sociodemographic characteristics and differences overall are unclear at this time, it does appear that specific phobias do affect children and adolescents across the socioeconomic and demographic spectrums (Davis and Ollendick 2011; Ollendick et al. 2010a, b).

Age of Onset The average age of onset for a specific phobia is in middle to late childhood: average ages of onset have been reported as young as nine (Stinson et al. 2007) to approximately 15 years of age (Kessler et al. 2012; Magee et al. 1996). Even so, a developmental progression in the onset of phobias appears to be present, akin to that seen of fear in children without phobias (Gullone 2000; Öst 1987a), and the actual age of onset of specific phobia is among the youngest of any disorder (Kessler et al. 2012). The onset of phobias has tended to follow the same cognitive-developmental trend of concrete to increasingly abstract thinking with animal phobias developing early (approximately 7 years of age), followed by blood (9 years), dentists (12 years), and small spaces (20 years of age; Öst 1987a). Unfortunately, specific phobias have also been found to be more than developmental phases of fear with the average duration of a phobia lasting more than 20 years (Stinson et al. 2007). Perhaps the most distressing fact is that fewer than 8–12% of those children and adolescents with specific

phobias have sought treatment, usually as adults in their 30s (Kessler et al. 1999; Stinson et al. 2007), despite specific phobia being one of the most researched disorders, one of the most prevalent disorders, and one of the disorders for which the most effective and brief treatments exist (Barlow 2002; Davis et al. 2011b; Davis et al. 2009, 2012c; Grills-Taquechel and Ollendick 2012; May et al. 2013; Zlomke and Davis 2008).

Comorbidity Specific phobias are also considered a gateway disorder with very high rates of comorbidity. In epidemiologic and treatment research across both community and clinical samples and from childhood to adulthood, comorbidity appears to be the rule rather than the exception: specific phobias tend to occur alongside one or more additional specific phobias (Davis and Ollendick 2011). In adults, specific phobias are commonly comorbid with other phobias, other anxiety disorders (especially panic disorder with agoraphobia and social phobia), personality disorders (especially dependent and avoidant personality disorders), bipolar II, and drug dependence (Stinson et al. 2007). As well, adults who had more than one specific phobia (regardless of type) were at significant risk of increased disability, impairment, and comorbidity compared to those who only had a single specific phobia: when multiple phobias were present, the most common comorbidities were other anxiety disorders, personality disorders, and nicotine dependence (Stinson et al. 2007). According to *DSM-5*, approximately 75% of individuals with a specific phobia will have a second, comorbid specific phobia.

Similar patterns are observed in children and adolescents with specific phobias. While differences in sample composition across studies make interpretation difficult, approximately half or more of all children with specific phobias in community samples have another comorbid specific phobia (Costello et al. 2004). In clinical samples, the rates of comorbidity have ranged from 42% of children having at least one comorbid disorder (Öst et al. 2001) to 95% of children having at least one disorder in addition to their specific phobia (Ollendick et al. 2009b). Between these extremes, Last et al. (1992) and Silverman et al. (1999) found comorbidity rates of 50 % and 72 %, respectively. A very rough comorbidity estimate averaged across the four studies then is that approximately 65 % of children and adolescents presenting to clinical studies have at least one comorbid disorder over and beyond their specific phobia. Similarly, summarizing across clinical trials, the most common comorbid diagnoses in children with specific phobias are other specific phobias, and then in no particular order, generalized anxiety disorder, separation anxiety disorder, social phobia, major depressive disorder, and attention-deficit/hyperactivity disorder (Davis and Ollendick 2011; Ollendick et al. 2010a, b, 2009b; Öst et al. 2001; Silverman et al. 1999). Between actual specific phobia types, differential comorbidity has been observed as well. Children with a natural environment-type specific phobia have been found to have higher comorbid rates of generalized anxiety disorder and separation anxiety disorder than children with an animal-type phobia (Ollendick et al. 2010a, b).

Fear and Specific Phobia in the Individual with ASD

Research on specific phobias in those with ASD is limited, which is surprising given the decades-old observation that those with ASD tend to have numerous, and at times unusual, fears. For example, Kanner (1943) repeats a mother's description of her son, "Frederick," as being "afraid of mechanical things; he runs from them. He used to be afraid of my egg beater, is perfectly petrified of my vacuum cleaner. Elevators are simply a terrifying experience to him. He is afraid of spinning toys" (pp. 222–223). As currently configured in the *DSM-5*, ASD is a broad spectrum of symptoms that collapses across, grandfathers in, or excludes the previous five *DSM-IV-TR* diagnoses of autistic disorder, Rett's disorder, childhood disintegrative disorder, Asperger's disorder, and pervasive developmental disorder—not otherwise specified (PDD-NOS; see Chap. 1, for a review of the history of ASD and current diagnostic criteria). While comorbidity in those with ASD

is quite common (*DSM-5*), and comorbidity with anxiety disorders more common still (White et al. 2009), relatively little research has looked at what may be the most common mental health disorder of all for typically and atypically developing individuals alike: specific phobia (Matson and Nebel-Schwalm 2007).

Diagnostic Criteria Overall, diagnostic criteria for a specific phobia are no different for an individual with or without an ASD, and no particular guidelines for differentiation are provided in the *DSM-5* along with that disorder (see the previous section on diagnostic criteria in the typically developing individual with specific phobia and Table 10.1; for a review of the diagnostic criteria for ASD, see Chap. 1). Similarly, there are no *DSM-5* diagnostic guidelines from the ASD criteria that would assist other than to suggest that ASD is comorbid with anxiety disorders and that those with ASD are prone to anxiety. For example, the discussion in the differential diagnosis section of *DSM-5* does not include specific phobia, obsessive–compulsive disorder, or similar disorders except selective mutism.

While one would expect little difficulty deciding between a diagnosis of ASD *or* specific phobia, the difficulty is deciding when and if an individual's symptoms merit ASD *and* a separate diagnosis of specific phobia. For example, when is hypersensitivity to sound actually a specific phobia of loud noises? Is an individual's refusal to wear a shirt or pants with buttons a phobia or excessive rigidity? When is an individual's refusal to consume particular food items rigidity, hypersensitivity to taste or texture, a phobia, or all of the above (e.g., refusal to eat yogurt or mushrooms). Is one's extensive interest in and learning about meteorology or archaeology a restricted interest or a specific phobia of thunderstorms or mummies, respectively, and the behaviors conceptualized as attempts to relieve anxiety? Again, the diagnostic determination is relatively easy in one direction: any of the preceding could be a specific phobia, but an ASD would require other more significant impairments that could easily rule out that diagnosis. However, the diagnostic determination in the other direction is more difficult: when are any of the preceding a specific phobia over and above symptoms of ASD? At least in the examples presented above, all of the stimuli were actual specific phobias seen in typically developing children and adolescents during randomized clinical trials: specific phobias of yogurt, mummies, thunderstorms, loud noises in Öst et al. 2001 and buttons, mushrooms, loud noises, and thunderstorms in Ollendick et al. 2009b). It is clear that the unusualness of the feared stimulus (e.g., mummies, buttons, or yogurt) is not necessarily the deciding factor in deciding between ASD and an additional specific phobia. As a result, the remaining sections of this chapter focus on what research exists that may be helpful in making this determination and what clinical recommendations might prove to be fruitful.

Phenomenology Similar to the literature examining specific phobias in typically developing children and adolescents, there has been little research on the phenomenology of specific phobia in those with an ASD. Leyfer et al. (2006) found the most common phobias in children and adolescents (i.e., 5–17 years) with autism were phobias of needles/injections and crowds; additionally, over 10 % had a phobia of loud noises. Specific phobias seen more commonly in typically developing children were not reported to occur at similarly high rates (Leyfer et al. 2006). Of note, full-scale intelligent quotient (IQ) scores ranged from 42 to 141 in the sample with most having a score above 70. The most frequent phobias diagnosed by Muris et al. (1998) were similar to those seen by Leyfer et al. (2006), with the two most common types related to the medical field: in decreasing frequency doctors, dentists, thunderstorms, darkness, water, insects, blood, heights, dogs, rabbits, and balloons. Potentially, this may reflect ASD children's more frequent, intensive, and possibly aversive experience with medical professionals—though this remains to be determined. In the work by Muris et al. (1998), most children with specific phobias had more than one, but almost every child with a phobia had a specific phobia of doctors or dentists. Their specific phobias included more of those seen in typically developing children; however, the IQ

range of their sample had a somewhat more constricted range from 59 to 116. Muris et al. (1998) also found that children with pervasive developmental disorder-not otherwise specified (PDD-NOS) more frequently met criteria for specific phobia than children with autistic disorder. At least one study as well has found that specific phobia is equally distributed across both high and low IQ individuals (defined as those above or below 70; IQ scores of individuals in the sample extended from the average range to the profound IQ range (Sukhodolsky et al. 2008). Interestingly, van Steensel et al. (2012) found that specific phobia was more common among a high-functioning ASD group of children than among a typically developing anxiety-disordered group.

Similar findings emerge when one examines fears in those with an ASD (i.e., not necessarily specific phobias). For example, Matson and Love (1990) found that children with an ASD have more fear than a group of age-matched typically developing children. They found the parents of ASD children endorsed their children as more fearful of thunderstorms, being punished, crowds, the dark, enclosed spaces, and dentists, but less fearful of failure or criticism (Matson and Love 1990). Evans et al. (2005) found that children with ASD had more medical and situational fears than children with Down's syndrome or two groups of typically developing controls (i.e., matched by chronological or mental age). Turner and Romanczyk (2012) had parents complete a fear questionnaire about their children who had an ASD. They found (in decreasing frequency) fears of getting blood drawn/an injection/a finger stick, making mistakes, getting teeth cleaned, taking tests, meeting peers, doctors, the dark, and insects to be the most common fears; though they also found poor correspondence between the parent questionnaire and the children's responses to pictures of the fear stimuli. Only about 12 % of parent-rated fears corresponded to the child's reactions based on observers' coding of the children's responses to the photos (Turner and Romanczyk 2012). Mayes et al. (2013) found 41 % of their sample had "unusual fears," with the most common fears being a fear of toilets and of mechanical devices. Of those with these more atypical fears, 60% had only one fear, 28% had two, and 10% had three unusual fears. Interestingly, Mayes et al. (2013) did not find differences between the children with and without unusual fears by age, IQ, mental age, or autism severity. Finally, in their meta-analysis, van Steensel et al. (2011) similarly found no relationship between IQ and specific phobia; however, higher rates of specific phobia were seen in studies that included a greater proportion of individuals with autistic disorder or a greater proportion of those with PDD-NOS. Studies with greater proportions of individuals with Asperger's disorder were actually associated with lower rates of specific phobia (in studies using *DSM-IV*).

Age of Onset Trends in the development of fear and anxiety in those with ASD are difficult to discern at present due to limited research on the topic. One cross-sectional study that has been done, however, found that anxious and avoidant behaviors may ebb and flow in those with ASD throughout the lifespan: rising during infancy only to decrease during childhood and young adulthood to then increase again during later adulthood (Davis et al. 2011a). Still, in as much as this study did not use a longitudinal design and was only based on a limited assessment of anxiety and avoidant symptoms, the results should be interpreted with caution. These findings did, however, lend credence to the possibility that anxiety and fear may have a developmental quality to their emergence in those with ASD, if somewhat delayed in onset compared to the trajectory expected in typically developing individuals (Davis et al. 2011a).

Comorbidity Approximately 70% of those with ASD have been suggested to have at least one comorbid disorder and 40% may have two or more comorbidities (*DSM-5*; see Chap. 4, for a review of disorders frequently comorbid with ASD). Further complicating the presentation of specific phobia in those with ASD is the likely presence of an ID. ID is a common comorbid concern in those with ASD; approximately 50–75% of those with ASD also have an ID (Matson and Shoemaker 2009; Rutter and Schopler 1987;

Wing 1981; Wing and Gould 1979). As well, the presence of ID and ASD may mask or overshadow additional comorbid diagnoses and at the very least make the determination of comorbidities more difficult and nuanced (for a complete review of how ID affects the presentation of ASD, see Chap. 2). Even so, in children and adolescents with an ASD and a specific phobia, it seems likely that a pattern similar to that seen in typically developing individuals may emerge: that one of the most common comorbid diagnoses is another specific phobia. For example, Muris et al. (1998) found that 15 children with specific phobias had a total of 54 specific phobia diagnoses (or approximately 3–4 phobias each).

Epidemiology

Epidemiological findings are particularly interesting when considering specific phobia, one of the most common disorders, and ASD, one of the less common but more severely impairing disorders. While less prevalent than specific phobia, recent estimates of the prevalence of ASD have increased over the last decade, from 1 in 150 children in 2000 to 1 in 88 children as of 2008 (Centers for Disease Control and Prevention [CDC] 2013). And while ASD occurs worldwide and across all races, ethnicities, and cultures, similar to specific phobias, ASD shows the opposite gender trend with ASD being five times more common in boys than girls (CDC 2013; for a more detailed discussion of the epidemiology of ASD, see Chap. 1).

Specific Phobias

In typically developing individuals, prevalence estimates for specific phobia frequently have specific phobias as one of the most prevalent disorders, if not the most prevalent disorder. Recent data indicate that prevalence rates for specific phobia are the highest of all disorders among those aged 13 years or older (15.6% lifetime, 12.1% 1-year prevalence; Kessler et al. 2012). Similarly, specific phobia carries one of the highest lifetime morbid risks (18.4 %; i.e., those who will have specific phobia at some point in their lives whether they have had it or not; Kessler et al. 2012): in other words, almost 20 % of individuals will develop specific phobia at some point in the future. These rates are similar to those previously reported (Kessler et al. 2005a, b; Stinson et al. 2007) indicating stability in clinical recognition and diagnosis patterns. In children, at the lower end of estimates, about 10 % of clinical samples of children and 5 % of community samples are thought to have fears intense and enduring enough to be considered specific phobias (*DSM-5*; Ollendick et al. 1997). Higher estimates exist, however, with possibly 17.6 % of parent-reported fears and 22.8 % of child-reported fears constituting cases of phobia (Muris and Merkelbach 2000; Muris et al. 2000).

Overall, girls and women are more likely than males to have most types of specific phobias (*DSM-IV-TR*; *DSM-5*; Kessler et al. 2012; Muris and Merckelbach 2012). Generally, twice as many females are affected as males; in addition, differences by type of phobia are present with females having more animal-, natural environment-, and situational-type phobias, and blood-injection-injury phobia being approximately equally distributed (*DSM-5*; Muris and Merckelbach 2012). Specific phobias are experienced worldwide, with rates in the USA and Europe approximately equal, but higher than those of Asian, African, or Latin American countries (*DSM-5*).

Specific Phobias in those with ASD

Specific phobias in those with ASD are common, with some researchers indicating it is the most common comorbid diagnosis for those with ASD (Leyfer et al. 2006; Muris et al. 1998). Leyfer et al. (2006) found that 44 % of a sample of children and adolescents with autism had comorbid specific phobia diagnoses based on a modified version of the *Kiddie Schedule for Affective Disorders and Schizophrenia* dubbed the *Autism Comorbidity Interview—Present and Lifetime Version*. In a study examining only the anxiety disorders, Muris et al. (1998) similarly found specific phobia to be the most common anxiety disorder among children and adolescents with either autistic disorder or PDD-NOS (i.e., 63.6 %). Sukhodolsky et al. (2008) also specifically examined anxiety in children and adolescents with a PDD using the *Child and Adolescent Symptoms Inventory*. Specific phobia symptoms, however, were only represented by a single item, "is overly fearful of specific objects." Based on their findings, specific phobia was the most common problem affecting 31 % of the total sample. van Steensel et al. (2011) similarly found specific phobia to be the most common diagnosis in children and adolescents with an ASD in their meta-analysis of 31 studies.

Assessment Recommendations

Assessing for comorbid fears and phobias in individuals with ASD is a complex endeavor that truly requires a multi-method, multi-informant assessment. Specifically, in both typically developing individuals and those with ASD, different fears and ratings of fears have been found depending on how one inquires and with whom one inquires (e.g., Lane and Gullone 1999; Muris and Merkelbach 2000; Muris et al. 2000; Turner and Romanczyk 2012; for a review, see Kerns and Kendall 2012 and Chap. 6). These differences have been especially apparent in comparisons between self- or parent-report and some form of in vivo or laboratory-based exposure or task (e.g., Turner and Romanczyk 2012). In addition, assessment recommendations are likely going to vary based upon the level of functioning of the individual with ASD. While there are currently very limited guidelines about assessing specific phobia in those with ASD, we are going to suggest a stepped, multi-method, multi-informant approach to ensure that the most complete information possible is obtained. As well, given that specific phobia has an early age of onset and ASD is generally identified in childhood, we focus on assessing (and later on treating) specific phobia in children and adolescents. Although we suggest this approach be taken with all clients with ASD, regardless of whether or not ID is present, our recommendations are generally geared toward working with individuals with perhaps mild ID to those who are higher, and even above average in, functioning (see Chap. 11 and Hagopian and Jennett 2008, for a review of behavioral assessment and treatment techniques for those who are lower functioning).

While extending the use of techniques that were developed for use with and validated with typically developing individuals to those with ASD should be done cautiously (Davis 2012), examining the typically developing literature for assessment suggestions can prove to be a good springboard for future research and development. In their review of evidence-based assessment for anxiety in children and adolescents, Silverman and Ollendick (2005) recommended using self-report scales to screen for disorders. In particular, they recommended the Fear Survey Schedule for Children-Revised (FSSC-R, Ollendick 1983) for specific phobia. In addition, they suggested the use of a semi-structured interview, the *Anxiety Disorders Interview Schedule for DSM-IV: Child and Parent Versions* (ADIS C/P; Silverman and Albano 1996), and some form of direct observation. Similarly, in their review of evidence-based assessment for specific phobia in particular, Ollendick et al. (2004) recommended using a clinical interview (i.e., both an open-ended interview and the ADIS C/P), the FSSC-R (among other instruments), and behavioral avoidance tasks (BAT) to directly observe how individuals react to their feared stimulus (e.g., Ollendick et al. 2012).

In general, the research on the assessment and treatment of specific phobia in those with ASD has mirrored these recommendations. Typically, individuals have been assessed with some form of fear survey schedule and behavioral observation (e.g., a BAT), and possibly an interview. Fear survey schedules have generally taken the form of either the FSSC-R by Ollendick (1983) or some derivative thereof, being administered to a parent or caregiver in some form (e.g., Davis et al. 2007; Evans et al. 2005; Matson and Love 1990; Turner and Romanczyk 2012). Unfortunately, these instruments are frequently adapted, modified, and administered in ways other than originally intended in attempts to better cap-

ture the unique ways individuals with ASD may experience fear. Unfortunately, however, this frequent adaptation and modification make outcomes difficult to evaluate and in need of additional research and replication (e.g., Turner and Romanczyk 2012 further adapted the measure from Evans et al. 2005 which was already adapted from Ollendick 1983). As well, the consistent use of a particular form of fear survey schedule is currently lacking. Similarly, a variety of diagnostic interviews have been used across studies. For example, interviews to assess specific phobia in those with ASD have included the parent portion of the ADIS C/P (e.g., in Davis et al. 2007), the *Diagnostic Interview Schedule for Children* (DISC version 2.3; e.g., in Muris et al. 1998), the *Checklist for Autism Spectrum Disorder* (CASD) as a means to identify topics and guide follow-up in a subsequent clinical interview (e.g., in Mayes et al. 2013), and the *Autism Comorbidity Interview—Present and Lifetime Version* (ACI-PL; Leyfer et al. 2006). A variety of behavioral tasks have also been used including more traditional BATs (e.g., Davis et al. 2007), direct observation (i.e., consistent with obtaining a baseline using applied behavior analytic techniques; Rapp et al. 2005), and other forms of assessment (e.g., observation of children's reactions to photos in Turner and Romanczyk 2012).

Also, the degree to which newer, indirect assessment methods may continue to be adapted to those with ASD remains to be investigated. For example, the *Motivation for Fear* (*MOTIF*; Nebel-Schwalm and Davis 2011) was originally adapted from the *Questions About Behavior Function* (*QABF*; Paclawskyj et al. 2000) to be a more anxiety-specific functional assessment tool in typically developing individuals. An indirect measure of behavioral avoidance has also been developed to approximate a BAT using a paper-and-pencil imaginal exposure task to minimize stressful, nontherapeutic exposures and the clinician's need to repeatedly arrange for assessment stimuli (Davis et al. 2013a, b). In fact, the *Behavioral Avoidance Task using Imaginal Exposure* (*BATIE*; Davis et al. 2013a, b) has been found to be an exceptionally good approximation of in vivo BATs; BATIE scores are highly correlated with actual BAT results, they predict approach better than other self-report measures, and they predict specific phobia diagnostic severity better than an in vivo BAT (Davis et al. 2013a, b).

At present, our recommendations for the assessment of a specific phobia in an individual with an ASD would be self-report (if possible independently or even with assistance) or parent-report on the FSSC-R, administration of the ADIS-P (and ADIS-C if possible), and a BAT. In addition, given the complexity of the presentation of anxiety and ASD and the varying levels of functioning of those with the disorder, a detailed assessment of the ASD symptoms themselves should also be conducted (see Chaps. 1–7 of this volume for detailed reviews of these issues). In particular, individuals' communication skills (Davis et al. 2011c, 2012b) and even their *DSM-IV-TR*-type of autism (Davis et al. 2010) have been found to impact anxiety levels. The assessment should also be multi-informant given researchers have found children with ASD and their parents may disagree about which fears are problematic (e.g., Turner and Romanczyk 2012). Finally, a detailed and thorough medical/physical examination should be conducted by an appropriately specialized practitioner to aid in the determination of specific phobia or other condition (e.g., hearing tests may help determine if there is an overall sensitivity to sound versus a phobia of particular noises, swallow studies and a gastroenterologist may help determine if there is an overall issue with an individual's ability to swallow or reflux versus a phobia of swallowing pills, choking, or eating particular foods). The use of these recommended assessments and many other instruments with those who have ASD, however, remains to be fully explored, and assessing those with ASD using instruments designed for typically developing individuals is an ongoing issue that needs resolution (Kerns and Kendall 2012).

Treatment Recommendations

Research investigating the treatment of specific phobia in those with ASD is still in its infancy. Various suggestions exist for modifying cogni-

tive-behavioral approaches for anxiety to use with those also having ASD (e.g., Moree and Davis 2010). Few suggestions, however, exist for applying known efficacious treatments for specific phobia to those with ASD (e.g., Rudy and Davis 2012) or provide evidence for having done so successfully (e.g., Davis et al. 2007). Although some guidelines exist for treating fear and phobia in those with ID (e.g., Jennett and Hagopian 2008), the individual effects of these interventions on ASD in particular have not been singled out.

In neurotypical individuals, exposure-based behavioral, and especially cognitive-behavioral, treatments are currently the best practice (Davis et al. 2011c; Davis and Ollendick 2005; Hood and Antony 2012). Behavioral techniques frequently used to treat specific phobia include reinforced practice, modeling (including participant modeling), and systematic desensitization, all in the context of gradual exposure to the feared stimulus or situation (Davis and Ollendick 2005); these techniques have been used across a wide age range and have even been done successfully with very young children (e.g., a 4- and 5-year-old in May et al. 2013). Reinforced practice is simply reinforcing successive steps along an exposure hierarchy until the individual is interacting with the stimulus or in the situation with minimal to no fear (Davis and Ollendick 2005). Modeling is simply having an individual observe another (the "model") interact with the feared stimulus or situation; participant modeling then involves having the model guide and interact with the observer during the exposure (Davis and Ollendick 2005). Finally, systematic desensitization involves pairing gradual exposure with a response (e.g., relaxation) that is incompatible with the experience of fear (Davis and Ollendick 2005). As it applies to those with ASD, reinforced practice and systematic desensitization have frequently been mischaracterized as "distraction," usually in the context of an individual receiving a preferred item for moving forward with an exposure or having a preferred item (e.g., a teddy bear), while being exposed because it lessens the intensity of the exposure (Davis 2009). As for cognitive-behavioral treatment (CBT), a massed,

3-hour form of cognitive-behavioral exposure therapy, one-session treatment (OST; Davis et al. 2009, 2012c; Öst 1987b, 1989, 1994; Ollendick et al. 2009b) has been found particularly quick, efficacious, and cost effective for children, adolescents, and adults (Davis et al. 2012a, b, c; Ollendick and Davis 2013; Zlomke and Davis 2008). During the massed session, OST uniquely incorporates reinforcement, participant modeling, skills training, and psychoeducation about the feared stimulus, and cognitive challenges all in the context of repeated behavioral experiments (Davis et al. 2009, 2012c). OST has also been found to have a unique benefit—in addition to treating the targeted specific phobia, it has also been found to have a positive impact on other comorbid anxiety disorders in children and adults (Davis et al. 2013b; Ollendick et al. 2010b).

While researchers and practitioners have been cautioned about relying upon downward (i.e., adult to child) and lateral (i.e., neurotypical to ASD or ID) extensions of anxiety and phobia research from those without an ASD to those with an ASD (Davis 2012), the use of behavioral and cognitive-behavioral therapies for specific phobia is not wholly without evidence or merit for those with an ASD (e.g., Davis et al. 2007; Love et al. 1990; Rapp et al. 2005). For example, Davis et al. (2007) were able to use unmodified OST to treat a high-functioning PDD-NOS child's specific phobias of water and heights (see Chap. 12, for a review of CBT and transdiagnostic treatments for anxiety in those with ASD). As well, exposure- and reinforcement-related treatments have been suggested to be well-established techniques for "phobic avoidance" in those with ID, though not necessarily those with ASD (Jennett and Hagopian 2008).

DSM-5: Implications and Thoughts on Changes to ASD and Specific Phobia Diagnoses

Determining the degree to which a new diagnostic criteria set for both specific phobia and ASD will impact the future rates, comorbidity, assessment, and treatment of these disorders is specu-

lative at best and remains an empirical question for the future. For specific phobia, the degree to which *DSM-5* changes indicate there can be fear *or* anxiety may lead to greater confusion with other anxiety disorders (e.g., generalized anxiety disorder). On the other hand, including anxiety and not just fear may promote recognition that often those with a phobia are anxious about and at times preoccupied with future encounters with the feared stimulus and experience those uncontrolled exposures more negatively than others do (Munson et al. 2010). In addition, the application of the 6-month duration criterion across the lifespan may help further distinguish normal fear or transient fear from brief, scary encounters from more stable phobia psychopathology. At the same time, changes in *DSM-5* did little compared to its predecessor to further clarify the developmental progression of fear (especially in children) and the discernment of "normal" developmental fears from childhood phobias.

For the intersection of specific phobia and ASD diagnoses, the impact will likely be felt more intensely. Problems with determining the degree to which phobia symptoms (and anxiety more broadly) are separable from ASD symptoms remain, and the degree to which those symptoms overlap is still poorly understood (Kerns and Kendall 2012). This may be a problem that is especially difficult for comorbidity with specific phobia compared to other disorders (e.g., social anxiety disorder—see Chap. 9—or obsessive-compulsive disorder—see Chap. 8) as the *DSM-5* specifically mentions that other comorbidities and clinicians may be more apt to question how obsessions or social worries are or are not related to an ASD. Given the heterogeneity of specific phobias, however, we would not be surprised to find a fair amount of diagnostic overshadowing as phobias of loud noises, crowds, swallowing pills, eating particular foods, and the like are simply construed as part of the ASD rather than comorbid disorders.

At present, most of the treatment trials and research that has been done with those having an anxiety disorder and ASD have occurred with those who are higher functioning. This will become a particularly difficult issue for the future as it has been suggested that changes from *DSM-5* may, in the worst-case scenario, lead to between one fourth and half of those with a *DSM-IV-TR* ASD diagnosis no longer being diagnosed in *DSM-5* (Davis 2012). While there is now a grandfathering in of those who previously met criteria, this is insufficient to address the increasing prevalence of ASD in the general population and those who have not yet been diagnosed (for more on this issue, see Chaps. 15–17). Of interest to the current discussion, it has been suggested that those who are higher functioning ASD may be disproportionately affected:

> Given research has shown it will likely be the individuals who are higher functioning and have diagnoses of PDD-NOS and Asperger's disorder who will no longer be included in *DSM-5*, at least in the autistic spectrum, this exclusion will have important and serious ramifications on how the study of anxiety in those with ASD will move forward (Davis 2012, p. 361).

Specific phobia is arguably *the* most common disorder overall in the population at large and certainly one of the most common comorbid disorders in those with ASD. Will higher-functioning individuals now just be diagnosed with specific phobia or possibly a piecemeal of diagnoses when they may have previously just been placed on the autism spectrum?

Conclusions

In this chapter, we have examined the role of fear in the typically developing and autistic individual. Current research indicates that fears are normal and typically arise in a predictable developmental progression consistent with cognitive-developmental milestones and life experience. Specific phobias, however, distinguish themselves from these fears by their stability, intensity, and the degree of interference they cause. While specific phobias are among the most prevalent disorders in those on or off the autism spectrum, there is a great deal to be learned in how research on normal fear and specific phobia in those without ASD can be applied and expanded upon for those with ASD. In addition, a number

of assessment and treatment options are available to help individuals with both an ASD and specific phobia; however, the research base for these options needs significant expansion and bolstering.

Davis (2012) points to a variety of challenges and areas for future study that remain for anxiety and ASD researchers to address. Researchers will continue to struggle with the degree to which downward and lateral extensions of the anxiety (and specific phobia) literature is appropriate for those with ASD. While they may remain a launching point for inquiry, we are encouraged to see ASD researchers moving beyond mere adaptations or modifications of existing assessments and treatments (though a great deal more work needs to be done). As well, the use of multiple informants using multiple techniques across multiple settings will need to remain the norm, but the wealth of information that can be obtained will remain a mixed blessing given issues with agreement and disagreement between reporters, techniques, and settings (Davis 2012). The degree to which an individual's intellectual functioning will impact findings is also an area that will need to be more fully explored. Finally, the transition to *DSM-5* will likely remain an issue for the near future as diagnostic criteria, assessment methodologies, treatments, and clinicians, researchers, and families alike adjust. In looking to the future adjustment and research to come, we are hopeful that these growing pains will not be as gloomy as some predict.

Acknowledgments The participation of Thompson E. Davis III was funded in part by the Manship Summer Research Award from the Louisiana State University College of Humanities and Social Sciences. The participation of Thomas H. Ollendick was funded in part by NIMH Grants 1R34MH096915 and 5R21MH094900. The authors are appreciative of this support.

References

American Psychiatric Association. (2000). *Diagnostic and statistical manual of mental disorders* (4th ed., Text revision ed.). Washington, DC: American Psychiatric Association.

American Psychiatric Association. (2013). *Diagnostic and statistical manual of mental disorders* (5th ed.). Arlington: American Psychiatric Publishing.

Barlow, D. H. (2002). *Anxiety and its disorders: The nature and treatment of anxiety and panic*. New York: Guilford.

Centers for Disease Control and Prevention. (2013). Autism spectrum disorders (ASD): Data & statistics. http://www.cdc.gov/ncbddd/autism/data.html Accessed 27 June 2013.

Costello, E. J., Egger, H. L., & Angold, A. (2004). Developmental epidemiology of anxiety disorders. In T. H. Ollendick & J. S. March (Eds.), *Phobic and anxiety disorders in children and adolescents: A clinician's guide to effective psychosocial and pharmacological interventions* (pp. 61–91). New York: Oxford University Press.

Davis, T. E. III (2009). PTSD, anxiety, and phobias. In J. Matson, F. Andrasik, & M. Matson (Eds.), *Treating childhood psychopathology and developmental disorders* (pp. 183–220). New York: Springer.

Davis, T. E. III (2012). Where to from here for ASD and anxiety? Lessons learned from child anxiety and the issue of DSM-5. *Clinical Psychology: Science and Practice, 19,* 358–363.

Davis, T. E. III, & Ollendick, T. H. (2005). Empirically supported treatments for specific phobia in children: Do efficacious treatments address the components of a phobic response? *Clinical Psychology: Science and Practice, 12,* 144–160.

Davis, T. E. III, & Ollendick, T. H. (2011). Specific phobia. In D. McKay & E. Storch (Eds.), *Handbook of child and adolescent anxiety disorders* (pp. 231–244). New York: Springer.

Davis, T. E. III, Kurtz, P., Gardner, A., & Carman, N. (2007). Cognitive-behavioral treatment for specific phobias with a child demonstrating severe problem behavior and developmental delays. *Research in Developmental Disabilities, 28,* 546–558.

Davis, T. E. III, Ollendick, T. H., & Öst, L. G. (2009). Intensive treatment of specific phobias in children and adolescents. *Cognitive and Behavioral Practice, 16,* 294–303.

Davis, T. E. III, Fodstad, J. C., Jenkins, W., Hess, J. A., Moree, B. N., Dempsey, T., & Matson, J. L. (2010). Anxiety and avoidance in infants and toddlers with autism spectrum disorders: Evidence for differing symptom severity and presentation. *Research in Autism Spectrum Disorders, 4,* 305–313.

Davis, T. E. III, Hess, J. A., Moree, B. N., Fodstad, J. C., Dempsey, T., Jenkins, W., & Matson, J. L. (2011a). Anxiety symptoms across the lifespan in people with autistic disorder. *Research in Autism Spectrum Disorders, 5,* 112–118.

Davis, T. E. III, May, A. C., & Whiting, S. E. (2011b). Evidence-based treatment of anxiety and phobia in children and adolescents: Current status and effects on the emotional response. *Clinical Psychology Review, 31,* 592–602.

Davis, T. E. III, Moree, B., Dempsey, T., Reuther, E., Fodstad, J., Hess, J., Matson, J. L., et al. (2011c). The relationship between autism spectrum disorders and anxiety: The moderating effect of communication. *Research in Autism Spectrum Disorders, 5,* 324–329.

Davis, T. E. III, Jenkins, W., & Rudy, B. (2012a). Empirical status of one-session treatment. In T. E. Davis III, T. Ollendick, & L. Öst (Eds.), *Intensive one-session treatment of specific phobias* (pp. 209–226). New York: Springer.

Davis, T. E. III, Moree, B., Dempsey, T., Hess, J., Jenkins, W., Fodstad, J., & Matson, J. L. (2012b). The effects of communication deficits on anxiety symptoms in infants and toddlers with autism spectrum disorders. *Behavior Therapy, 43,* 142–152.

Davis, T. E. III, Ollendick, T. H., & Öst, L. G. (Eds.). (2012c). *Intensive one-session treatment of specific phobias.* New York: Springer.

Davis, T. E. III, Reuther, E., May, A., Rudy, B., Munson, M., Jenkins, W., & Whiting, S. (2013a). The behavioral avoidance task using imaginal exposure (BATIE): A paper- and-pencil version of traditional in vivo behavioral avoidance tasks. *Psychological Assessment, 25,* 1111–1119.

Davis, T. E. III, Reuther, E., & Rudy, B. (2013b). One-session treatment of a specific phobia of swallowing pills: A case study. *Clinical Case Studies, 12,* 399–410.

Evans, D., Canavera, K., Kleinpeter, L., Maccubbin, E., & Taga, K. (2005). The fears, phobias and anxieties of children with autism spectrum disorders and Down syndrome: Comparisons with developmentally and chronologically age matched children. *Child Psychiatry and Human Development, 36,* 3–26.

Gibson, E. J., & Walk, R. D. (1960). The "visual cliff." *Scientific American, 202,* 64–71.

Grills-Taquechel, A. E., & Ollendick, T. H. (2012). *Phobic and anxiety disorders in youth.* Cambridge: Hogrefe & Huber.

Gullone, E. (2000). The development of normal fear: A century of research. *Clinical Psychology Review, 20,* 429–451.

Hagopian, L., & Jennett, H. (2008). Behavioral assessment and treatment of anxiety in individuals with intellectual disabilities and autism. *Journal of Developmental and Physical Disabilities, 20,* 467–483.

Hodgson, R., & Rachman, S. (1974). Desynchrony in measures of fear. *Behaviour Research and Therapy, 12,* 319–326.

Hood, H. K., & Antony, M. M. (2012). Evidence-based assessment and treatment of specific phobias in adults. In T. E. Davis III, T. H. Ollendick, & L.-G. Öst (Eds.), *Intensive one-session treatment of specific phobias* (pp. 19–42). New York: Springer.

Jennett, H., & Hagopian, L. (2008). Identifying empirically supported treatments for phobic disorders in individuals with intellectual disabilities. *Behavior Therapy, 39,* 151–161.

Kanner, L. (1943). Autistic disturbances of affective contact. *Nervous Child, 2,* 217–250.

Kerns, C. M., & Kendall, P. C. (2012). The presentation and classification of anxiety in autism spectrum disorder. *Clinical Psychology: Science & Practice, 19,* 323–347.

Kessler, R. C., Zhao, S., Katz, S., Kouzis, A., Frank, R., Edlund, M., & Leaf, P. (1999). Past-year use of outpatient services for psychiatric problems in the National Comorbidity Survey. *American Journal of Psychiatry, 156,* 115–123.

Kessler, R., Berglund, P., Demler, O., Jin, R., Merikangas, K. R., & Walters, E. E. (2005a). Lifetime prevalence and age-of-onset distributions of DSM-IV disorders in the National Comorbidity Survey Replication. *Archives of General Psychiatry, 62,* 593–602.

Kessler, R., Chiu, W. T., Demler, O., Merikangas, K. R., & Walters, E. E. (2005b). Prevalence, severity and comorbidity of 12-month DSM-IV disorders in the National Comorbidity Survey Replication. *Archives of General Psychiatry, 62,* 617–627.

Kessler, R., Petukhova, M., Sampson, N., Zaslavsky, A., & Wittchen, H. (2012). Twelve-month and lifetime prevalence and lifetime morbid risk of anxiety and mood disorders in the United States. *International Journal of Methods in Psychiatric Research, 21,* 169–184.

King, N. J., Hamilton, D. I., & Ollendick, T. H. (1988). *Children's phobias: A behavioural perspective.* London: Wiley.

Lane, B., & Gullone, E. (1999). Common fears: A comparison of adolescents' self-generated and fear survey schedule generated fears. *The Journal of Genetic Psychology, 160,* 194–204.

Lang, P. (1979). A bio-informational theory of emotional imagery. *Psychophysiology, 16,* 495–512.

Last, C. G., Perrin, S., Hersen, M., & Kazdin, A. (1992). DSM-III-R anxiety disorders in children: Sociodemographic and clinical characteristics. *Journal of the American Academy of Child & Adolescent Psychiatry, 31,* 1070–1076.

Leyfer, O. T., Folstein, S. E., Bacalman, S., Davis, N. O., Dinh, E., Morgan, J., Lainhart, J., et al. (2006). Comorbid psychiatric disorders in children with autism: Interview development rates of disorders. *Journal of Autism and Developmental Disorders, 36,* 86–97.

Love, S., Matson, J. L., & West, D. (1990). Mothers as effective therapists for autistic children's phobias. *Journal of Applied Behavior Analysis, 23,* 379–385.

Magee, W. J., Eaton, W. W., Wittchen, H. U., McGonagle, K. A., & Kessler, R. C. (1996). Agoraphobia, simple phobia, and social phobia in the National Comorbidity Survey. *Archives of General Psychiatry, 53,* 159–168.

Mason, J., & Scior, K. (2004). "Diagnostic overshadowing" amongst clinicians working with people with intellectual disabilities in the UK. *Journal of Applied Research in Intellectual Disabilities, 17*(2), 85–90.

Matson, J. L., & Love, S. R. (1990). A comparison of parent-reported fear for autistic and non-handicapped age-matched children and youth. *Australian and New Zealand Journal of Developmental Disabilities, 16,* 349–357.

Matson, J. L., & Nebel-Schwalm, M. (2007). Comorbid psychopathology with autism spectrum disorder in children: An overview. *Research in Developmental Disabilities, 28,* 341–352.

Matson, J. L., & Sevin, J. (1994). Theories of dual diagnosis in mental retardation. *Journal of Consulting and Clinical Psychology, 62,* 6–16.

Matson, J. L., & Shoemaker, M. (2009). Intellectual disability and its relationship to autism spectrum disorders. *Research in Developmental Disabilities, 30,* 1107–1114.

May, A., Rudy, B., Davis, T. E. III, & Matson, J. (2013). Evidence-based behavioral treatment of dog phobia with young children: Case examples. *Behavior Modification, 37,* 143–160.

Mayes, S. D., Calhoun, R. A., Aggarwal, R., Baker, C., Mathapati, S., Molitoris, S., & Mayes, R. (2013). Unusual fears in children with autism. *Research in Autism Spectrum Disorders, 7,* 151–158.

Milne, J. M., Garrison, C. Z., Addy, C. L., McKeowen, R. E., Jackson, K. L., Cuffe, S. P., & Waller, J. L. (1995). Frequency of phobic disorder in a community sample of young adolescents. *Journal of the American Academy of Child and Adolescent Psychiatry, 34,* 1202–1211.

Mineka, S., & Zinbarg, R. (2006). A contemporary learning theory perspective on the etiology of anxiety disorders. *American Psychologist, 61,* 10–26.

Moree, B., & Davis, T. E. III (2010). Cognitive-behavioral therapy for anxiety in children diagnosed with autism spectrum disorders: Modification trends. *Research in Autism Spectrum Disorders, 4,* 346–354.

Munson, M., Davis, T. E. III, Grills-Taquechel, A., & Zlomke, K. (2010). The effects of Hurricane Katrina on females with a preexisting fear of storms. *Current Psychology, 29,* 307–319.

Muris, P., & Merkelbach, H. (2000). How serious are common childhood fears? II. The parent's point of view. *Behaviour Research and Therapy, 38,* 813–818.

Muris, P., & Merckelbach, H. (2012). Specific phobia: Phenomenology, epidemiology, and etiology. In T. E. Davis III, T. H. Ollendick, & L.-G. Öst (Eds.), *Intensive one-session treatment of specific phobias* (pp. 3–18). New York: Springer.

Muris, P., Steerneman, P., Merckelbach, H., Holdrinet, I., & Meesters, C. (1998). Comorbid anxiety symptoms in children with pervasive developmental disorders. *Journal of Anxiety Disorders, 12,* 387–393.

Muris, P., Merkelbach, H., Mayer, B., & Prins, E. (2000). How serious are common childhood fears? *Behaviour Research and Therapy, 38,* 217–228.

Nebel-Schwalm, M., & Davis, T. E. III (2011). Preliminary factor and psychometric analysis of the Motivation for Fear (MOTIF) Survey. *Journal of Anxiety Disorders, 25,* 731–740.

Nebel-Schwalm, M., & Davis, T. E. III (2013). Nature and etiological models of anxiety disorders. In E. Storch & D. McKay (Eds.), *Handbook of treating variants and complications in anxiety disorders* (pp. 3–21). New York: Springer.

Ollendick, T. H. (1983). Reliability and validity of the Revised Fear Survey Schedule for Children (FSSC-R). *Behaviour Research and Therapy, 21,* 395–399.

Ollendick, T. H., & Davis, T. E. III (2013). One-session treatment for specific phobias: A review of Öst's single-session exposure with children and adolescents. *Cognitive Behaviour Therapy, 42,* 275–283.

Ollendick, T. H., Hagopian, L. P., & King, N. J. (1997). Specific phobias in children. In G. C. L. Davey (Ed.), *Phobias: A handbook of theory, research and treatment* (pp. 201–223). London: Wiley.

Ollendick, T. H., Davis, T. E. III, & Muris, P. (2004). Treatment of specific phobia in children and adolescents. In P.

Barrett & T. H. Ollendick (Eds.), *The handbook of interventions that work with children and adolescents: Prevention to treatment* (pp. 273–300). West Sussex: Wiley

Ollendick, T. H., Davis, T. E. III, & Sirbu, C. V. (2009a). Specific phobias. In D. McKay & E. Storch (Eds.), *Cognitive behavior therapy for children: Treating complex and refractory cases* (pp. 171–199). New York: Springer.

Ollendick, T. H., Öst, L. G., Reuterskiöld, L., Costa, N., Cederlund, R., Sirbu, C., Jarrett, M., et al. (2009b). One-session treatment of specific phobias in youth: A randomized clinical trial in the USA and Sweden. *Journal of Consulting and Clinical Psychology, 77,* 504–516.

Ollendick, T. H., Raishevich, N., Davis, T. E. III, Sirbu, C. V., & Öst, L. G. (2010a). Specific phobia in youth: Phenomenology and psychological characteristics. *Behavior Therapy, 41,* 133–141.

Ollendick, T. H., Öst, L. G., Reuterskiöld, L., & Costa, N. (2010b). Comorbidity in youth with specific phobias: Impact of comorbidity on treatment outcome and the impact of treatment on comorbid disorders. *Behaviour Research and Therapy, 48,* 827–831.

Ollendick, T. H., Allen, B., Benoit, K., & Cowart, M. J. (2011). The tripartite model of fear in children with specific phobias: Assessing concordance and discordance using the behavioral approach test. *Behaviour Research and Therapy, 49,* 459–465.

Ollendick, T. H., Lewis, K., Cowart, M., & Davis, T. E. III (2012). Prediction of child performance on a parent-child behavioral approach test with animal phobic children. *Behavior Modification, 36,* 509–524.

Öst, L. G. (1987a). Age of onset in different phobias. *Journal of Abnormal Psychology, 96,* 223–229.

Öst, L.-G. (1987b). One-session treatments for a case of multiple simple phobias. *Scandinavian Journal of Behavior Therapy, 16,* 175–184.

Öst, L.-G. (1989). One-session treatment for specific phobias. *Behaviour Research and Therapy, 27,* 1–7.

Öst, L.-G., Svensson, L., Hellström, K., & Lindwall, R. (2001). One-session treatment of specific phobias in youths: A randomized clinical trial. *Journal of Consulting and Clinical Psychology, 69,* 814–824.

Paclawskyj, T. R., Matson, J. L., Rush, K. S., Smalls, Y., & Vollmer, T. R. (2000). Questions about behavioral function (QABF): A behavioral checklist for functional assessment of aberrant behavior. *Research in Developmental Disabilities, 21,* 223–229.

Rachman, S. (1998). *Anxiety.* East Sussex: Psychology Press.

Rachman, S., & Hodgson, R. (1974). Synchrony and desynchrony in fear and avoidance. *Behaviour Research and Therapy, 12,* 311–318.

Rapp, J., Vollmer, T., & Hovanetz, A. (2005). Evaluation and treatment of swimming pool avoidance exhibited by an adolescent girl with autism. *Behavior Therapy, 36,* 101–105.

Rudy, B., & Davis, T. E. III (2012). Interventions for specific phobia in special populations. In T. E. Davis III, T. H. Ollendick, & L.-G. Öst (Eds.), *Intensive one-session treatment of specific phobias* (pp. 177–193). New York: Springer.

Rutter, M., & Schopler, E. (1987). Autism and pervasive developmental disorders: Concepts and diagnostic issues. *Journal of Autism and Developmental Disorders, 17,* 159–186.

Silverman, W. K., & Albano, A. M. (1996). *Anxiety disorders interview schedule for DSM-IV, child and parent versions.* San Antonio: Psychological Corporation.

Silverman, W. K., & Ollendick, T. H. (2005). Evidence-based assessment of anxiety and its disorders in children and adolescents. *Journal of Clinical Child and Adolescent Psychology, 34,* 380–411.

Silverman, W. K., Kurtines, W. M., Ginsburg, G. S., Weems, C. F., Rabian, B., & Serafini, L. T. (1999). Contingency management, self-control, and education support in the treatment of childhood phobic disorders: A randomized clinical trial. *Journal of Consulting and Clinical Psychology, 67,* 675–687.

Stinson, F. S., Dawson, D. A., Chou, S. P., Smith, S., Goldstein, R. B., Ruan, W. J., & Grant, B. (2007). The epidemiology of DSM-IV specific phobia in the USA: Results from the National Epidemiologic Survey on alcohol and related conditions. *Psychological Medicine, 37,* 1047–1059.

Sukhodolsky, D. G., Scahill, L., Gadow, K. D., Arnold, L. E., Aman, M. G., McDougle, C. J., Vitiello, B., et al. (2008). Parent-rated anxiety symptoms in children with pervasive developmental disorders: Frequency and association with core autism symptoms and cognitive functioning. *Journal of Abnormal Child Psychology, 36,* 117–128.

Turner, L. B., & Romanczyk, R. G. (2012). Assessment of fear in children with an autism spectrum disorder. *Research in Autism Spectrum Disorders, 6,* 1203–1210.

van Steensel, F., Bögels, S., & Perrin, S. (2011). Anxiety disorders in children and adolescents with autism spectrum disorders: A meta-analysis. *Clinical Child and Family Psychology Review, 14,* 302–317.

van Steensel, F., Bögels, S., & Dirksen, C. (2012). Anxiety and quality of life: Clinically anxious children with and without autism spectrum disorders compared. *Journal of Clinical Child & Adolescent Psychology, 41,* 731–738.

White, S. W., Oswald, D., Ollendick, T. H., & Scahill, L. (2009). Anxiety in children and adolescents with autism spectrum disorders. *Clinical Psychology Review, 29,* 216–229.

Wing, L. (1981). Asperger's syndrome: A clinical account. *Psychological Medicine, 11,* 115–129.

Wing, L., & Gould, J. (1979). Severe impairments of social interaction and associated abnormalities in children: Epidemiology and classification. *Journal of Autism and Developmental Disorders, 9,* 11–30.

Zlomke, K., & Davis, T. E. III (2008). One-session treatment of specific phobias: A detailed description and review of treatment efficacy. *Behavior Therapy, 39,* 207–223.

Part III

Assessment and Treatment

Behavioral Assessment and Treatment for Anxiety for Those with Autism Spectrum Disorder

11

Louis Hagopian and Heather Jennett

Introduction

Anxiety has been described as a constellation of responses to a potential threat that includes behaviors from multiple response domains—specifically, behavioral, physiological, verbal/cognitive, and subjective (Davis and Ollendick 2005). In contrast to adaptive anxiety, where a potentially harmful stimulus is avoided, an anxiety disorder is said to exist when the avoided stimulus poses little actual risk, or when the avoidance generalizes to a broader class of stimuli to the extent that the individual's functioning is impaired. Traditional two-factor learning models of anxiety posit that anxiety disorders are established and maintained though a conditioning process involving Pavlovian and operant conditioning (Mowrer 1960). This process involves the pairing of a neutral stimulus with an aversive event (via Pavlovian conditioning); and then escape and avoidance of the conditioned aversive stimulus is maintained through negative reinforcement. Among higher functioning individuals, conditioning or associations between aversive events and neutral stimuli do not need be directly experienced but may emerge via transfer of function

(Friman et al. 1998) or higher-order conditioning. The extent to which the individual's functioning is impaired due to avoidance depends on several factors, including how ubiquitous the avoided stimulus is in everyday life, the negative consequences or "costs" of avoiding it, and subjective distress associated with the experience (though this latter factor may not be difficult to determine in some individuals).

Special Considerations for ASD

Autism spectrum disorder (ASD) represents a heterogeneous diagnostic category in terms of intellectual functioning, communication skills, repetitive behavior, and psychiatric comorbidities (Myers and Johnson 2007). Limited communication skills and social impairments commonly present in ASD limit the extent to which the individual can self-report thoughts, affective states, and physiological sensations—making it more challenging to identify the subjective experiences of fear and anxiety. Therefore, it is important to have a working definition of anxiety that is applicable across the ASD continuum. We define anxiety here as a constellation of responses (including avoidant behavior, facial expressions indicative of fear and distress, and increased physiological arousal) that are occasioned by stimuli that signal potential punishment, and maintained by escape or avoidance of those stimuli. For persons with ASD who are able to verbally describe internal events (thoughts, feelings, physiological

L. Hagopian (✉)
The Kennedy Krieger Institute and Johns Hopkins University School of Medicine, Baltimore, MD, USA
e-mail: hagopian@kennedykrieger.org

H. Jennett
Little Leaves Behavioral Services, Silver Spring, MD, USA

responses), these would be self-characterized as being aversive themselves and self-labeled using terms such as fear, anxiety, panic, etc.

Another challenge to determining the presence of anxiety in a person with ASD arises from the fact that anxiety and ASD share some common features, making it difficult to determine if behaviors typically thought of as symptomatic of anxiety (e.g., avoidance of certain situations) are actually secondary to ASD itself or indicative of the presence of anxiety (see Chaps. 7, 8, 9, and 10 for a detailed discussion of these issues). For example, avoidance of social interaction and other specific situations are the primary features of certain anxiety disorders (e.g., social phobia and specific phobia)—yet these behaviors are commonly seen in many individuals with ASD, including those who are not suspected of being anxious (Kuusikko et al. 2008). Similarly, repetitive and ritualistic behaviors that are the hallmarks of obsessive–compulsive disorder (OCD) are also commonly observed in many persons with ASD (McDougle et al. 1995; Zandt et al. 2007)—including those individuals that are not suspected of being anxious.

Another issue that complicates the assessment of anxiety in persons with ASD is that individuals with ASD are at increased risk for engaging in problem behavior (e.g., aggression, self-injury, and property destruction)—often to avoid or escape situations. This occurs in approximately 25 % of cases (Hagopian et al. 2013; Hanley et al. 2003), and can be associated with emotional distress—which can raise questions about whether anxiety may be present. Determining whether this is indicative of anxiety or simply the avoidance of nonpreferred or mildly aversive situations, such as academic tasks, can sometimes be challenging. We use the term *simple avoidance* to refer to avoidance of nonpreferred stimuli or situations (e.g., wearing shoes, participating in certain instructional tasks) that is not associated with seemingly anxious or fearful behavior—based on observation of facial expressions, affect, and physiological arousal traditionally associated with anxiety (and the absence of self-report indicative of anxiety in those who are able to communicate this). In contrast, we use the term

anxious avoidance to refer to avoidant behavior that is associated with traditional indicators of anxiety (including facial expressions indicative of fear, increased physiological arousal, and self-reported anxiety in those who are able to report). Thus, the distinction between these two types of avoidant behavior is based on the presence or absence of some indicator of emotional distress and subjective states characteristic of anxiety. When anxious avoidance markedly interferes with functioning, then this would constitute an *anxiety disorder* (which particular diagnosis obviously depends on the nature of the feared stimulus and the response). This most often occurs when the avoided stimulus is encountered frequently (e.g., riding in a car, going into a restroom), and/or when avoidance comes at a high cost (e.g., avoiding examinations by a physician, getting a medically indicated injection). Thus, we argue that not all avoidant behavior in ASD is associated with anxiety, and not all anxiety in ASD would constitute an anxiety disorder per se.

Behavioral Assessment

The overarching goal of behavioral assessment is to formulate hypotheses regarding the controlling antecedent and consequent variables. Obviously, this must be done within the broader social and developmental context. The issues previously noted suggest one must consider the following: (1) social avoidance and ritualistic behaviors indicative of anxiety disorders in typically developing persons are routinely observed in ASD, including among those not suspected of being anxious; and (2) individuals with ASD (and intellectual disabilities; ID) often engage in avoidant behavior that may not necessarily be associated with anxiety. Another consideration is that both children and adults with ASD are more dependent on care providers (Shattuck et al. 2012) than typically developing peers—so behavioral assessment must include an analysis of the interactions between the individual with ASD and care providers.

In light of the unique challenges to the assessment of anxiety in ASD, the clinician's first goal upon encountering a person with ASD referred for treatment of possible anxiety should be to ascertain whether the presenting problems are indeed due to anxiety (i.e., anxious avoidance), or represent simple avoidance. Caution should be taken to not assume the presence of anxiety (or dismiss it) based on how the presenting complaint is labeled by care providers (or even by the individual himself or herself). Rather, multimodal, multi-informant behavioral assessment should be initiated to determine this. Multimodal assessment includes a range of assessment modalities, including direct observation of behavior, observation of affect, and measurement of physiological responding, as well as self-reported cognitions and affective states. (King et al. 1997; MacNeil et al. 2009; Velting et al. 2004)

For individuals with ASD (or other developmental disorders), one must also consider this information in the context of the individual's skills and skills deficits related to ASD (as well as the level of intellectual functioning). In the case of ASD in particular, core skills deficits may contribute to the development of both simple avoidance and anxious avoidance. For example, communication deficits that limit one's ability to ask for assistance with work or to request a break from work can lead to the establishment of escape-maintained problem behavior (i.e., simple avoidance). Deficits in social skills may result in embarrassing social interactions for higher functioning individuals with ASD, which then may result in social anxiety (White et al. 2010; see Chap. 9). Sensory stimulation may be experienced differently by people who have ASD, to the extent that stimuli that would be neutral or benign to most individuals (e.g., certain noises, the touch of water) appear to be highly aversive to some with ASD.

For many parents, observing one's child in an anxious or upset state is often unpleasant and anxiety inducing itself. A parent reacting to an anxious child in a way that reduces child anxiety (e.g., by permitting the child to avoid the feared situation) may also reduce the parent's anxiety and thus reinforce those parent behaviors that inadvertently reinforced the child's avoidant behavior—resulting in a maladaptive self-sustaining parent–child interaction. Although avoidant behavior is, by definition, maintained by negative reinforcement, behavioral assessment must also attempt to determine what, if any, other reinforcing consequences may be obtained. Understanding these parent–child interactions is important for understanding the broader context in which anxiety occurs, and has important implications for designing treatment in a way that will increase the probability of parental adherence to recommendations. That is, it might be necessary to include treatment components aimed at minimizing and managing parental anxiety during the child's treatment in cases where a parent has a very low tolerance for his/her child becoming anxious. An understanding of the antecedents, behavioral skills and deficits, and controlling consequences—including interactions with care providers—is important not only for guiding the development of an individualized treatment plan but also for adherence to recommendations (Reaven & Hepburn 2006). Behavioral assessment methods described below include screening and diagnostic instruments, behavioral interviews, direct observation of behavior, and physiological measures.

Behavioral Interviews

Interviews should be conducted with individuals with ASD to the extent possible with consideration of the individual's cognitive and language capabilities (Blakeley-Smith et al. 2012). For some individuals with ASD, cognitive and communication deficits and difficulties identifying emotions may make the assessment of cognitions, and affective and physiological states through self-report very challenging, and in some cases not possible at all (Baron-Cohen 2002; Ollendick et al. 1993). Consequently, when assessing possible anxiety in ASD, interviews may rely mostly, or completely, on the report of other informants (typically, parents and other care providers). Information should be gathered on the nature of the anxiety response, collateral behaviors (including other problem behaviors such as aggression and self-injury), the relevant antecedents that occasion anxiety, as well as the consequences the behavior produces. Information provided by respondents regarding the individual's affective states can help determine whether the behavior of concern is simple avoidance or anxious avoidance.

When interviewing care providers, it is important to distinguish between the respondent's observation of events versus his or her interpretation of what the individual with ASD may be experiencing and why. In light of limited communication skills and overlapping features of ASD and anxiety, care providers are subject to the same challenges as clinicians in making attributions about behavior. For example, a parent may characterize a child as having "OCD" based on observations of repetitive, ritualistic behavior. While care providers' own hypotheses about the individual's anxiety may be useful, the clinician must also gather descriptive information and form his or her own hypotheses. In particular, it is important to identify what situations or stimuli the child avoids, elicit escape, and occasion negative emotional states suggesting anxiety (e.g., fearful facial expressions, crying, shaking, and panic-like states). For individuals who are unable to verbally express fear or a desire to avoid a situation, avoidance sometimes occurs in the form of dropping or running off, and may co-occur with problem behavior such as aggression, property destruction, and self-injury—particularly when initial attempts to avoid or escape are ineffective (Hagopian et al. 2001; Ricciardi et al. 2006). Although avoidant and escape responses are generally maintained by negative reinforcement, it is important to also determine how care providers respond. Reactions on the part of care providers, including attention (in the form of consoling the individual or talking about his/her anxiety), as well as providing access to preferred activities, can further reinforce these behaviors. Thus, in some cases, avoidant behaviors may be maintained by negative reinforcement in the form of escape/avoidance of the feared stimulus and by positive reinforcement in the form of attention or access preferred activities. The interview can also provide information about how the individu-

al's anxiety affects the care provider and how he/she might respond.

Screening and Diagnostic Instruments

In general, screening and diagnostic instruments can be important tools to use in order to assess whether the individual meets formal diagnostic criteria for an anxiety disorder. However, there are multiple issues to consider when using these measures with individuals with ASD as well as limited guidance from the literature to date (White and Roberson-Nay 2009). Currently, there are two categories of instruments available for the assessment of anxiety in individuals with ASD. These include (1) instruments designed to assess a broad range of psychopathology, including anxiety disorders, in individuals with ASD and (2) instruments originally designed to assess anxiety in typically developing individuals, which have been extended to individuals with ASD.

Instruments Designed to Assess a Broad Spectrum of Psychopathology in Individuals with ASD There are only a few instruments that have been developed specifically for the ASD population. These involve both semi-structured interviews and rating scales. All of these instruments are in their infancy and require additional study of their psychometric properties.

The Autism Comorbidity Interview—Present and Lifetime Version (ACI-PL; Leyfer et al. 2006) is a semi-structured diagnostic interview based on the Kiddie Schedule for Affective Disorders and Schizophrenia (KSADS; Ambrosini 2000). It was modified to make it appropriate for use with individuals having ASD; and has been designed to distinguish whether impairment is due to a comorbid psychiatric disorder or due to the core features of ASD. Some of the modifications include questions to establish the child's emotions and behaviors at his/her best in order to obtain a baseline, as well as additional screening questions about common observable features and presenting concerns of parents of children with

ASD to determine whether the potential comorbid disorder is applicable. Thus far, the ACI-PL has been found to be reliable and valid only for certain psychiatric disorders, with OCD as the only anxiety disorder (Leyfer et al. 2006). However, in relation to other commonly used scales to assess for psychiatric comorbities in ASD, the ACI-PL yielded the fewest false positives (Mazefsky et al. 2011).

The Autism Spectrum Disorders—Comorbidity for Children (ASD-CC; Matson and Wilkins 2008) and the Baby and Infant Screen for Children with Autism Traits (BISCUIT—Part 2; Matson et al. 2009b) are informant-based rating scales used to examine comorbid psychopathology, including anxiety in children with ASD. Both scales were designed to be part of a comprehensive assessment battery for diagnosing ASD, comorbid psychopathology, and challenging behavior in children and adolescents. Parents or other caregivers are asked to endorse items on a 3-point Likert scale. The ASD-CC was designed for children with ASD aged 3–17, and the BISCUIT was designed for toddlers with ASD aged 17–37 months. Factor analyses of each scale have yielded factors specifically related to anxiety and avoidance behaviors (Matson et al. 2009a; Matson et al. 2011). Both scales have good reliability (Matson and Wilkins 2008; Matson et al. 2009b) and the ASD-CC has good validity (Matson et al. 2009a).

Instruments Designed for Typically Developing Children and Extended to Individuals with ASD There are several well-established instruments developed to assess anxiety in typically developing children. Although many of these instruments have been extended to individuals with ASD, few have been tested for reliability or validity in this population. One possible limitation in using these instruments is the presence of overlapping symptoms between ASD and anxiety disorders. A couple of studies have looked at whether a clinical diagnosis of an anxiety disorder can be identified after eliminating the items targeted the overlapping symptoms or making other modifications (e.g., Kuusikko et al. 2008; Sukhodolsky et al. 2008) and have yielded

improved validity. However, this research is still in its infancy and great caution still needs to be taken when using these tools (Davis 2012). Further, as with typically developing children, they should never be used in isolation to make a diagnosis of an anxiety disorder.

The most common instruments in this category involve semi-structured interviews, self-report measures, and informant-based rating scales. The Anxiety Disorders Interview Schedule Child and Parent Version (ADIS-C/P; Silverman and Albano 1996) is a commonly utilized semi-structured interview based on *DSM-IV* (APA 2000) criteria. Its reliability and validity are well established with typically developing children (Silverman et al. 2001; Wood et al. 2002) but not with children with ASD. Aside from this interview, there are many rating scales available for the assessment of anxiety in typically developing children, but the ones most widely adapted to this population include the Revised Children's Manifest Anxiety Scale (RCMAS; Reynolds and Richmond 1985), the Multidimensional Anxiety Scale for Children (MASC; March 1997), the Spence Children's Anxiety Scale (SCAS; Spence 1997), and the Screen for Child Anxiety and Related Emotional Disorders (SCARED; Birmaher et al. 1999). The latter three scales also have parent versions available.

Although the self-report versions of these scales generally have good psychometric properties for typically developing children (Silverman and Ollendick 2005), they should be used with caution with individuals with ASD who have cognitive challenges (White and Roberson-Nay 2009), as well as difficulties with emotion recognition (Baron-Cohen 2002). Very little research has been conducted on the accuracy of self-report in this population and the research that does exist has mixed results (Farrugia and Hudson 2006; Russell and Sofronoff 2005). A recent study suggested that there may be better agreement between child and parent report on some anxiety symptoms in more verbal individuals with ASD (Blakeley-Smith et al. 2012). However, questions still remain about agreement between parent and child report about anxiety symptoms, as well as whose report is the most accurate (Davis

2012). Until more research has been conducted to determine the validity of self-report in individuals with ASD, caution should be exercised (Mazefsky et al. 2011). Nevertheless, since these instruments are designed to obtain self-report of subjective states, the information they provide could help distinguish between simple and anxious avoidance.

Direct Observation of Behavior

Though more effortful and time consuming than other methods of assessment, direct observation of the apparently anxious or avoidant behavior is essential. Findings from the interviews with the individual and care providers and from self- and other-report measures will help one determine the appropriate methods for conducting direct observation. Once the stimuli that occasion avoidant behavior have been identified, it will be necessary to distinguish between those that can be presented in a controlled manner from those that cannot. For example, some studies have described cases in which anxiety was elicited by specific stimuli such as water, needles, or dental care (Conyers et al. 2004; Rapp et al. 2005; Shabani and Fisher 2006). Certain anxiety disorders, such as specific phobias, social phobia, and separation anxiety disorder, and OCD are characterized by anxiety that is elicited by a specific stimulus or classes of stimuli (APA 2013). In these cases, presentation of the avoided stimulus in a controlled fashion may be possible. In other cases, however, the stimuli that occasion avoidance may be difficult to identify or control. For example, individuals with generalized anxiety disorder may not be able to identify specific stimuli that reliably elicit fear. Some stimuli may be identifiable but difficult to present and terminate with the level of control required in treatment—such as the behavior of peers and certain internal stimuli (e.g., physiological sensations). Another consideration, which may be more relevant for higher functioning individuals with ASD, is whether the individual may be reactive to contrived presentation conditions.

Behavioral Monitoring In cases where the avoided stimulus cannot be readily presented in a controlled manner (or in cases where the individual may behave differently when being observed), enlisting care providers to conduct behavioral monitoring in the natural setting can be highly effective. In contrast to self- and other-report measures, which involve standard questions and the retrospective reporting of behavioral patterns or tendencies, behavioral monitoring involves the observation and recording of behaviors targeted for that particular individual—ideally, in real time. For example, behavioral monitoring may involve a care provider recording each time the individual engages in an avoidant or apparently anxious behavior that has been operationally defined a priori (e.g., dropping to the floor and crying). The monitoring form would allow the care provider to record observable antecedents and consequences for this behavior; describe the behavior itself; provide some rating of the apparent level of distress based on observable indices of affect such as crying, trembling, or facial expressions (which is important to determining the presence of anxious avoidance); and record the date and time of the event. In addition to helping to identify antecedents and consequences during the assessment phase, data obtained using behavioral monitoring during the assessment phase can be used to establish a pretreatment baseline for the purpose of evaluate treatment outcomes. Parental monitoring of anxiety in children without ASD has been reported in several studies (Chorpita et al. 1996; Hagopian and Slifer 1993; Hagopian et al. 1990). Although all of these examples involved children without ASD, a similar type of monitoring can also be used with children with ASD, and in cases where the avoided stimulus cannot be readily controlled (or the individual may be reactive to contrived in-clinic sessions) may be the only source of direct behavioral observation data.

Behavioral Avoidance Test In cases where the avoided stimulus is identifiable and can be presented in a controlled fashion (e.g., insects), it may be possible to arrange conditions to directly observe the response in vivo. This could involve creating a behavioral avoidance test (BAT; Dadds et al. 1994) which is a highly structured method of assessing avoidant behavior associated with the avoided stimulus. Generally, this procedure involves progressively exposing the individual to the stimulus along some dimension (e.g., physical distance between person and stimulus, time person can remain near the stimulus), and recording the point at which the avoidant response is displayed, and/or anxiety is reported. BATs can be highly individualized based on the specific stimuli that elicit avoidance in the person being observed. In addition to the benefit of observing the individual's responses (including avoidance/escape, facial expressions, physiological arousal, and self-report that would suggest anxious avoidance) directly and in a controlled manner, one can use the same method of stimulus presentation during graduated exposure treatment (see the following section on treatment). For individuals with ASD who are unable to self-report, some form of BAT is essential during assessment and in treatment evaluation. Many of the available clinical case studies that report on the assessment and treatment of anxiety in this population describe the use of a BAT (Davis et al. 2007; Erfanian and Miltenberger 1990; Matson 1981).

Assessment of Skills and Skills Deficits In light of the social impairments that define ASD, assessment of social skills and skills deficits must be undertaken when anxiety related to social interactions is suspected. As previously noted, relative to their more intellectually disabled peers, higher functioning individuals with ASD may be more aware of skills deficits and more sensitive to embarrassing social interactions. This can establish social interaction as a conditioned aversive stimulus that induces anxiety, which in turn, can further impair social performance (White et al. 2010). The reader is referred to Chap. 9 for a more detailed discussion-related assessment and treatment of social skills deficits concurrently with social anxiety. In addition to addressing social skills deficits, it is also important to consider other adaptive skills deficits when assessing and treating anxiety in persons with ASD. This includes communication deficits, lei-

sure skills deficits, the presence of restricted and stereotyped patterns of behavior, stimulus overselectivity, and deficits in varying behavior in the context of changing situations—all of which are commonly observed in ASD. Indeed, deficits in adaptive behavior and the severity of autism have been shown to be correlated with the presence of problem behavior such as aggression and self-injury (McClintock et al. 2003). Although those findings are correlational, it is possible that deficits in adaptive behavior may establish otherwise neutral or simply nonpreferred situations as aversive to the extent that they can lead to the emergence of escape-maintained problem behavior (i.e., simple avoidance). In some cases, this same process could lead to the emergence of anxious avoidance and ultimately an anxiety disorder. As noted at the outset, understanding the broader context of the individual's skills and skills deficits is important to developing a treatment that addresses both the presenting problem and the deficits that may have predisposed its emergence.

Physiological Measures

The use of psychophysiological measurement for the assessment of anxiety is commonly recommended by researchers (King et al. 1997; Silverman and Lopez 2004) but rarely used in practice. The studies (Chok et al. 2010; Jennett et al. 2011) that have included physiological measures for assessment of anxiety in individuals with ASD have provided some support for the feasibility and utility of using heart rate monitors with this population. However, knowledge is still limited with regard to the selection of measures, appropriate conditions under which to measure physiological responding, and the validity of this measure (Turpin 1991). Moreover, for some individuals with ASD, physiological measurement may be even more challenging because they may have difficulty tolerating the equipment and procedures. Despite these limitations, the potential use of physiological measures should continue to be explored as these could provide additional information regarding the situations that cause increased arousal in individuals with ASD, especially for those individuals who are unable to reliably verbalize or report on internal sensations not readily observable. In combination with more subjective sources of data suggesting distress, the objective measurement of increased physiological arousal associated with exposure to the avoided stimulus would make a more compelling case in favor of anxious avoidance over simple avoidance.

Behavioral Treatment

Although the literature on the treatment of anxiety in persons with ASD is quite limited, the available findings suggest that behavioral treatments demonstrated to be effective with other populations appear applicable to persons with ASD—though with some modifications (it should be noted that the focus of the current chapter is on behavioral treatment for anxiety in ASD; cognitive-behavioral treatment (CBT), which has been utilized for a wide variety of anxiety diagnoses for higher functioning individuals with ASD, is discussed in detail in Chap. 12 see also Reaven & Hepburn 2006). Behavioral interventions used for treatment of escape-maintained problem behavior that could be described as simple avoidance provide indirect support for these types of interventions. A review by Jennett and Hagopian (2008) identified behavioral treatment as an evidence-based treatment for "phobic avoidance" in individuals with ID. The term phobic avoidance was used in that review because few studies reported on formal diagnoses (only Ricciardi et al. 2006 reported a diagnosis of Specific Phobia), but did report avoidant behavior of a particular stimulus that was associated with phobic-like emotional responses (characteristic of specific phobia). The authors identified 38 studies published over a 35-year period which included case reports, single-case experimental designs, and a few uncontrolled group studies. Among the studies were 12 well-designed, single-case, experimental studies. Four of these studies included five participants who were reported to have an ASD diagnosis, and ranged from having mild to profound ID (Love et al. 1990; Rapp et al. 2005;

Ricciardi et al. 2006; Shabani and Fisher 2006). The main components of behavioral treatment for anxiety included graduated exposure and reinforcement for approach behavior. The review revealed that behavioral treatment, involving the use of graduated exposure and reinforcement, has been sufficiently researched to characterize this class of interventions as a "well-established" evidence-based treatment for individuals with ID based on APA Division 12 and 16 criteria for empirically supported treatments (Chambless and Hollon 1998; Chambless et al. 1998; Krotochwill and Stoiber 2002). Since this chapter, an additional two high-quality studies have been published that used single-case experimental studies to evaluate treatments for avoidance of a particular stimulus (i.e., "phobic avoidance") in individuals with ASD (Chok et al. 2010; Schmidt et al. 2013; only Chok et al. 2010 reported a diagnosis of Specific Phobia). To date, there are a total of six studies utilizing good single-case design and showing an effect of graduated exposure plus reinforcement in individuals with ASD (see Table 11.1). Thus, this treatment can also be characterized as a "probably efficacious" treatment for individuals with autism according to the same guidelines.

Graduated Exposure

Graduated exposure is most appropriate for anxiety disorders in which there is an identifiable and controllable stimulus that is avoided (and therefore is most applicable to disorders such as specific phobia, social phobia, and OCD). Graduated exposure involves presenting the avoided stimulus in progressively more intense forms along one or more physical dimensions—such as size, proximity, mode of presentation (pictorial to actual); ideally, while maintaining low levels of anxiety. This technique aims to extinguish any associations between the avoided stimulus and aversive events (such as intense physiological arousal) by presenting the avoided stimulus in the absence of those aversive events (i.e., Pavlovian extinction); and to extinguish negative reinforcement

Table 11.1 Behavioral treatments for anxious avoidance in individuals with autism spectrum disorders

Author (year)	N	Participant characteristics	Stimulus avoided	Anxiety characteristics	Treatment components	Treatment outcomes
Chok et al. (2010)	1	15 y.o. male with ASD, mod ID, specific phobia	Dogs	Running away (including into running into street or woods), screaming, self-injury, elevated heart rate	Graduated exposure, positive reinforcement, prompting	Participant approached and touched 4 different dogs without elevated heart rate; results maintained at 6 mo follow-up
Love et al. (1990)	2	4.5 y.o. and 6 y.o. males with ASD	Going outside alone, water	Shaking, wide eyes, grimacing, crying, physical resistance, running away	Graduated exposure, positive reinforcement, participant modeling, prompting	Both participants showed increase in approach, decrease in fear verbalizations, and decrease in ratings of appearance of fear
Rapp et al. (2005)	1	14 y.o. female with ASD, severe ID	Swimming pools	Screaming, running away, flopping, self-injury, and choking	Graduated exposure, positive reinforcement, extinction (response prevention)	Participant entered pool without problem behavior and remained in 4 ft water
Ricciardi et al. (2006)	1	8 y.o. male with ASD, specific phobia	Animatronic objects	Screaming, attempts to run away, aggression when blocked from leaving area	Graduated exposure, positive reinforcement	Participant approached animatronic objects and remained within a meter distance without negative behavior
Schmidt et al. (2013)	1	16 y.o. male with ASD, severe ID	Particular school settings	Appearance of distress, agitation, physical resistance, running away, aggression, self-injury, destructive behavior	Graduated exposure, positive reinforcement	Participant attended activities with classmates in these settings without problem behavior for at least 5 min at a time
Shabani and Fisher (2006)	1	18 y.o. male with ASD, ID, diabetes	Blood draws/needles	Crying, screaming, running away, self-injury, aggression, pulling hand away; this resulted in no blood draws for 2 years	Graduated exposure, positive reinforcement	Participant remained still for blood draws; results maintained over 2 mos on daily glucose measures

associated with escape or avoidance (i.e., operant extinction). For exposure to be therapeutic, it is critical that the avoided stimulus is not paired with any aversive events (including extreme anxiety), and that encountering the stimulus not result in anxious escape/avoidance from the stimulus in a manner that could strengthen avoidance and produce counter-therapeutic effects. The intensity of exposure is arranged in a graduated fashion to maximize the likelihood that the participant will not become too anxious and eventually habituate to the stimulus.

For individuals with ASD who may not be able to generate a hierarchy of stimuli based on verbal report, the hierarchy may be developed based on interviews with care providers, or the results of a BAT. It is advisable to consider a range of stimulus variations by altering the avoided stimulus along a physical dimension, such as its distance from the individual, the duration of contact, or size of the stimulus. Regardless of how the hierarchy is developed, graduated exposure involves systematically exposing the participant to variations of the avoided stimulus that progress to closer approximations of the actual stimulus. Progression along the hierarchy is based on the participant successfully completing the previous step, ideally with minimal anxiety. Based on the participant's progress, the hierarchy can be changed by including intermediate stimulus variations.

Supplementing Graduated Exposure

Obviously, the primary maintaining consequence for anxious avoidance is negative reinforcement in the form or either avoidance or escape from the feared situation. Therefore, it is important to impose reinforcement procedures targeting approach responses that are strong enough to counter or compete with the negative reinforcement produced by escape or avoidance. Although typically developing individuals may be able to identify and verbalize powerful reinforcers, for lower functioning individuals with ASD, a systematic preference assessment to identify potential reinforces should be conducted to identify preferred

items that may potentially serve as reinforcers (see Hagopian et al. 2004 for a comprehensive summary of preference assessment procedures for individuals with ASD and other developmental disabilities).

For nonverbal individuals who might not understand instructions, it may be necessary to program learning trials without using the avoided stimulus to establish compliance with the general procedures. That is, one could initiate exposure sessions using a neutral stimulus (instead of the feared stimulus) for the purpose of ensuring the individual contacts the programmed reinforcement contingencies for cooperation. For lower functioning individuals, numerous simulated exposure sessions may be necessary before initiating graduated exposure. For individuals who can understand verbal instructions, however, much time can be saved through informing the individual about the procedures, including the contingencies for approach behavior and appropriate ways to request termination of exposure.

Other Treatment Components

Prompting may be needed to assist the individual to comply with the steps of the exposure hierarchy and come into contact with the reinforcement contingencies in place; however, caution should be taken to not "force" compliance. This may be especially important when the individual appears to exhibiting signs of distress. For individuals who can understand verbal prompts, it may be helpful to prompt the individual how to approach the avoided stimulus—and how to appropriately request pausing at the current hierarchy step (Runyan et al. 1985). Modeling approach behavior and reinforcement consumption may facilitate learning the contingencies, and demonstrate successful approach behaviors (Erfanian and Miltertenberger 1990; Love et al. 1990). Video modeling may be appropriate for some individuals with ASD who prefer watching videos to observing live models. Response prevention is another component that has been reported (Rapp et al. 2005), but most studies published to date that describe the behavioral treatment of anxiety in individuals with ASD do not include response prevention or escape extinction. Finally, use of distracting stimuli, particularly free access to preferred activities and reinforcers may be used in conjunction with graduated exposure and contingent reinforcement (Luscre and Center 1996). The use of distracting stimuli might be helpful for several possible reasons including to help focus attention away from the feared stimulus, to increase the overall level of reinforcement in the context of exposure, and to pair otherwise anxiety-provoking exposure with a preferred stimulus. However, some caution should also be taken when providing free access to reinforcers, especially when using contingent reinforcement, because this has the potential to weaken programmed reinforcement for successful approach behavior. The combination of the specific treatment components listed above can be highly individualized based on the functioning level and needs of the individual. For higher functioning individuals, cognitive-behavioral treatment components may be used as well (see Chap. 12).

Caregiver Involvement

For individuals with ASD who are often supported by care providers (e.g., parents, aides), their involvement in treatment is essential. The more the individual is dependent on care providers, the more the care provider can support or degrade behavioral treatment. As noted previously, parent–child interactions can establish and maintain both simple and anxious avoidance. Therefore, it is essential to include an analysis of parent–child interactions that may reinforce anxiety and avoidant behavior, as well as evaluate parental anxiety. When developing interventions, one should provide parents with information regarding the nature of anxiety, how their interactions may inadvertently reinforce anxious and avoidant behavior, and how behavioral treatment will progress in a graduated fashion for the purpose of extinguishing avoidant behaviors. In many cases,

it will be important to have parents conduct exposure exercises outside of therapy sessions to enhance generalization of the skills learned in session.

Skills Training

Skills training involves a focus on deficits specific to children with ASD that may impact the efficacy of treatment. Skills training is an explicit part of some CBT treatment packages (e.g., White et al. 2010; White and Roberson-Nay 2009; Wood et al. 2009), but it can also be an important component of behavioral treatment. For example, White and Roberson-Nay (2009) and White et al. (2010) have hypothesized that social deficits in individuals with high functioning autism (HFA) may contribute to the promotion of social anxiety in this population. Adolescents with HFA may develop and maintain social anxiety because of their awareness of their own social difficulties. As a result, they may avoid social situations, and therefore, have few opportunities to practice appropriate social skills. Thus, White and her colleagues have developed a comprehensive treatment package that contains the components described above plus the use of social skills training through the use of modeling, feedback, and reinforcement. Targeted social skills may include initiating interaction with peers, conversational skills, flexibility, recognizing the cues of others, and handling rejection. In another example, Wood et al. (2009), have included skills training on areas such as self-help skills and increasing interest in areas as an adjunct to the traditional components of treatment. These researchers hypothesize that skill deficits in such areas may make the completion of graduated exposure exercises more difficult and lead to diminished efficacy of treatment. White and Roberson-Nay (2009), White et al. (2010) and Wood et al. (2009) have shown promising results with their treatment packages for children with HFA. Although skills training has not been included as a primary component of the behavior treatment packages described in this chapter, there are decades of research showing that behavioral treatments are effective for skills training across all functioning levels on the autism spectrum (e.g., Carr and Durand 1985; Horner and Keilitz 1975; Lovaas 1987). Thus, the addition of skills training, such as functional communication training, social skills training, and self-help skills, should be considered as an adjunctive behavioral treatment whenever necessary.

Conclusions

Anxiety is a prominent associated feature in ASD; however, determining the presence of anxiety in this population can be especially challenging for several reasons. Overlapping features between anxiety and ASD (e.g., social avoidance and repetitive, seemly compulsive behavior) can make it difficult to determine if seemly anxious and avoidant behaviors are due to anxiety or a component of the autism. In addition, limited communication skills and social impairments common to ASD may limit the extent to which the individual can self-report, making it more challenging to identify the subjective experiences of fear and anxiety. Another issue that complicates the assessment of anxiety in persons with ASD is that these individuals are at increased risk for engaging in problem behavior (e.g., aggression, self-injury, and property destruction), some of which occurs to avoid or escape certain situations. We use the term *simple avoidance* to refer to avoidance of nonpreferred stimuli or situations (e.g., wearing shoes, participating in certain instructional tasks), and the term *anxious avoidance* to refer to avoidant behavior that is associated with traditional indicators of anxiety (including facial expressions indicative of fear, increased physiological arousal, and self-reported anxiety in those who are able). When the anxious avoidance markedly interferes with functioning, then this would constitute an *anxiety disorder* (which particular disorder obviously depends on the nature of the feared stimulus and the response). Caution should be taken to not assume the presence of

anxiety (or dismiss it) based on how the presenting complaint is labeled by care providers (or even by the individual him or herself). Rather, multimodal, multi-informant behavioral assessment should be initiated.

Review of the existing literature suggests that many of the behavioral assessment strategies traditionally employed with non-ASD populations may be applicable to individuals with ASD, despite the communication deficits that may limit or prevent self-report. Interviews and direct behavioral observation via behavioral avoidance tests and behavioral monitoring in natural settings may be the primary sources of information during both the assessment and treatment evaluation phases. Treatment should be individualized based on the characteristics and functioning level of the individual. The core components of behavioral treatment procedures include graduated exposure and reinforcement, but these are often supplemented with other components. Despite significant gaps in the literature, research conducted thus far is sufficient to guide clinicians on how to proceed clinically with assessment and treatment of anxiety in individuals with ASD. Nevertheless, additional research designed to examine the presence of other types of anxiety disorders, to develop additional assessment strategies, and to further examine treatment efficacy for anxiety in individuals with ASD is needed.

References

American Psychiatric Association. (2000). *Diagnostic and statistical manual of mental disorders* (4th ed.). Washington, D.C.: Author.

American Psychiatric Association. (2013). *Diagnostic and statistical manual of mental disorders* (5th ed.). Washington, D.C.: Author.

Ambrosini, P. J. (2000). Historical development and present status of the schedule for affective disorders and schizophrenia for school-age children (K-SADS). *Journal of the American Academy of Child and Adolescent Psychiatry, 39,* 49–58.

Baron-Cohen, S. (2002). The extreme male brain theory of autism. *Trends in Cognitive Sciences, 6,* 248–254,

Birmaher, B., Brent, D. A., Chiappetta, L., Bridge, J., Monga, S, & Baugher, M. (1999). Psychometric properties of the Screen for Child Anxiety Related Emotional Disorders (SCARED): A replication study. *Journal of the American Academy of Child and Adolescent Psychiatry, 38,* 1230–1236.

Blakeley-Smith, A., Reaven, J., Ridge, K., & Hepburn, S. (2012). Parent-child agreement of anxiety symptoms in youth with autism spectrum disorders. *Research in Autism Spectrum Disorders, 6*(2), 707–716.

Carr, E. G., & Durand, V. M. (1985). Reducing behavior problems through functional communication training. *Journal of Applied Behavior Analysis, 18,* 111–126.

Chambless, D. L., & Hollon, S. D. (1998). Defining empirically supported therapies. *Journal of Consulting and Clinical Psychology, 66,* 7–18.

Chambless, D. L., Baker, M. J., Baucom, D. H., Beutler, L. E., Calhoun, K. S., Crits-Christoph, P., et al. (1998). Update on empirically validated therapies, II. *The Clinical Psychologist, 51,* 3–16.

Chok, J. T., Demanche, J., Kennedy, A., & Studer, L. (2010). Utilizing physiological measures to facilitate phobia treatment with individuals with autism and intellectual disability: A case study. *Behavioral Interventions, 11,* 325–337.

Chorpita, B. F., Albano, A. M., Heimberg, R. G., & Barlow, D. H. (1996). A systematic replication of the prescriptive treatment of school refusal behavior in a single subject. *Journal of Behavior Therapy and Experimental Psychiatry, 27,* 281–290.

Conyers, C., Miltenberger, R. G., Peterson, B., Gubin, A., Jurgens, M., Selders, A., et al. (2004). An evaluation of in vivo desensitization and video modeling to increase compliance with dental procedures in persons with mental retardation. *Journal of Applied Behavior Analysis, 37,* 233–238.

Dadds, M., Rapee, R., & Barrett, P. (1994). Behavioral Observation. In T. Ollendick, N. King, & W. Yule (Eds.), International handbook of phobic and anxiety disorders in children and adolescents (pp. 349–364). New York: Plenum.

Davis III, T. E. (2012). Where to from here for ASD and anxiety? Lessons learned from child anxiety and the issue of DSM-5. *Clinical Psychology: Science and Practice, 19,* 358–363. doi:10.1111/cpsp.12014.

Davis, T. E., & Ollendick, T. H. (2005). Empirically supported treatments for specific phobia in children: Do efficacious treatments address the components of a phobic response? *Clinical Psychology: Science and Practice, 12,* 144–160.

Davis III, T. E., Kurtz, P., Gardner, A., & Carman, N. (2007). Cognitive-behavioral treatment for specific phobias with a child demonstrating severe problem behavior and developmental delays. *Research in Developmental Disabilities, 28,* 546–558. doi:10.1016/j.ridd.2006.07.003.

Erfanian, N., & Miltenberger, R. G. (1990). Contact desensitization in the treatment of dog phobias in persons who have mental retardation. *Behavioral Interventions, 5,* 55–60.

Farrugia, S., & Hudson, J. (2006). Anxiety in adolescents with Asperger Syndrome: Negative thoughts, behavioral problems, and life interference. *Focus on Autism and Other Developmental Disabilities, 21,* 25–35.

Friman, P. C., Hayes, S. C., & Wilson, K. G. (1998). Why behavior analysts should study emotion: The example for anxiety. *Journal of Applied Behavior Analysis, 31,* 137–156.

Hagopian, L. P., & Slifer, K. J. (1993). Treatment of separation anxiety disorder with graduated exposure and reinforcement targeting school attendance: A controlled case study. *Journal of Anxiety Disorders, 7,* 271–280.

Hagopian, L. P., Weist, M. D., & Ollendick, T. H. (1990). Cognitive-behavior therapy with an 11- year-old girl fearful of AIDS infection, other diseases, and poisoning: A case study. *Journal of Anxiety Disorders, 4,* 257–265.

Hagopian, L. P., Crockett, J. L., & Keeney, K. M. (2001). Multicomponent treatment for blood- injury-injection phobia in a young man with mental retardation. *Research in Developmental Disabilities, 22,* 141–149.

Hagopian, L. P., Long, E. S., & Rush, K. S. (2004). Preference assessment procedures for individuals with developmental disabilities. *Behavior Modification, 28,* 668–677.

Hagopian, L. P., Rooker, G. W., Jessel, J., & Deleon, I. G. (2013). Initial functional analysis outcomes and modifications in pursuit of differentiation: A summary of 176 inpatient cases. *Journal of Applied Behavior Analysis, 46,* 88–100.

Hanley, G. P., Iwata, B. A., & McCord, B. E. (2003). Functional analysis of problem behavior: A review. *Journal of Applied Behavior Analysis, 36,* 147–185.

Horner, R. D., & Keilitz, I. (1975). Training mentally retarded adolescents to brush their teeth. *Journal of Applied Behavior Analysis, 8,* 301–309.

Jennett, H. K., & Hagopian, L. P. (2008). Identifying empirically supported treatments for phobic avoidance in individuals with intellectual disabilities. *Behavior Therapy, 39,* 151–161.

Jennett, H., Hagopian, L. P., & Beaulieu, L. (2011). Analysis of heart rate and self-injury with and without restraint in an individual with autism. *Research in Autism Spectrum Disorders, 5,* 1110–1118.

King, N. J., Ollendick, T. H., & Murphy, G. C. (1997). Assessment of childhood phobias. *Clinical Psychology Review, 17,* 667–687.

Krotochwill, T. R., & Stoiber, K. C. (2002). Evidence-based interventions in school psychology: conceptual foundations of the procedural and coding manual of division 16 and the society for the study of school psychology task force. *School Psychology Quarterly, 17,* 341–389.

Kuusikko, S., Pollock-Wurman, R., Jussila, K., Carter, A. S., Mattila, M. L., Ebeling, H., et al. (2008). Social anxiety in high-functioning children and adolescents with Autism and Asperger syndrome. *Journal of Autism and Developmental Disorders, 8,* 1697–1709.

Leyfer, O. T., Folstein, S. E., Bacalman, S., Davis, N. O., Dinh, E., Morgan, J., et al. (2006). Comorbid psychiatric disorders in children with autism: Interview development and rates of disorders. *Journal of Autism and Developmental Disorders, 36*, 849–861.

Lovaas, O. I., (1987). Behavioral treatment and normal educational and intellectual functioning in young autistic children. *Journal of Consulting and Clinical Psychology, 55*, 3–9.

Love, S. R., Matson, J. L., & West, D. (1990). Mothers as effective therapists for autistic children's phobias. *Journal of Applied Behavior Analysis, 23*, 379–385.

Luscre, D. M., & Center, D. B. (1996). Procedures for reducing dental fear in children with autism. *Journal of Autism and Developmental Disorders, 26*, 547–556.

MacNeil, B. M., Lopes, V. A., & Minnes, P. M. (2009). Anxiety in children and adolescents with autism spectrum disorders. *Research in Autism Spectrum Disorders, 3*, 1–21.

March, J. S. (1997). *Multidimensional Anxiety Scale for Children (MASC)*. Toronto: Multi-Health Systems.

Matson, J. L. (1981). Assessment and treatment of clinical fears in mentally retarded children. *Journal of Applied Behavior Analysis, 14*, 287–294.

Matson, J., & Wilkins, J. (2008). Reliability of the autism spectrum disorders-comorbid for children (ASD-CC). *Journal of Developmental & Physical Disabilities, 20*, 327–336.

Matson, J. L., LoVullo, S. V., Rivet, T. T., & Boisjoli, J. A. (2009a). Validity of the autism spectrum disorder-comorbid for children (ASD-CC). *Research in Autism Spectrum Disorders, 3*, 345–357.

Matson, J. L., Wilkins, J., Sevin, J. A., Knight, C., Boisjoli, J. A., & Sharp, B. (2009b). Reliability and item content of the baby and infant screen for children with autism traits (BISCUIT): Parts 1–3. *Research in Autism Spectrum Disorders, 3*, 336–344.

Matson, J. L., Boisjoli, J. A., Hess, J. A., & Wilkins, J. (2011). Cormorbid psychopathology factor structure on the baby and infant screen for children with autism traits-Part 2 (BISCUIT-Part 2). *Research in Autism Spectrum Disorder, 5*, 426–432.

Mazefsky, C. A., Kao, J., & Oswald, D. P. (2011). Preliminary evidence suggesting caution in the use of psychiatric self-report measures with adolescents with high-functioning autism spectrum disorders. *Research in Autism Spectrum Disorders, 5*, 164–174.

McClintock, K., Hall, S., & Oliver, C. (2003). Risk markers associated with challenging behaviours in people with intellectual disabilities: A meta-analytic study. *Journal of Intellectual Disability Research, 47*, 405–416.

McDougle, C. J., Kresch, L. E., Goodman, W. K., Naylor, S. T., Volkmar, F. R., Cohen, D. J., & Price, L. H. (1995). A case-controlled study of repetitive thoughts and behavior in adults with autistic disorder and obsessive-compulsive disorder. *American Journal of Psychiatry, 152*, 772–777.

Mowrer, O. H. (1960). *Learning theory and behavior*. New York: Wiley.

Myers, S. M., & Johnson, C. P. (2007). American Academy of Pediatrics Council on Children with Disabilities. Management of children with Autism Spectrum Disorders. *Pediatrics, 120*, 1162–1182.

Ollendick, T. H., Oswald, D. P., & Ollendick, D. G. (1993). Anxiety disorders in mentally retarded persons. In J. L. Matson & R. P. Barrett (Eds.), *Psychopathology in the mentally retarded* (pp. 41–85). Needham Heights: Allyn & Bacon.

Reaven, J. (2011). The treatment of anxiety symptoms in youth with high-functioning autism spectrum disorders: Developmental considerations for parents. *Brain research, 1380*, 255–263.

Reaven, J., & Hepburn, S. (2006). The Parent's Role in the Treatment of Anxiety Symptoms In Children With High-Functioning Autism Spectrum Disorders. *Mental Health Aspects of Developmental Disabilities*.

Rapp, J. T., Vollmer, T. R., & Hovanetz, A. N. (2005). Evaluation and treatment of swimming pool avoidance exhibited by an adolescent girl with autism. *Behavior Therapy, 36*, 101–105.

Reynolds, C. R., & Richmond, B. O. (1985). *Revised Children's Manifest Anxiety Scale: RCMAS Manual*. Los Angeles: Western Psychological Services.

Ricciardi, J. N., Luiselli, J. K., & Camare, M. (2006). Shaping approach responses as intervention for specific phobia in a child with autism. *Journal of Applied Behavior Analysis, 39*, 445–448.

Runyan, M. C., Stevens, D. H., & Reeves, R. (1985). Reduction of avoidance behavior of institutionalized mentally retarded adults through contact desensitization. *American Journal of Mental Deficiency, 90*, 222–225.

Russell, E., & Sofronoff, K. (2005). Anxiety and social worries in children with Asperger syndrome. *Australian and New Zealand Journal of Psychiatry, 39*, 633–638.

Shabani, D. B., & Fisher, W. W. (2006). Stimulus fading and differential reinforcement for the treatment of needle phobia in a youth with autism. *Journal of Applied Behavior Analysis, 39*, 449–452.

Schmidt, J. D., Luiselli, J. K., Rue, H., & Whalley, K. (2013). Graduated exposure and positive reinforcement to overcome setting and activity avoidance in an adolescent with autism. *Behavior Modification, 37*, 128–142.

Shattuck, P. T., Roux, A. M., Hudson, L. E., Taylor, J. L., Maenner, M. J., & Trani, J. F. (2012). Services for adults with an autism spectrum disorder. *Canadian Journal of Psychiatry, 57*, 284–291.

Silverman, W., & Albano, A. (1996). *Anxiety disorders interview schedule for children for DSM-IV: (Child and Parent Versions)*. San Antonio: Psychological Corporation/Graywind.

Silverman, W., & Lopez, B. (2004). Anxiety disorders. In M. Hersen (Ed.), *Psychological assessment in clinical practice: A pragmatic guide* (pp. 269–296). New York: Psychology.

Silverman, W. K., & Ollendick, T. H. (2005). Evidence-based assessment of anxiety and its disorders in children and adolescents. *Journal of Clinical Child and Adolescent Psychology, 34*, 380–411.

Silverman, W. K., Saavedra, L. M., & Pina, A. A. (2001). Test-retest reliability of anxiety symptoms and diagnoses with the anxiety disorders interview schedule for DSM-IV: Child and parent versions. *Journal of the American Academy of Child and Adolescent Psychiatry, 40*, 937–944.

Spence, S. H. (1997). Structure of anxiety symptoms among children: A confirmatory factor-analytic study. *Journal of Abnormal Psychology, 106*, 280–297.

Sukhodolsky, D. G., Scahill, L., Gadow, K. D., Arnold, L. E., Aman, M. G., McDougle, C. J., et al. (2008). Parent-rated anxiety symptoms in children with Pervasive Developmental Disorders: Frequency and association with core autism symptoms and cognitive functioning. *Journal of Abnormal Child Psychology, 36*, 117–128.

Turpin, G. (1991). The psychophysiological assessment of anxiety disorders: Three-systems measurement and beyond. Psychological Assessment: *A Journal of Consulting and Clinical Psychology, 3*, 366–375.

Velting, O. N., Setzer, N. J., & Albano, A. M. (2004). Update on and advances in assessment and cognitive-behavioral treatment of anxiety disorders in children and adolescents. *Professional Psychology: Research and Practice, 35*, 42–54.

White, S. W., & Roberson-Nay, R. (2009). Anxiety, social deficits, and loneliness in youth with autism spectrum disorders. *Journal of Autism and Developmental Disorders, 39*, 1006–1013.

White, S. W., Albano, A. M., Johnson, C. R., Kasari, C., Ollendick, T., Klin, A., et al. (2010). Development of a cognitive-behavioral intervention program to treat anxiety and social deficits in teens with high-functioning autism. *Clinical Child and Family Psychology Review, 13*, 77–90.

Wood, J. J., Piacentini, J. C., Bergman, R. L., McCracken, J., & Barrios, V. (2002). Concurrent validity of the anxiety disorders section of the Anxiety Disorders Interview Schedule for DSM-IV: Child and parent versions. *Journal of Clinical Child and Adolescent Psychology, 31*, 335–342.

Wood, J. J., Drahota, A., Sze, K., Har, K., Chiu, A., & Langer, D. A. (2009). Cognitive behavioral therapy for anxiety in children with autism spectrum disorders: A randomized, controlled trial. *Journal of Child Psychology and Psychiatry, 50*, 224–234.

Zandt, F., Prior, M., & Kyrios, M. (2007). Repetitive behaviour in children with high functioning autism and obsessive compulsive disorder. *Journal of Autism and Developmental Disorders, 37*, 251–259.

Kate Sofronoff, Renae Beaumont and Jonathan A. Weiss

Treating Transdiagnostic Processes in ASD: Going Beyond Anxiety

Cognitive behavioral therapy (CBT) for anxiety is an extremely well-validated approach and is considered to be the best practice (Davis et al. 2011; Kendall et al. 2003; Ollendick et al. 2006). While there is quite a long history of successful behavioral interventions for children with autism spectrum disorders (ASD; e.g., Hastings et al. 2009; Lovaas 1987), the history of success with cognitive-behavioral interventions for the ASD population is relatively recent (Chalfant et al. 2007; Sofronoff et al. 2005; Wood et al. 2009; White et al. 2013). We have learned many important lessons from these early trials of CBT for anxiety on children with ASD that now inform the development of new innovations in intervention with the population.

Moree and Davis (2010) provided a review of the types of modifications to CBT programs for anxiety that have proven successful. The major trends in modification are consistent with our current knowledge of ASD and take account of the cognitive profile of children with a diagnosis on the autism spectrum. We have learned that it is important to use more concrete and visual strate-gies to explain new concepts, to create disorder-specific hierarchies, and to include each child's specific interest when possible in order to build rapport, increase motivation, and as a metaphor to explain concepts. It is also important to actively engage with parents as those who can reinforce the child for efforts and remind the child of what has been learned. Donoghue et al. (2011) also published an approach to CBT for children with ASD. These researchers use the acronym PRECISE to encapsulate the necessary modifications to CBT required to work effectively with children with ASD. Within the acronym, "P" represents the collaborative partnership that is needed to accommodate a child's individual profile of strengths and difficulties; "R" for right developmental level, using visual cues, involving parents; "E" for the empathy required; "C" for creativity in the approach used that may need to include a special interest; "I" for investigation and experimentation—behavioral experiments likely to be more effective than verbally based restructuring; "S" for self-discovery to encourage the child to see what they already know and do and then add to this; and "E" to underline the need to make the process enjoyable to the child. It is clear that the modifications encompassed in the acronym are congruent with the direction that the research is currently taking.

An anxiety intervention developed for children with ASD may, on the surface, not appear to be so different from a program developed for typically developing children. It will still include the active ingredients of psychoeducation about

K. Sofronoff (✉) · R. Beaumont
School of Psychology, University of Queensland,
McElwain Building, St. Lucia, QLD 4072, Australia
e-mail: kate@psy.uq.edu.au

J. A. Weiss
York University, Toronto, ON, Canada

T. E. Davis III et al. (eds.), *Handbook of Autism and Anxiety,* Autism and Child Psychopathology Series,
DOI 10.1007/978-3-319-06796-4_12, © Springer International Publishing Switzerland 2014

anxiety, exposure, and challenging of unhelpful thoughts. The delivery of the intervention, however, may be quite different and it is important that the clinician not assume that any "out-of-the-box" anxiety interventions will work simply by slowing down the pace—as long as you take it slowly. While the slower pace is likely necessary, if this is the only modification, it will also likely be insufficient.

An essential component will involve an assessment process that gathers data about the individual child's cognitive profile—strengths and difficulties—so that it is possible to develop hierarchies that take the profile into account. In most cases, this will include taking account of social and communication factors that may impede success if not addressed. The issue of motivation can be significant and it is important to take a strengths-based approach, to celebrate the child's successes, to include special interests, and to foster positivity and confidence. Many children will find perspective taking to be challenging and managing this can require creativity on the part of the therapist.

Review of the Current Literature

Lang et al. (2010) completed a systematic review of anxiety treatments in ASD that used CBT and their review focused on the modifications reported. All of their included trials had recruited children with a diagnosis of Asperger syndrome or high-functioning autism. The review found five individual case studies (Cardaciotto and Herbert 2004; Greig and MacKay 2005; Reaven and Hepburn 2003; Sze and Wood 2007, 2008) and four randomized controlled trials (Chalfant et al. 2007; Reaven et al. 2009; Sofronoff et al. 2005; Wood et al. 2009). The types of modifications described are those that accommodate the cognitive profile of high-functioning ASD (HF/ASD). Several of these studies actively included components to increase the use of social interaction skills and some mentioned the increased use of visual aides to teach important concepts. The child's special interest was incorporated into some programs either to explain concepts during

psychoeducation (e.g., incorporation of the interest in learning metaphors) or to increase engagement with the program and some programs included the child's parents as well as providing reinforcers for appropriate behaviors.

Since this review, there have been several more trials of CBT for anxiety. Reaven et al. (2012) conducted a randomized trial with 47 children using a family-focused group program (Facing Your Fears). The program had 12 sessions of 1.5 h and used a manual for participants and facilitators. This program was developed specifically for children with ASD and it contains CBT components such as graded exposure and strategies for emotional regulation. Modifications included many of those described above—additionally there was opportunity for video modeling and the creation of movies, with a focus on the child's interest, and specific program content for parents. On parent and child report, the intervention group showed significant reduction in anxiety symptoms at post intervention. These findings are consistent with previous findings (Chalfant et al. 2007; Sofronoff et al. 2005; Wood et al. 2009).

Storch et al. (2013) also conducted a randomized trial of a 16-week CBT intervention for children with HF/ASD and clinically significant anxiety. This program was based on an intervention for typically developing anxious children and allowed for a flexible format so that modules could be selected based on individual child needs. Parents were included in the program to assist with task completion within session but also to ensure that exposure tasks were completed at home. The program demonstrated large effect sizes post intervention with significant reduction in anxiety symptoms reported.

McNally Keehn et al. (2013) ran a randomized pilot trial of the modified Coping Cat Program for children with anxiety and ASD. Modifications were made to the programs that were consistent with those recommended in earlier interventions—inclusion of parents, longer sessions, more use of visuals, integrating special interests, and so on. This program was delivered to the children individually. The results provide promising evidence for the effectiveness of the modified program.

When we look at the consistent findings from these trials, the evidence is mounting to suggest that CBT approaches are likely to be effective with children with HF/ASD and anxiety when specific modifications are included. It is also clear that there is no one program that has all the answers and that there are different ways of addressing the needs of these children and their families.

Lickel et al. (2012) raised an interesting question in their study about the prerequisite skills for successful CBT in children with ASD. They suggested that the cognitive skills required to participate in CBT include skills that might be especially difficult for children with ASD, namely emotion recognition, self-reflection, metacognition, perspective taking, and so on. The study compared children with ASD to typically developing children on tasks that assessed emotion recognition, ability to differentiate between thoughts, behaviors, and feelings, and cognitive mediation. Results from the study demonstrated that the children with ASD were comparable on all tests except the emotion recognition task. The authors suggested that CBT programs should contain affect education—teaching about emotions. There is evidence that children can learn emotion recognition and emotion awareness (Golan et al. 2010) and this is certainly an important component in the program evaluated by Sofronoff et al. (2005).

Another consideration that has started to emerge in the literature is that of whether developing disorder-specific programs for the ASD population is the best way to serve the population. When we look at the types of modifications that are suggested above, it is clear that within any group of children with ASD we are likely to be dealing with multiple and diverse problems—issues of emotion recognition certainly but also significant emotion dysregulation, anxiety, anger management, sensory sensitivities, and depression. There is evidence to suggest that children with ASD have an increased likelihood of behavior problems and noncompliance, and it may be preferable for parents to participate in a parenting program before the child undertakes an intervention for anxiety (Whittingham et al. 2009). Any

program that purports to deal with social interaction skills will necessarily need to include components that target emotion management since the difficulties inherent in social interaction will likely increase anxiety and/or anger.

A Transdiagnostic Approach

There is in fact evidence of substantial co-occurrence of emotional problems in youth with ASD, across internalizing and externalizing symptoms (Gadow et al. 2006; Lecavalier et al. 2008; Leyfer et al. 2006; Weisbrot et al. 2005). There is also considerable overlap of sadness, anger, and anxiety in typically developing individuals with anxiety disorders and in youth with ASD (Hurtig et al. 2009; Quek et al. 2012; Rohde 2012). Many clinical scientists search for common explanations for problems with emotional coping across diagnostic categories (Trosper et al. 2009), known as the "transdiagnostic approach," which may be particularly useful in addressing multiple emotional disorders in youth with ASD.

In the general population, a number of authors have designed CBT programs that aim to address transdiagnostic factors common across presenting problems (Boisseau et al. 2010; Ehrenreich et al. 2009; Norton 2012). The most central aspect of these transdiagnostic models is the importance of emotion regulation (McLaughlin et al. 2011). The *Unified Protocol for the Treatment of Emotional Disorders* (UP) is one well-known transdiagnostic cognitive-behavioral intervention for adults with anxiety or depression (Barlow et al. 2011). The UP combines familiar cognitive-behavioral techniques, such as extinction, exposure, and cognitive reappraisal, with a focus on an individual's emotional experience and their emotion regulation (see Ellard et al. 2010). Recently, the UP was adapted for youth (UP-Y; Bilek and Ehrenreich-May 2012; Ehrenreich et al. 2009; Trosper et al. 2009) to help children with a range of emotional problems. Ehrenreich-May and colleagues' application of an emotion regulation framework (Gross and Thompson 2007) to CBT in youth has direct relevance to addressing anxiety in youth with ASD through a transdiagnostic lens.

Emotion regulation can be defined as "the extrinsic and intrinsic processes responsible for monitoring, evaluating, and modifying emotional reactions, especially their intensive and temporal features, to accomplish one's goals" (Thompson 1994, pp. 27–28). Emotion regulation is adaptive when it helps us to successfully achieve an appropriate emotion or intensity of emotion. In contrast, it can be maladaptive when regulating emotion results in long-term negative outcomes. Gross and Thompson (2007) describe five associated components of emotion regulation: situation selection, situation modification, attentional deployment, cognitive change, and response modulation. Each component is briefly described below, followed by a discussion of how an intervention based on such a transdiagnostic framework might help children with ASD build the skills required to promote adaptive emotion regulation. Understanding the underlying emotion regulation deficits in children with ASD can help to develop more effective interventions that target a host of related symptoms (Mazefsky et al. 2013).

Situation selection involves the control we exert over the choice of the situations we enter into or avoid (Trosper et al., 2009). For example, seeking out someone to talk to when upset or avoiding dangerous situations are examples of adaptive situation selection. It requires a good understanding of situations and the ability to predict likely outcomes and is something that, in children, is greatly assisted by parental guidance. Maladaptive situation selection often appears as the avoidance of situations that are feared but for which, in reality, there is no real danger that exists, as well as when such avoidance leads to long-term problems for the individual or family. For example, avoiding an uncomfortable social situation over fear of embarrassment relieves anxiety in the short term (emotion regulation) but increases the likelihood of avoidance in the future and a stronger situation-avoidant response. Avoidance is readily seen in anxiety disorders (Aldao et al. 2010; Rapee 2002) and in individuals who are depressed and withdraw from pleasurable activities and social situations (Mash and Wolfe 2002). Helping children choose to face

problem situations is the hallmark of exposure-based CBT for children with and without ASD and highlights how CBT already addresses a key preliminary aspect of emotion regulation—helping children to make better choices about experiencing distressing situations (Munoz-Solomando et al. 2008; Reaven et al. 2012; Wood et al. 2009)

There are times when we have no choice about the situations we enter into, yet still manage to regulate our emotions (e.g., recall the last time you sat in a dentist's chair). *Situation modification* involves altering the situation once we are faced with it, in order to modulate our emotional responses. Problem solving of distressing situations is a form of adaptive situation modification, as we aim to alter our context in a helpful way that also helps regulate how we feel. Youth with ASD are known to struggle in social and "real-world" problem solving (Channon et al. 2001), making this emotion regulation step particularly challenging. For example, an effective solution to a problem with a school situation that is leading to stress could be to speak to the teacher about the issue in a calm but assertive manner and determine how a situation could change. A maladaptive situation modification strategy would be to lose one's temper to achieve the same end of altering the stressful experience. Improving a child's ability to problem solve effectively, by developing skills to generate, evaluate, and adapt potential solutions, can help them regulate their emotions (Magyar and Pandolfi 2012).

How we choose to focus on or, conversely, distance our attention from the emotional aspects of a situation also matters on with respect to how we regulate, even in situations that cannot be modified. Successful *attentional deployment* involves emotional awareness and being able to shift our attention when needed to focus on helpful information or emotions. Emotional awareness has been defined "as an attentional process that serves to monitor and differentiate emotions, locate their antecedents, but ignore the physical arousal that is part of the emotion experience" (Rieffe et al. 2011, p. 656). Children with ASD are known to struggle with emotional awareness of themselves and others (Tanaka et al. 2012; Williams and Happé 2010). By helping youth with ASD learn about the cognitive, behavioral, and physiological aspects of emotional signals, we can serve to improve their emotion regulation ability. As a result of a predisposition toward perseveration, youth with ASD are also at risk for rumination (Rieffe et al. 2011). It is critical that we help them to learn how to shift their attention to focus on distressing topics in an acceptable way and to shift toward positive topics when needed. In children with ASD, mindfulness-based strategies that focus on shifting from aversive stimuli and negative emotions to neutral topics can lead to decreases in aggressive behavior (Singh et al. 2011).

Our emotional reactions can further be regulated through our appraisal of the distressing stimuli (i.e., the meaning and importance we ascribe to a situation) and our capacity to manage it, known as *cognitive control* (Gross & Thompson 2007). A reappraisal of the distressing situation, or intentionally editing our view of a situation or the meanings we place on the emotions that result, are common adaptive cognitive control strategies (Aldao et al. 2010; Gross and Thompson 2007). Traditionally, this takes the form of using evidence to reinterpret experiences (including the situation, our thoughts, feelings, and behaviors) to alter either the valence or the intensity of the experience. All CBT interventions for anxiety in youth with ASD appear to build coping statements and helpful ways to think about distressing situations (Beaumont and Sofronoff 2008; Reaven et al. 2012; Sofronoff et al. 2005). Although abstract reappraisal strategies may be challenging for youth with ASD who apply a concrete cognitive style (such as Socratic dialogue or weighing the evidence for and against negative thoughts), reappraisal continues to be effective when using the more concrete strategy of developing positive statements to counteract negative ones.

The preceding emotion regulation components are viewed as "antecedent" processes (Gross and Thompson 2007) because they are implemented in ways to help us prior to experiencing the emotional distress. If we have been unable to apply these antecedent processes and we experience tremendous distress, we still have options in how we regulate that affect. Known as *response mod-*

ulation, it involves the physiological and behavioral ways of addressing an experienced emotion. Problematic behaviors often occur as a result of experiencing a distressing emotion, in an attempt to suppress or reduce it, whether it be withdrawal (in the case of depression), aggression (in the case of anger), or escape (in the case of anxiety; Barlow et al. 2004). These "emotion-driven behaviors" serve to maintain the contingency linking the negative emotion to the situation (Barlow et al. 2004; Trosper et al. 2009). Relaxation strategies are often intended to address arousal at a physiological level, thus dampening an emotional response (Weersing et al. 2012). If used appropriately, relaxation strategies can help children with ASD who are experiencing negative emotions to manage the emotion at an appropriate level while remaining in those emotion-eliciting situations to benefit from exposure (Sofronoff et al. 2005; Sofronoff et al. 2007). The intention is to regulate the experience, rather than to stifle or remove it altogether. Another aspect of response modulation is how we choose to express the emotion, which is partly moderated by one's awareness of social context and by how such expression is modeled by others (Gross and Thompson 2007; Zeman and Shipman 1998). Youth with ASD are particularly prone to missing social cues regarding appropriate behavior and emotions (Loveland et al. 2001), and helping them to understand how best to express their feelings in a social context can be an important aspect of helping them behaviorally control negative affect.

The Secret Agent Society: Features that Fit with a Transdiagnostic Approach and the PRECISE Model

Program Description

The Secret Agent Society (SAS; Beaumont 2010) is a multimedia social–emotional skills training program for 8–12-year-old children with HF/ASD. The program applies the PRECISE model in treating the core emotion regulation deficits that appear to underlie multiple psychological problems in youth with ASD. The espionage-themed group intervention teaches children how to recognize emotions in themselves and others, express their feelings in appropriate ways, piece together face, voice, body, and situational clues to correctly interpret social situations and introduces step-by-step skill codes for talking and playing with others and preventing and managing bullying and teasing. The program features a four-level computer game to introduce the social–emotional skills featured in the program to children. Children practice these skills through games and activities played at nine weekly child group meetings with the support of their group "mentors" (trained program facilitators). Parent group meetings, a school staff information session, and parent and teacher program resources help to boost parents' and teachers' skills and confidence in supporting children to apply the social–emotional skills that they learn in the program at home and at school.

Results from an initial randomized controlled trial showed the SAS program to be effective in improving children's social–emotional skills at home and at school as rated by parents and teachers, with treatment gains maintained at 5-month follow-up (Beaumont and Sofronoff 2008). On one of the parent-report measures used in the trial, 76% of the children who experienced significant social–emotional difficulties at the beginning of the program improved to within the range of typically developing children at the end of the program and/or at the 5-month follow-up. A recent evaluation of a parent-delivered variant of the program showed that, in addition to improved social skills, the program resulted in a reduction in child behavior problems and anxiety (Sofronoff, Silva, & Beaumont, submitted).

The Application of PRECISE (Donoghue et al. 2011) to SAS

SAS exemplifies many of the modifications to CBT for children with ASD that are recommended in the PRECISE acronym by Donoghue et al. (2011) previously described. Program facilitators develop a collaborative *partnership* with children from the outset. In Child Group Meeting 1,

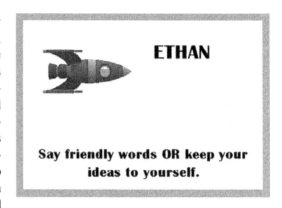

Fig. 12.1 Example behavior card

children select individualized rewards that they would like to receive for following the group rules in each session and for displaying target behaviors described on an individualized behavior card. A behavior card is created for each child group member that features a picture related to their special interest and lists one or two behaviors the child is to display to help group sessions run smoothly (see Fig. 12.1). For example, the target behavior for an over-talkative child might be, "Keep comments brief and on topic" or "Listen quietly to other group members." For a child who is reluctant to participate in group activities, the target behavior rewarded with session tokens might be, "Try your best at SAS club activities."

The program content and resources also cater to children's different learning styles (verbal, visual, and/or action-based). Concepts are taught in a variety of ways—verbal discussion and written descriptions in the child Cadet Handbook, animated examples and explanations in the SAS computer game, full-color illustrations of skill steps on pocket-sized "Code Cards" and in the child Cadet Handbook, and role plays and games that involve practicing skills. For example, the SAS Challenger Board Game features role plays of skills taught in the program and fun "physical challenges" where children use relaxation strategies ("gadgets") to stay calm and in control when competing against each other. Weekly home practice tasks ("home missions") are also tailored to the skill level and specific social–emotional difficulties faced by each child. For example, children decide on the anxiety- or anger-provoking situations where they will practice using their chosen relaxation gadgets (with parent and/or school staff support).

To ensure that the program is pitched at the *right* developmental level, printed text in the SAS computer game is narrated to cater to children with reading difficulties and each skill taught in the program is broken down into simple step-by-step instructions that are illustrated with pictures (with more detailed guidelines written in fine print). Blank skill "Code Cards" and stickers are provided to allow facilitators to create customized, simplified illustrations of skills and concepts where needed. To optimize the enjoyment and learning experience of all children involved, program facilitators are also encouraged to try to match children in a group on developmental level and verbal comprehension skills where possible.

Parent group meetings, a school staff information session, and parent and teacher program resources help parents and school staff to support children to apply their social–emotional skills at home and at school and to complete their weekly home missions. The SAS Parent Workbook and Teacher Tip Sheet Pack provides succinct summaries of weekly session activities and tips on how parents and school staff can help children to put their social–emotional skills into action through preplanning, skill modeling, prompting, and reviewing. The teacher resources also include recommendations on class- and school-based policies and procedures to create a caring, compassionate school community where bullying (especially as it relates to students with ASD) is effectively prevented and managed. A customized home–school diary and rewards system is also used by parents and school staff to monitor and reward children's skill usage between sessions.

The central principle underlying the SAS program is to set every child and family up for success. Thus, program facilitators are trained to take an *empathic* approach to understanding each child's social–emotional difficulties and to work with children, parents, and school staff to determine the specific emotion regulation strategies and social skill steps each child will focus on as they move through the program. If a child is reluctant to try a specific skill or strategy, facilitators are encouraged to explore the reasons with them and adapt the skill or strategy where possible. Facilitators are also advised that not all strategies will be appropriate for all children. For example, imagining a relaxing or happy memory is a powerful relaxation strategy for some children, but unfavorable for others where theory of mind impairments may make recalling past memories challenging (even with evocative imagery scripts and relevant sensory aids, such as smelling a beach-scented candle and looking at a beach holiday photograph).

The SAS uses a variety of *creative* games and activities to engage children to crack the code of emotions and "solve the mystery of social encounters." For example, the SAS computer game and Secret Message Transmission Device walkie-talkie game appeal to the special interest that children with ASD often have in technology. A variety of other games are also used to help children learn and practice the social–emotional skills taught in the program (e.g., the Body Clues Freeze Game, Helpful Thought Missile Game, and Challenger Board Game). Children can also use a picture-creation device in the computer game (the "Scene Generator") to illustrate how they have used target skills during the week and are encouraged to use smart phones or tablets (where available) to take pictures and audio recordings of the "evidence" they collect when completing their home missions. If children are not engaged by the detective theme of the program, facilitators are encouraged to use a child's area of special interest as a metaphor to teach social–emotional concepts where possible.

The SAS program encourages children to use their powers of *investigation* to practice detecting how other people feel from face, voice, body, and situational clues, to be on high alert for the thoughts and body clues that signal the nature and intensity of their own feelings, and to discover for themselves the benefits of using their SAS skills by completing home mission questions in a "Secret Agent Journal." Thus, a *self-discovery* approach is used to boost children's motivation to use the skills that they learn in the program, as these approaches typically lead to better outcomes than less appropriate alternatives.

Children also discover for themselves the consequences of using helpful strategies (e.g., breathing slowly and thinking helpful thoughts) and ineffective ways of coping with feelings (e.g., running away and hitting others) in the virtual reality missions in Level 3 of the SAS computer game. These missions are similar to choose-your-own-adventure style story books, where the player's character in the game is required to navigate common social challenges for children with ASD (e.g., trying a new activity, group work, losing a game or competition, coping with teasing). Exploring the consequences of choosing different solutions to social problems for their game character in a virtual world is initially less confronting and more engaging for individuals with ASD than being told by a practitioner or parent how to express their feelings and solve problems (Kandalaft et al. 2013). This initial engagement and normalization process helps children to be more open to discussing their own social–emotional challenges and exploring possible ways of coping with them. The use of therapeutic games and activities related to common special interests, the opportunity to connect with other children like themselves, and the provision of individualized within- and between-session rewards help to make the SAS program an *enjoyable* experience for children with ASD.

Teaching Emotion Regulation with the SAS Program: The Application of Gross and Thompson's (2007) Five-Factor Model

A core objective of the SAS program is to improve children's social competence. The social impairments that characterize children with ASD are often exacerbated by emotion regulation difficulties. Therefore, SAS teaches foundational skills in emotion recognition and emotional expression first, before introducing social interaction skills. Please see the following summary of the intervention elements that illustrate Gross and Thompson's (2007) five-factor model of emotion regulation.

Situation Selection

A cornerstone of the SAS program is children facing situations that they find anxiety provoking or frustrating and using their relaxation gadgets to cope. Through their home missions, children confront successively more challenging situations that they may have previously avoided. The program concludes with them joining a new club or team (often related to their special interest) and using their social–emotional skills to make new friends and cope with challenges (e.g., team work, compromising, losing, and so on). Children are also taught how to decipher social situations by focusing their attention on clues that may indicate how other people are feeling and what they may be thinking. This helps them to more accurately detect and define social problems that they may need to solve.

Situation Modification

Within the SAS program, children are taught a step-by-step problem-solving formula (D.E.C.O.D.E.R) that helps them to *detect* and *define* a social problem, *explore* possible solutions, *consider* the *consequences* and *choose* a solution, *organize* a plan, *do* it, *evaluate* how it went, and *reward* themselves for trying their best. They are encouraged to work through the D.E.C.O.D.E.R steps with the help of an adult and practice their chosen solution with an adult before putting it into action. This problem-solving formula integrates the emotion recognition and regulation skills that they learn in the first four sessions of the program to optimize the likely success of their chosen methods for coping with social challenges.

Attentional Deployment

Within the program, children learn about the physical sensations, behaviors, and thoughts that

Fig. 12.2 Relaxation gadget Code Card from SAS program (front and back view)

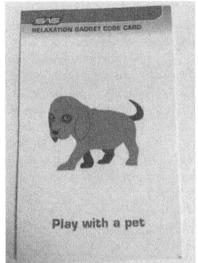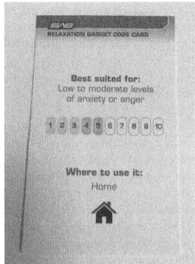

signal when they feel mildly, moderately, and very anxious and angry. They are encouraged to be on "high alert" for these clues (especially *early* warning signs of anxiety and anger) and to use contextually appropriate relaxation gadgets to cope. In a new program variant soon to be evaluated, children will also be taught the "relaxation radar" technique, which involves focusing on happy or friendly things around them when they feel distressed. This new program variant also teaches them to observe their breath, body, and surroundings ("enviro-body scan") to calm their mind and boost their brain power.

Cognitive Control

One of the relaxation gadgets that children learn in the SAS program is the Helpful Thought Missile. This involves them detecting unhelpful "enemy" thoughts that go through their mind when they feel upset and shooting these down and replacing them with more helpful alternatives. Recent trials of the program have included an alternative to this activity for children who are resistant to changing their unhelpful thoughts. Consistent with Acceptance and Commitment Therapy principles, this alternative exercise involves children just being aware of the unhelpful thoughts they think when they feel upset and defusing from these thoughts by imagining them

printed on a blimp or airplane that flies around them (Twohig et al. 2008).

Response Modulation

Throughout the SAS program, children are taught a range of cognitive behavioral relaxation gadgets to help regulate their emotions. They are advised that relaxing activities work best for low-to-moderate levels of anxiety or anger, whereas physical activities work best for high levels of distress. Some of the relaxation gadgets featured in the program include the O_2 Regulator gadget (slow breathing), the Fire Engine (doing a physical activity when very distressed), and the Helpful Thought Missile (as described in the previous section). Children choose a range of pocket-sized full-color "Code Cards" illustrating their chosen relaxation gadgets. These cards feature a picture of the relaxation gadget on the front and a description of what the strategy involves (if needed), what level of anxiety or anger it is best suited for, and where it is best used on the back. An example Relaxation Gadget Code Card is shown in Fig. 12.2.

These cards capitalize on the common interest in collecting items among children with ASD, motivating them to consider several different relaxation strategies rather than perseverating on just one or two. Children are also encouraged to "spy" on others when completing their home missions to learn contextually appropriate ways of expressing their feelings in different situations.

Conclusions

In reviewing the programs that have aimed to address anxiety in children with ASD through CBT approaches, it is clear that many of these have included material that is typically not used in a traditional anxiety program. We have reviewed the modifications that are recommended but, in looking at these more closely, we face the question of whether it makes sense to develop programs that are narrowly focused on just one psychological domain (for example anxiety or social skills) when working with this population. The fact that emotional dysregulation is a central feature in this population means that there will be significant overlap and diversity in presentations of anxiety, anger, behavioral problems, and depressive symptoms. Indeed, we already have evidence to demonstrate this (Quek et al. 2012) as well as demographic characteristics of children in the studies that indicate overlapping symptoms.

Some programs have been developed to manage presentations of emotion dysregulation other than anxiety (e.g., anger; Sofronoff et al. 2007) and appropriate expression of affectionate behavior (Sofronoff et al. 2011). What is important to note here is that these programs use essentially the same format and content as the anxiety program evaluated by this group (Sofronoff et al. 2005) but focus on a different target. Including the modifications to CBT that have been shown to be useful, there is also a focus on teaching emotion recognition from the outset, accounting for individual differences in learning style, and an awareness of other issues that may present in the context of program delivery—e.g., behavioral issues, restlessness, the need to incorporate a special interest, and so on.

Finally, it is important to recognize that many of the programs that we are developing and evaluating are already moving in a transdiagnostic direction. The example of the SAS program illustrates this and also shows that, along with the in-novative approaches used, there still remains a fidelity to the central components of CBT. The trial by Reaven et al. (2012) shows similar innovation within the context of a CBT intervention and the Storch et al. (2013) trial demonstrates how modules can be flexibly delivered to address the multiple additional problems with which children with ASD and anxiety typically present. Clearly, we are moving to recognize that even within a good anxiety program we must go beyond anxiety in this population.

References

Aldao, A., Nolen-Hoeksema, S., & Schweizer, S. (2010). Emotion-regulation strategies across psychopathology: A meta-analytic review. *Clinical Psychology Review, 30*(2), 217–237. http://dx.doi.org/10.1016/j.cpr.2009.11.004.

Barlow, D. H., Allen, L. B., & Choate, M. L. (2004). Toward a unified treatment for emotional disorders. *Behavior Therapy, 35*(2), 205–230. doi:10.1016/S0005-7894(04)80036-4.

Barlow, D. H., Farchione, T. J., Fairholme, C. P., Ellard, K. K., Boisseau, C. L., Allen, L. B., et al. (2011). *The unified protocol for transdiagnostic treatment of emotional disorders: Therapist guide.* New York: Oxford University Press.

Beaumont, R. (2010). *Secret Agent Society: Solving the mystery of social encounters—Facilitator kit.* Queensland: The Social Skills Training Institute.

Beaumont, R., & Sofronoff, K. (2008). A multi-component social skills intervention for children with Asperger syndrome: The Junior Detective Training Program. *Journal of Child Psychology and Psychiatry, 49,* 743–753.

Bilek, E. L., & Ehrenreich-May, J. (2012). An open trial investigation of a transdiagnostic group treatment for children with anxiety and depressive symptoms. *Behavior Therapy, 43*(4), 887–897. doi:10.1016/j.beth.2012.04.007.

Boisseau, C. L., Farchione, T. J., Fairholme, C. P., Ellard, K. K., & Barlow, D. H. (2010). The development of the Unified Protocol for the transdiagnostic treatment of emotional disorders: A case study. *Cognitive and Behavioral Practice, 17*(1), 102–113. doi:10.1016/j.cbpra.2009.09.003.

Cardaciotto, L., & Herbert, J. D. (2004). Cognitive Behavior Therapy for social anxiety disorder in the context of Asperger's syndrome: A single subject report. *Cognitive and Behavioral Practice, 11,* 75–81.

Chalfant, A. M., Rapee, R., & Carroll, L. (2007). Treating anxiety disorders in children with high functioning autism spectrum disorders: A controlled trial. *Jour-*

nal of Autism and Developmental Disorders, 37(10), 1842–1857. doi:10.1007/s10803-006-0318-4.

Channon, S., Charman, T., Heap, J., Crawford, S., & Rios, P. (2001). Real-life-type problem-solving in Asperger's syndrome. *Journal of Autism and Developmental Disorders, 31*(5), 461–469. doi:10.1023/A:1012212824307.

Davis, T. E. III, May, A. C., & Whiting, S. E. (2011). Evidence-based treatment of anxiety and phobia in children and adolescents: Current status and effects on the emotional response. *Clinical Psychology Review, 31*, 592–602. doi:10.1016/j.cpr.2011.01.001.

Donoghue, K., Stallard, P., & Kucia, J. (2011). The clinical practice of Cognitive Behavioural Therapy for children and young people with a diagnosis of Asperger's syndrome. *Clinical Child Psychology and Psychiatry, 16*(1), 89–102. doi:10.1177/1359104509355019.

Ehrenreich, J. T., Goldstein, C. R., Wright, L. R., & Barlow, D. H. (2009). Development of a unified protocol for the treatment of emotional disorders in youth. *Child & Family Behavior Therapy, 31*(1), 20–37. doi:10.1080/07317100802701228.

Ellard, K. K., Fairholme, C. P., Boisseau, C. L., Farchione, T. J., & Barlow, D. H. (2010). Unified protocol for the transdiagnostic treatment of emotional disorders: Protocol development and initial outcome data. *Cognitive and Behavioral Practice, 17*(1), 88–101. doi:10.1016/j.cbpra.2009.06.002.

Gadow, K. D., DeVincent, C. J., & Pomeroy, J. (2006). ADHD symptom subtypes in children with pervasive developmental disorder. *Journal of Autism and Developmental Disorders, 36*(2), 271–283. doi:10.1007/s10803-005-0060-3.

Golan, O., Ashwin, E., Granader, Y., McClintock, S., Day, K., Leggett, V., et al. (2010). Enhancing emotion recognition in children with autism spectrum conditions: An intervention using animated vehicles with real emotional faces. *Journal of Autism and Developmental Disorders, 40*, 269–279. doi:10.1017/s0954579406060305.

Greig, A., & MacKay, T. (2005). Asperger's syndrome and Cognitive Behavior Therapy: New applications for educational psychologists. *Educational and Child Psychology, 22*, 4–15.

Gross, J. J., & Thompson, R. A. (2007). *Emotion regulation: Conceptual foundations. Handbook of emotion regulation.* New York, NY: Guilford Press.

Hastings, R. P., Hughes, J. C., Jahr, E., Eikeseth, S., & Cross, S. (2009). Met-analysis of early intensive behavioral intervention for children with autism. *Journal of Clinical Child and Adolescent Psychology, 38*(3), 439–450. doi:10.1080/15374410902851739.

Hurtig, T., Kuusikko, S., Mattila, M. L., Haapsamo, H., Ebeling, H., Jussila, K., et al. (2009). Multi-informant reports of psychiatric symptoms among high-functioning adolescents with Asperger syndrome or autism. *Autism: The International Journal of Research and Practice, 13*(6), 583–598. doi:10.1177/1362361309335719.

Kandalaft, M. R., Didehbani, N., Krawczyk, D. C., Allen, T. T., & Chapman, S. B. (2013). Virtual reality social cognition training for young adults with high-functioning autism. *Journal of Autism and Developmental Disorders, 43*(1), 34–44. doi:10.1007/s10803-012-1544-6.

Kendall, P. C., Aschenbrand, S. G., & Hudson, J. L. (2003). Child-focused treatment of anxiety. In A. E. Kazdin & J. R. Weisz (Eds.), *Evidence-based psychotherapies for children and adolescents* (pp. 81–100). New York: Guilford Press.

Lang, R., Regester, A., Lauderdale, S., Ashbaugh, K., & Haring, A. (2010). Treatment of anxiety in autism spectrum disorders using cognitive behavior therapy: A systematic review. *Developmental Neurorehabilitation, 13*(1), 53–63. doi:10.3109/17518420903236288.

Lecavalier, L., Gadow, K. D., DeVincent, C. J., & Edwards, M. C. (2008). Validation of DSM-IV model of psychiatric syndromes in children with autism spectrum disorders. *Journal of Autism and Developmental Disorders, 39*(2), 278–289. doi:10.1007/s10803-008-0622-2.

Leyfer, O. T., Folstein, S. E., Bacalman, S., Davis, N. O., Dinh, E., Morgan, J., et al. (2006). Comorbid psychiatric disorders in children with autism: Interview development and rates of disorders. *Journal of Autism and Developmental Disorders, 36*(7), 849–861. doi:10.1007/s10803-006-0123-0.

Lickel, A., Maclean, W. E. Jr., Blakeley-Smith, A., & Hepburn, S. (2012). Assessment of the prerequisite skills for Cognitive Behavioral Therapy in children with and without autism spectrum disorders. *Journal of Autism and Developmental Disorders, 42*, 992–1000. doi:10.1007/s10803-011-1330-x.

Lovaas, O. I. (1987). Behavioral treatment and normal educational and intellectual functioning in young autistic children. *Journal of Consulting and Clinical Psychology, 55*, 3–9.

Loveland, K. A., Pearson, D. A., Tunali-Kotoski, B., Ortegon, J., & Gibbs, M. C. (2001). Judgments of social appropriateness by children and adolescents with autism. Journal of Autism and Developmental Disorders, 31(4), 367–376. doi:10.1023/A:1010608518060.

Magyar, C. I., & Pandolfi, V. (2012). Considerations for establishing a multi-tiered problem-solving model for students with autism spectrum disorders and comorbid emotional-Behavioral disorders. *Psychology in the Schools, 49*(10), 975–987. doi:10.1002/pits.21645.

Mash, E. J., & Wolfe, D. A. (2002). *Abnormal child psychology.* Belmont: Wadsworth.

Mazefsky, C. A., Herrington, J., Siegel, M., Scarpa, A., Maddox, B. B., Scahill, L., et al. (2013). The role of emotion regulation in autism spectrum disorder. *Journal of the American Academy of Child & Adolescent Psychiatry, 52*(7), 679–688.

McLaughlin, K. A., Hatzenbuehler, M. L., Mennin, D. S., & Nolen-Hoeksema, S. (2011). Emotion dysregulation and adolescent psychopathology: A prospective study. *Behaviour Research and Therapy, 49*(9), 544–554. doi:10.1016/j.brat.2011.06.003.

McNally Keehn, R. H., Lincoln, A. J., Brown, M. Z., & Chavira, D. A. (2013). The Coping Cat Program for children with anxiety and autism spectrum disorder: A pilot randomized controlled trial. *Journal of Autism and Developmental Disorders, 43,* 57–67. doi:10.1007/210803-012-1541-9.

Moree, B. N., & Davis, T. E. (2010). Cognitive-behavioral therapy for anxiety in children diagnosed with autism spectrum disorders: Modification trends. *Research in Autism Spectrum Disorders, 4,* 346–354. doi:10.1016/j.rasd.2009.10.015.

Munoz-Solomando, A., Kendall, T., & Whittington, C. J. (2008). Cognitive behavioural therapy for children and adolescents. *Current Opinion in Psychiatry, 21*(4), 332–337. http://dx.doi.org.ezproxy.library.yorku.ca/10.1097/YCO.0b013e328305097c.

Norton, P. J. (2012). A randomized clinical trial of transdiagnostic cognitve-behavioral treatments for anxiety disorder by comparison to relaxation training. *Behavior Therapy, 43*(3), 506–517. doi:10.1016/j.beth.2010.08.011.

Ollendick, T. H., King, N. J., & Chorpita, B. F. (2006). Empirically supported treatments for children and adolescents. In P. C. Kendall (Ed.), *Child and adolescent therapy: Cognitive-behavioral procedures* (3rd ed., pp. 492–520). New York: Guilford Press.

Quek, L.-H., Sofronoff, K., Sheffield, J., White, A., & Kelly, A. (2012). Co-occurring anger in young people with Asperger's syndrome. *Journal of Clinical Psychology, 68*(10), 1142–1148. doi:10.1002/jclp.21888.

Rapee, R. M. (2002). The development and modification of temperamental risk for anxiety disorders: Prevention of a lifetime of anxiety? Biological Psychiatry, 52(10), 947–957. doi:10.1016/S0006-3223(02)01572-X.

Reaven, J. A., Blakeley-Smith, A., Nichols, S., Dasari, M., Flanigan, E., & Hepburn, S. (2009). Cognitive-behavioral group treatment for anxiety symptoms in children with high-functioning autism spectrum disorders: A pilot study. *Focus on Autism and Other Developmental Disabilities, 24,* 27–37.

Reaven, J. A., Blakeley-Smith, A., Culhane-Shelburne, K., & Hepburn, S. (2012). Group Cognitive Behavior Therapy for children with high-functioning autism spectrum disorders and anxiety: A randomized trial. *Journal of Child Psychology and Psychiatry, 53*(4), 410–419. doi:10.1111/j.1469-7610.2011.02486.x.

Reaven, J., & Hepburn, S. (2003). Cognitive-behavioral treatment of obsessive-compulsive disorder in a child with Asperger syndrome: A case report. *Autism: The International Journal of Research and Practice, 7,* 145–164.

Rieffe, C., Oosterveld, P., Terwogt, M. M., Mootz, S., van Leeuwen, E., & Stockmann, L. (2011). Emotion regulation and internalizing symptoms in children with autism spectrum disorders. *Autism: The International Journal of Research and Practice, 15*(6), 655–670. doi:10.1177/1362361310366571.

Rohde, P. (2012). Applying transdiagnostic approaches to treatments with children and adolescents: Innovative models that are ready for more systematic evaluation.

Cognitive and Behavioral Practice, 19(1), 83–86. doi:10.1016/j.cbpra.2011.06.006.

Singh, N. N., Lancioni, G. E., Manikam, R., Winton, A. S. W., Singh, A. N. A., Singh, J., et al. (2011). A mindfulness-based strategy for self-management of aggressive behavior in adolescents with Autism. *Research in Autism Spectrum Disorders, 5*(3), 1153–1158. http://dx.doi.org/10.1016/j.rasd.2010.12.012.

Sofronoff, K., Attwood, T., & Hinton, S. (2005). A randomized controlled trial of a CBT intervention for anxiety in children with Asperger syndrome. *Journal of Child Psychology and Psychiatry, 4*(11), 1152–1160. doi:10.1111/j.1469-7610.2005.00411.x.

Sofronoff, K., Attwood, T., Hinton, S., & Levin, I. (2007). A randomized controlled trial of a cognitive behavioural intervention for anger management in children diagnosed with Asperger syndrome. *Journal of Autism and Developmental Disorders, 37*(7), 1203–1214. doi:10.1007/s10803-006-0262-3.

Sofronoff, K., Eloff, J., Sheffield, J., & Attwood, T. (2011). Increasing the understanding and demonstration of appropriate affection in children with Asperger syndrome. *Autism Research and Treatment.* doi:10.1155/2011/214317.

Sofronoff, K., Silva, J., & Beaumont, R. (submitted). Parent delivery of the Secret agent Society social-emotional skills training program for children with high-functioning autism spectrum disorders. Focus on Autism and other Developmental disorders.

Storch, E. R., Arnold, E. B., Lewin, A. B., Nadeau, J. M., Jones, A. M., De Nadai, A. S., et al. (2013). The effect of Cognitive-Behavioral Therapy versus treatment as usual for anxiety in children with autism spectrum disorders: A randomized controlled trial. *Journal of the American Academy of Child and Adolescent Psychiatry, 52*(2), 132–142.

Sze, K. M., & Wood, J. J. (2007). Cognitive Behavioral treatment of comorbid anxiety disorders and social difficulties in children with high functioning autism: A case report. *Journal of Contemporary Psychotherapy, 37,* 133–143.

Sze, K. M., & Wood, J. J. (2008). Enhancing CBT for the treatment autism spectrum disorders and concurrent anxiety. *Behavioural and Cognitive Psychotherapy, 36,* 403–409.

Tanaka, J. W., Wolf, J. M., Klaiman, C., Koenig, K., Cockburn, J., Herlihy, L., et al. (2012). The perception and identification of facial emotions in individuals with autism spectrum disorders using the let's face it! Emotion skills battery. *Journal of Child Psychology and Psychiatry, 53*(12), 1259–1267. http://dx.doi.org/10.1111/j.1469-7610.2012.02571.x.

Thompson, R. A. (1994). Emotion regulation: A theme in search of definition. *Monographs of the Society for Research in Child Development, 59,* 25–52.

Trosper, S. E., Buzzella, B. A., Bennett, S. M., & Ehrenreich, J. T. (2009). Emotion regulation in youth with emotional disorders: Implications for a unified treatment approach. *Clinical Child and Family*

Psychology Review, 12(3), 234–254. doi:10.1007/s10567-009-0043-6.

Twohig, M. P., Hayes, S. C., & Berlin, K. S. (2008). Acceptance and commitment therapy for childhood externalizing disorders. In L. A. Greco & S. C. Hayes (Eds.), *Acceptance and mindfulness treatments for children and adolescents—A practitioner's guide* (pp. 163–186). Oakland: New Harbinger Publications.

Weersing, V. R., Rozenman, M. S., Maher-Bridge, M., & Campo, J. V. (2012). Anxiety, depression, and somatic distress: Developing a transdiagnostic internalizing toolbox for pediatric practice. *Cognitive and Behavioral Practice, 19*(1), 68–82. doi:10.1016/j.cbpra.2011.06.002.

Weisbrot, D. M., Gadow, K. D., DeVincent, C. J., & Pomeroy, J. (2005). The presentation of anxiety in children with pervasive developmental disorders. *Journal of Child & Adolescent Psychopharmacology, 15*(3), 477–496. doi:10.1089/cap.2005.15.477.

White, S. W., Ollendick, T., Albano, A. M., Oswald, D., Johnson, C., Southam-Gerow, M. A., et al. (2013). Randomized controlled trial: Multimodal anxiety and social skill intervention for adolescents with autism spectrum disorder. *Journal of Autism and Developmental Disorders, 43*, 382–394. doi:10.1007/s10803-012-1577-x.

Whittingham, K., Sofronoff, K., Sheffield, J., & Sanders, M. (2009). Stepping stones triple P: A randomized controlled trial with parents of a child diagnosed with an autism spectrum disorder. *Journal of Abnormal Child Psychology, 37*, 469–480.

Williams, D., & Happé, F. (2010). Representing intentions in self and other: Studies of autism and typical development. *Developmental Science, 13*(2), 307–319. doi:10.1111/j.1467-7687.2009.00885.x.

Wood, J., Drahota, A., Sze, K., Kim, H., Chui, A., & Langer, D. (2009). Cognitive Behavioral Therapy for anxiety in children with autism spectrum disorders: A randomized controlled trial. *Journal of Child Psychology and Psychiatry, 50*, 224–234. doi:10.1111/j.1469-7610.2008.01948.x.

Zeman, J., & Shipman, K. (1998). Influence of social context on children's affect regulation: A functionalist perspective. *Journal of Nonverbal Behavior, 22*(3), 141–165. doi:10.1023/A:1022900704563.

Bridging the Research to Practice Gap in Autism Research: Implementing Group CBT Interventions for Youth with ASD and Anxiety in Clinical Practice

Judy Reaven, Audrey Blakeley-Smith and Susan Hepburn

Introduction

Over the past 10 years, researchers and clinicians have shown increasing interest in the assessment and treatment of co-occurring clinical anxiety in individuals with autism spectrum disorder (ASD). Although still a relatively new area of research, much attention has been devoted to the development of efficacious treatments in efforts to ameliorate the debilitating impact of anxiety symptoms. At least eight randomized controlled trials have been conducted with children and adolescents with ASD and anxiety, using modified cognitive behavior therapy (CBT) approaches (Chalfant et al. 2007; Keehn et al. 2013; Reaven et al. 2012a; Sofronoff et al. 2005; Storch et al. 2013; Sung et al. 2011; White et al. 2013; Wood et al. 2009). Individual treatment (e.g., Wood et al. 2009), group treatment (e.g., Reaven et al. 2012a, 2012b), and combined individual/group treatment programs (White et al. 2013) have all yielded promising results.

Notably, these treatment programs have occurred primarily in tightly controlled university-based research environments and have not yet been systematically delivered in real-world clinical settings. Furthermore, the participants in these studies were typically recruited and selected based on specific inclusion and exclusion criteria, leading to fairly homogeneous samples. The homogeneity among participants in clinical trials, while critical in the initial stages of treatment development and efficacy research, may contribute to the substantial gap between research environments and the "real world" (Storch and Crisp 2004; Weisz et al. 2004). For example, variability in participant characteristics (e.g., motivation to improve, parental involvement, or socioeconomic status) may not be fully represented by subjects who participate in clinical trials. That is, psychiatric comorbidity or serious behavioral challenges may be seen as criteria for exclusion in some studies. Thus, the factors that comprise exclusion criteria and influence participation in treatment trials may inadvertently thwart the inclusion of many of the families that the treatment protocols are designed to reach. Similarly, financial constraints, inflexible parent work schedules, or limitations in transportation may prevent some youth and their families from participating in lengthy assessments to determine eligibility and/or consistently attending treatment sessions.

Therefore, a key component in the development of new interventions is to examine the sustainability and portability of the intervention from the "lab" setting to existing clinical practice (Schoenwald and Hoagwood 2001). If the ultimate goal of treatment development is for widespread dissemination and implementation of novel interventions, then systematic approaches for moving evidence-based approaches from

J. Reaven (✉) · A. Blakeley-Smith · S. Hepburn
Departments of Psychiatry and Pediatrics, School of Medicine, JFK Partners, University of Colorado Anschutz Medical Campus, Aurora, CO, USA
e-mail: judy.reaven@ucdenver.edu

T. E. Davis III et al. (eds.), *Handbook of Autism and Anxiety,* Autism and Child Psychopathology Series,
DOI 10.1007/978-3-319-06796-4_13, © Springer International Publishing Switzerland 2014

research settings to clinical practice must be put in place. Introducing treatment programs into new clinical settings *early* in the development process has the potential to inform protocol development, increase acceptability of the intervention, and ultimately maximize success for clinical practice with real-world populations (Beidas et al. 2011; Weisz et al. 2004).

As treatment development for ASD has burgeoned in recent years, work groups comprised of experts in the field were formed and charged with developing guidelines for the systematic and rigorous development of psychosocial interventions (Lord et al. 2005; Smith et al. 2007). A primary purpose of the guidelines was to provide careful and systematic standards for validating and disseminating evidence-based psychosocial interventions for youth with ASD (Smith et al. 2007). Smith et al. (2007) delineated a step-by-step approach to treatment development comprised of four phases: (1) formulation and systematic application of a new intervention, (2) manualization and protocol development, (3) conducting efficacy studies using randomized clinical trials, and (4) exploring community effectiveness. Although proposed for treatment research with individuals with ASD, these principles and other rubrics for developing evidence-based practice (e.g., Reichow 2011) have guided research in childhood psychopathology more broadly, as well as in ASD. The degree to which evidence-based treatments that were developed in controlled research settings can be transported to clinical settings *and* yield the same positive impact remains an empirical question (Weisz et al. 2004).

This chapter concentrates on bridging the research-to-practice gap in autism research, with special attention paid to interventions targeting anxiety symptoms in children and adolescents with ASD. Barriers to the dissemination of evidence-based interventions and strategies for fostering the implementation of novel interventions are discussed. A review of clinical training models geared towards instructing community practitioners in how to deliver evidence-based treatments is also described. Given the limited research on the dissemination of evidence-based interventions for youth with ASD, examples of

successful dissemination efforts in mental health interventions for children with other psychiatric disorders, as well as a sampling of the progress to date of dissemination treatment research for youth with ASD, are provided. The final section of this chapter includes descriptions of the initial implementation efforts of our group CBT program for youth with ASD and anxiety (Facing Your Fears (FYF): Group Therapy for Managing Anxiety in Children with High-Functioning Autism Spectrum Disorders; Reaven et al. 2011). We present efforts to deliver FYF beyond the traditional research setting to new clinic settings and school environments, and explore telehealth applications as an additional forum for delivering the intervention.

Barriers to Dissemination

There are many potential barriers to dissemination of evidence-based treatment, beginning with basic issues of access. Research suggests that empirically supported treatments are not frequently available to youth who need them most (Beidas et al. 2011; Elkins et al. 2011). Patient-level factors such as geographic location, socioeconomic status, ethnicity (i.e., minorities are underserved), easy access to transportation, time to search for and participate in affordable services, and the stigma associated with seeking interventions (such as psychiatric care) are some of the variables that interfere with participation in empirically supported programs (Elkins et al. 2011; Kendall et al. 2012).

Perhaps most discouraging is that even when research-based treatment curricula (e.g., treatment programs for ASD) become available to clinicians in the community, they are rarely adopted (Dingfelder and Mandell 2011). For practitioners working with individuals with ASD, access to scientifically based treatments may be limited, and practitioners may rely on outdated information to select the most effective interventions (Volkmar et al. 2011). Additionally, community administrators are charged with sorting through numerous autism treatment programs and determining which programs have the best research support, even though they may not have the background or knowledge to assess which programs represent truly evidence-based practice. The sheer volume of information (and misinformation) about intervention programs for ASD, coupled with anecdotal reports of "cures" as well as the emotional investment of key stakeholders, all contribute to the challenge in selecting evidence-based treatments. Compounding the problem is that once programs are selected for use in community settings, practitioners delivering the proposed intervention programs may not be qualified to deliver the specialized treatment. Finally, because autism interventions may be delivered by professionals from different disciplinary backgrounds (e.g., psychology, speech/language pathology, occupational and physical therapy) across a variety of settings (e.g., autism centers, schools, and home), establishing clear guidelines for evidence-based practice has been challenging. Together, these factors have contributed to the gap separating research from practice (Volkmar et al. 2011).

Importantly, when evidence-based approaches are identified and efforts are made for community clinicians to deliver the selected intervention, treatment programs may be only partially implemented by practitioners in community settings, or rejected altogether. Clinicians may be skeptical of evidence-based approaches because they view them as too resource intensive or inflexible for their setting and question whether they can be modified for their clientele (Elkins et al. 2011). Contributing to the perception of evidence-based programs as inflexible is the common misperception that a particular model must be implemented in its original form; that is, the entire treatment protocol must be delivered exactly as it was delivered in a research context, without regard for the contextual differences between community and "lab" environments (Beidas et al. 2011). This perceived lack of compatibility (e.g., inconsistency with the organization's values and beliefs, lack of cultural sensitivity, and failure to target the population's most pressing needs) contributes to the potential rejection of a novel intervention. Treatments that are cost-effective, that include practical guidelines for training professionals to effectively deliver the intervention, and that allow for bidirectional discussions and dialogue regarding the intervention may be most successful in community contexts. Thus, it is critical that the factors influencing the rejection or adoption of evidence-based approaches be outlined, and that any potential challenges to adoption and sustainability be directly addressed (Beidas et al. 2011).

Fostering Dissemination and Adoption of Novel Interventions

Dingfelder and Mandell (2011) have proposed an approach to improve the dissemination of interventions for individuals with ASD that complements the guidelines outlined above (Lord et al. 2005; Smith et al. 2007), integrating their stepwise schemas with Rogers's (2003) "diffusion of innovations" theory. Rather than working from the traditional model of treatment development that reserves the dissemination of interventions to community settings for the final step in the development process, the model brings treatments into clinical practice early in the development process and examines effectiveness in practice settings recurrently throughout development (Dingfelder and Mandell 2011; Rogers 2003; Weisz et al. 2004). Thus, it is the integration of traditional treatment development approaches with diffusion of innovation theory that may increase the probability that effective interventions will be adopted and sustained in real-world clinical settings. To improve dissemination of treatments for ASD, Dingfelder and Mandell (2011) focus on three of Rogers's (2003) original five attributes that are most likely to influence the adoption of an innovative intervention: *relative advantage* (the degree to which an innovation is thought to be better than an existing program), *compatibility* (the extent to which an innovative treatment is compatible with an organization's values, priorities, and resources), and *complexity* (the extent to which the innovation is viewed as difficult to use). In order to maximize the perceptions of a receiving population towards acceptance of an innovative treatment program, they must view the intervention as compatible with organizational values, superior to existing programs, and feasible.

A bidirectional model of science and practice may be optimal for maximizing the relative advantage, compatibility, and feasibility of an innovation, thus facilitating the adoption of innovation (Brookman-Frazee et al. 2012a; Teachman et al. 2012). A bidirectional model suggests that in order to develop interventions that are cost-effective, feasible, and sustainable in the long term, partnerships and collaborations between clinicians and researchers must be formed. Field testing evidence-based interventions in naturalistic settings, emphasizing reciprocity and interaction between researchers and practitioners, and obtaining feedback from participants regarding "goodness of fit" may promote interventions' long-term sustainability (Brookman-Frazee et al. 2012a).

Community-based participatory research is an example of a collaborative and bidirectional effort among community members, organizations, and researchers where key stakeholders work together towards a shared goal (Brookman-Frazee et al. 2012a). It is through the collaboration between researchers and nonresearchers that broad social changes can occur (Denis and Lomas 2003). Collaborative research allows the "researcher" to appreciate the approach of the "practitioner" and vice versa. In fact, some note that knowledge acquired solely in the laboratory environment may not be "real" knowledge at all (Denis and Lomas 2003). Only by inserting investigators into contextually valid environments can "knowledge" with real-life, practical consequences result (Denis and Lomas 2003). Therefore, a potential benefit of community/university collaborations may be that they commonly lead to projects that are community-driven, useful, and culturally appropriate, thereby increasing the chances that communities will ultimately adopt innovative programming (O'Fallon and Dearry 2002).

Dingfelder and Mandell (2011) use the tenets of participatory collaborative research and diffusion of innovation to youth with ASD in the following recommendations for maximizing the adoptability of evidence-based ASD interventions: (1) target interventions that address public priorities, (2) include heterogeneous samples in more naturalistic settings to increase generalizability, (3) involve stakeholders in research from the beginning of protocol development so that treatment programs are tailored to the values and priorities of key stakeholders, (4) include comprehensive formal data collection and follow-up to monitor implementation fidelity, and (5) include a systematic plan for maintaining *independent* delivery of the intervention, so that the intervention is sustainable long after the developers have left.

Studying the specific organizational factors, therapist and client characteristics, and features of service delivery, as well as establishing best practice training procedures, is also key in the adoption of novel interventions (Schmidt and Taylor 2002; Schoenwald and Hoagwood 2001). When a new intervention is introduced to an organization, the degree of agency "buy-in" towards the approach and assessment of the real impact on employee workload naturally occur. In addition, organizations informally examine the extent to which the new intervention is congruent with organizational beliefs. If the new model excessively challenges existing perceptions and staff believe that the new model cannot be sufficiently adapted for their environment, then even when an organization has formally chosen to "adopt" a model, they can also choose to "un-adopt" (either explicitly or unintentionally) an innovative program (Massatti et al. 2007). Factors that may cause an innovative intervention to be "un-adopted" include lack of staff commitment, insufficient staff training, and inability for staff to access appropriate assistance to deliver the intervention (Massatti et al. 2007). Staff attitudes towards the adoption of new interventions are particularly crucial to understand, as they may be especially influential as to whether an innovation will be considered for adoption (Stahmer and Aarons 2009). For example, the intuitive appeal of the intervention, staff openness towards adopting new practices, concerns about practitioner competence to administer the intervention, and beliefs as to whether the intervention will address client needs are important to consider and may represent potential barriers to implementation (Gunter and Whittal 2010; Stahmer and Aarons 2009). Further, freeing up time for training, providing high-quality supervision, and establishing peer-learning work groups may be essential in translating evidence-based interventions to community environments (Schmidt and Taylor 2002).

Training Considerations

Training for clinical effectiveness trials under ideal circumstances generally consists of the selection of clinicians who are experienced in and committed to the type of treatment they will ultimately implement, provision of an intensive didactic seminar, and opportunity for ongoing and close supervision (Carroll 2013; Sholomskas et al. 2005). While this may represent a gold standard "classic" clinical training model, efforts to disseminate treatments to the community have typically consisted of widespread distribution of manuals, only occasionally paired with brief didactic training (Sholomskas et al. 2005). Reading treatment manuals may be necessary, but not sufficient, for skill acquisition, particularly when learning novel interventions (Herschell et al. 2010). The same may be said for attending brief didactic workshops without additional consultation. That is, although short-term increases in knowledge of a novel intervention may occur after attending didactic workshops, the increases in knowledge generally do not translate to the long-term implementation of novel interventions (Herschell et al. 2010).

Even though best practice training procedures are recommended for providers who may be implementing new interventions, the format and content of trainings may vary considerably, in terms of both session material as well as duration of trainings. Training length may range from as little as an hour-long seminar, to half-day trainings, to full-day workshops, to weeklong intensive training experiences. The content and format of trainings vary as well, with some centering on theoretical content and conceptual understanding of the intervention, and others focusing on a systematic review of a treatment manual session-by-

session "how-to" procedures (Sholomskas et al. 2005). Some treatment programs for youth with ASD have used multiday workshops as a vehicle for obtaining "certification" signifying that the participant has achieved high treatment fidelity for a particular program (e.g., PEERS; Laugeson et al. 2012); Relationship Developmental Intervention (RDI; Gutstein et al. 2007); Early Start Denver Model (ESDM; Rogers and Dawson 2010). However, there continues to be much variability across intervention programs about *how,* or *whether,* it is essential to obtain specialized certification.

Ideal training formats are typically active, experiential, and behaviorally oriented. The most effective training techniques provide opportunities for direct feedback, behavioral rehearsal, and role-play for all participants (Beidas et al. 2011; Kendall and Beidas 2007; Sholomskas et al. 2005; Vismara et al. 2013). Although didactic training combined with direct and ongoing coaching/supervision may be most ideal for creating treatment adherence, balancing cost-effectiveness with the direct impact of treatment outcomes is also important (Carroll 2013; Vismara et al. 2013; Webb et al. 2010).

The extent to which strong adherence and clinician competence are necessary to obtain improved child outcomes is unclear (Beidas et al. 2011). Some researchers state that the correct practice and delivery of a manualized treatment is critical for optimal outcomes. However for children with autism (Vismara et al. 2013) a recent meta-analysis of adherence and competence outcome indicated that neither adherence nor clinician competence was significantly related to patient outcomes in studies of individual psychotherapy (Webb et al. 2010). The lack of a relationship may be because of the variability in how adherence and clinician competence are rated, or because the relationship is curvilinear, with extremely low and high adherence related to poorer outcome, and moderate adherence (indicative of flexible and individualized implementation) possibly related to the best outcomes (Webb et al. 2010). It may be that strict adherence to protocol may be most critical for treating specific disorders or delivering interventions within certain modalities, but may not be required for all treatment modalities and all disorders (Beidas et al. 2011). Perhaps it is the "transfer of training" that is most critical to examine; that is, a successful adoption occurs when clinicians continue to implement a new intervention even after training has concluded, strong intervention fidelity (without drift) is maintained, and clinically significant treatment outcomes are achieved (Beidas et al. 2011; Carroll 2013).

Creating an appropriate balance between treatment fidelity and the flexible adaptation of a particular treatment for community settings may be important to determine as evidence-based programs move towards dissemination (McHugh et al. 2009). Achieving excellent treatment fidelity may be meaningless in the presence of limited patient receptivity or progress. Towards this end, emphasizing "flexibility within fidelity" (Kendall and Beidas 2007) may be key when delivering manualized interventions. "Breathing life" into manualized interventions typically balances adherence to the treatment protocol with individualization of concepts and techniques to account for variation among clients. Transdiagnostic treatments provide one example of how psychotherapeutic interventions can be individualized (Kendall et al. 2012). These treatments allow for flexibility in treatment delivery and are comprised of protocols that treat related disorders based on similar underlying processes (e.g., negative affect, emotion regulation, somatic management). Transdiagnostic approaches acknowledge high rates of psychiatric comorbidity and so may be flexible enough to tailor treatments according to individual symptom presentation (Kendall et al. 2012; McHugh et al. 2009).

Dissemination of Evidence-Based Interventions

A primary focus of this chapter is on bridging the research to practice gap in autism research, with a particular emphasis on interventions targeting anxiety symptoms in youth with ASD. To address the paucity of research in this area and to inform the dissemination process for treatments tailored to the needs of children with ASD, we begin by examining successful dissemination efforts in related fields. In the section that follows, dissemination efforts of psychiatric treatments for children are presented first, followed by a summary of dissemination treatment research in autism. Finally, examples of dissemination efforts in our research program are described.

Psychiatric Interventions

One of the most successful dissemination efforts in mental health research involves multisystemic therapy (MST), an empirically supported treatment that addresses antisocial behavior in adolescents (Henggeler 2011; Kazdin and Weisz 1998; McHugh and Barlow 2010). MST has been widely adopted nationally and internationally. Contributing to the success of these dissemination efforts were the developers' initial steps to enhance the adoption of MST via a comprehensive needs and barriers assessment. They assessed financial resources, long-term sustainability, and compatibility with existing organizational infrastructure and included advocates and key stakeholders in these efforts to inform the implementation process (McHugh and Barlow 2010). Once community partners decided to adopt MST, the developers provided intensive didactic training that was both educational and experiential, along with regular supervision, written materials, and quarterly booster training sessions. The developers created web-based materials to facilitate treatment fidelity and trained on-site supervisors to further promote the sustainability of the intervention (McHugh and Barlow 2010).

CBT for the treatment of childhood anxiety is perfectly positioned for dissemination and implementation, as this approach has been found to be more efficacious than other active treatments (Kendall et al. 2012). Extending the accessibility of CBT for childhood anxiety disorders to other settings (e.g., schools, camps, computer-based programs) and moving beyond the traditional clinic to reach large numbers of youth represent important steps in treatment delivery and dissemination (Elkins et al. 2011; Kendall et al. 2012).

School-based CBT

Researchers have generally clustered school-based CBT interventions under three categories: (1) universal prevention programs, (2) prevention programs specifically targeting students at risk for developing an anxiety disorder, and (3) intervention programs supporting students who are already evidencing symptoms consistent with an anxiety disorder. One universal prevention program, the FRIENDS program (Barrett and Turner 2001), has undergone extensive evaluation. Results from the implementation of the FRIENDS program has been consistently positive, as remission rates have ranged between 65 and 90 % following participation in the intervention, with treatment effects maintained up to 6 years post intervention (Barrett et al. 2001; Shortt et al. 2001). Other researchers have suggested that prevention programs (i.e., "selective programs") and intervention programs result in greater symptom change than universal programs alone, due in part to more elevated symptoms (and thus more potential to see change) in these students (Reivich et al. 2005).

Camp-based CBT

A creative extension of CBT to natural environments is the development of camps that combine recreational programming with group-based, intensive CBT approaches. Benefits of embedding CBT into camp environments include the normalization of receiving mental health services, opportunities for group cohesion, and multiple opportunities throughout the day to practice and reinforce strategy use (Santucci et al. 2009). An additional advantage of camp-based interventions is that they provide families the opportunity to access evidence-based mental health supports that may be impossible to access during the academic year (Walker et al. 2010). Similar to school-based CBT programs, camp-based CBT programs include universal and specific intervention programs. For example, Pelham and Hoza's (1996) Summer Treatment Program, developed specifically for children with ADHD, has been well researched and has paved the way for the exploration of other CBT approaches in camp settings. Camp programs specifically targeting

anxiety symptoms are also emerging. Ehrenreich-May and Bilek (2011) examined a universal prevention program using CBT to target symptoms of anxiety and depression during a preexisting recreational program. Their CBT intervention, the Emotion Detectives Prevention Program, is a transdiagnostic approach that yielded mixed findings however; significant reductions in anxiety, but not in depressive symptoms were found.

Computer-based CBT

Computerized CBT is an emerging field that examines the delivery of CBT through the Internet and computer-based programs. Computerized CBT provides opportunities for enhancing dissemination of evidence-based treatments through reduced cost of services, increased convenience (e.g., increased availability of computers and reduced need to manage transportation challenges), privacy, and standardization of intervention techniques (Kendall et al. 2012). Transportability challenges of computerized CBT may include limited adaptability and individualization of the program to client needs, loss of the therapist–client relationship, and concerns about computer security/privacy (Elkins et al. 2011; Kendall et al. 2012).

Computerized CBT can be clustered within two domains: (1) computer-based services (i.e., the computer intervention is online and either does not include clinician contact or has minimal clinician contact) and (2) computer-assisted delivery of services (i.e., computer intervention that includes clinician contact). Two computer-based CBT programs targeting anxiety and depression include Stressbusters (Abeles et al. 2009) and Cool Teens CD-Rom (Cunningham et al. 2006, 2009). Results from these studies yielded mixed results, as reductions in depression and anxiety ranged from 40 (Cunningham et al. 2009) to 75 % (Abeles et al. 2009) of the samples no longer meeting diagnostic criteria for psychiatric disorders post intervention.

Several randomized controlled trials have been conducted examining the use of computer-assisted CBT targeting anxiety reduction in youth. The BRAVE-Online program (March et al. 2009; Spence et al. 2006) is a manualized evidenced-based program for childhood anxiety; half of the treatment is delivered via the Internet, while the other half is delivered in a group therapy format. Camp Cope-a-Lot (CCAL; Khanna and Kendall 2010), a similar program, is a computer-assisted CBT program based on Coping Cat (Kendall 1994). It was compared to individual CBT and a control condition where psychoeducation was delivered via computer. Results of both studies indicated high participant satisfaction with the programs and significant reductions in anxiety compared to wait-list controls or other active control conditions. Currently, computer-assisted delivery of services appears to result in more significant symptom reduction than computer-based delivery.

Telehealth and Mental Health Interventions

Telehealth, or the provision of medical/mental health care via videoconferencing (either to clinics, schools, or homes), has been shown to be a feasible and potentially efficacious modality for mental health support for adults (Cowain 2001; Maheu et al. 2005; Smith et al. 1998) and youth (Baggett et al. 2010; Marcin et al. 2004; Pesämaa et al. 2004) in the general population. There is empirical support for the feasibility and efficacy of telehealth delivery of psychosocial interventions targeting a variety of psychiatric conditions, including anxiety (Bouchard et al. 2004; Day and Schneider 2002), depression (Nelson et al. 2003), anorexia (Goldfield and Boachie 2003), and psychosis (Nelson and Palsbo 2006). Manualized protocols, such as those commonly seen in cognitive-behavioral treatments, are used in the majority of published telehealth studies (Griffiths et al. 2006). Most published work focuses on using telehealth to connect local practitioners and patients with specialists from far away; however, with the advent of commercially available and secure videoconferencing platforms, more specialists are connecting directly to patients at home (Nesbitt et al. 2006).

There are several potential advantages to delivering mental health care through telehealth. Costs of videoconferencing sessions have been shown to be significantly lower than in-person care, particularly if the patient and provider are geographically distant from one another (Dávalos et al. 2009; Kelso et al. 2009). Patient satisfaction is generally high, with patients and their families reporting benefits in access to qualified practitioners, convenience, and efficiency (Myers et al. 2008). Technological obstacles that initially compromised timely access to effective care via this new modality have largely been eliminated (or at least reduced) by improved hardware, software, and bandwidth capability, even in most rural areas of the USA (Stout and Martinez 2011). User readiness has also improved substantially, as more adults and youth have acquired experience communicating via video chat technologies (PEW Internet and American Life Project 2010). Importantly, the provision of psychological services through telehealth requires careful attention to ethical issues such as practicing within state of licensure, informing clients of potential risks to confidentiality, and defining the scope of practice where telehealth is an appropriate modality for service delivery (Reed et al. 2000). Fortunately, progress in establishing practice guidelines, anticipating potential ethical dilemmas, and developing practical billing protocols all contribute to the prospect of telehealth becoming a sustainable method of psychological service delivery (AACAP Practice Parameters 2008; Reed et al. 2000).

Dissemination of ASD Interventions

Efforts to transport and implement evidence-based psychosocial interventions for youth with ASD from research to community settings have begun with the dissemination of early intervention treatment models (Bryson et al. 2007—Pivotal Response Training (PRT); Vismara et al. 2012—Early Start Denver Model (EDSM)). In both studies, community providers participated in intensive trainings, and adherence to treatment protocol was assessed. Results indicated that community providers could be trained to fidelity on the intervention models, with positive results in child outcome (Bryson et al. 2007; Vismara et al. 2009).

The dissemination of interventions for school-aged children and adolescents with ASD has occurred more recently. In one of the initial studies in this area, Brookman-Frazee et al. (2012b) examined the preliminary feasibility, acceptability, and outcomes of training community mental health therapists with limited ASD experience to deliver evidence-based interventions targeting challenging behaviors in school-aged children with ASD. Results indicated that the therapists were able to deliver the intervention to fidelity; furthermore, child treatment outcomes reflected reduced problem behaviors (Brookman-Frazee et al. 2012b).

Several treatment programs for youth with ASD have occurred in classroom settings. In a teacher-led study, Bauminger (2007) trained teachers to deliver a multimodal social skills curriculum (cognitive-behavioral-ecological model; CB-E) to children and adolescents with ASD. Results indicated that youth who participated in the treatment demonstrated significant improvements in overall social behaviors, improved problem solving, and increased emotional knowledge. In another study focusing on school-aged youth with ASD in school settings, a comparison of the relative effectiveness of two contextually based interventions occurred (Kenworthy et al. 2013). Children with ASD were randomized either to an executive functioning program targeting inflexibility and insistence on sameness ("Unstuck and On Target," Cannon et al. 2011) or to a social skills intervention (Baker 2003). In this study, both interventions were delivered by school staff; classroom teachers and parents attended brief trainings on how to reinforce the lessons taught in the treatment conditions. Youth who were randomized to the Unstuck and On Target treatment condition demonstrated significantly greater improvements in measures of problem solving,

flexibility, planning/organizing, and classroom behavior relative to participants who participated in the specific social skills intervention. Interestingly, youth in both groups made equivalent improvement in social skills (Kenworthy et al. 2013).

Telehealth applications to support intervention with persons with ASD and other developmental disabilities (DD) are not as well developed as those reported in the general psychiatric literature; however, current work supports the potential feasibility and efficacy of pursuing this dissemination strategy. Most of the published studies of telehealth in DD/ASD focus on assessment (Barretto et al. 2006; Elford et al. 2000; Slone et al. 2012), family support/parent education (Baharav and Reiser 2010; Ferdig et al. 2009; Kelso et al. 2009), personnel preparation (Machalicek 2008; Vismara et al. 2009), and school consultation (Gibson et al. 2010; Machalicek et al. 2009; Rule et al. 2006; see Boisvert et al. 2010 for review). Investigations of telehealth interventions designed to target psychological outcomes for persons with ASD/DD are relatively rare.

Although the provision of direct intervention to persons with ASD via telehealth is an understudied area, there are several compelling reasons to pursue this dissemination strategy, particularly when treating psychiatrically complex persons with ASD. First, access to evidence-based mental health intervention is significantly limited for persons with ASD and their families, regardless of geographic proximity to specialty clinics (Chen et al. 2008; Liptak et al. 2008). Families who live in rural settings face even greater access problems, given the lack of skilled practitioners outside of urban centers (Graef-Martins et al. 2007; Symon 2001). Second, without treatment, co-occurring mental health challenges in persons with ASD/DD often worsen, becoming more intractable and severe over time (Myers and Johnson 2007). In the absence of support or intervention, caregivers also become increasingly stressed when caring for a dually diagnosed person over time (McIntyre et al. 2002), and the risk of expensive hospitalizations and out-of-home placements is exceedingly high in this population (Brannan et al. 2003; Seltzer et al. 1997).

Third, technologically based interventions may be a particularly good fit for persons with ASD. Several researchers have suggested that the use of computers to mediate social interaction is likely to appeal to the social preferences and learning style of many persons with ASD (Bernard-Opitz et al. 2001; Bölte et al. 2010; Goodwin 2008). In fact, results from our pilot treatment study of adolescents with high-functioning autism and anxiety indicate that when teens were given the use of an Apple iPod touch as part of the treatment program, they were significantly more likely to use this device for purposes of self-monitoring symptoms than were teens who were given a more technologically limiting device (Reaven et al. 2012b). A Palm Z22 PDA was used for the first half of the study ($n=12$) and an Apple iPod touch was used for the second half of the study ($n=12$). The Apple iPod touch was added halfway through the study because of changes made by the software company. Although the handheld devices served similar functions for the project, teens preferred the Apple device over the Palm Z22 PDA due to its visual appeal and broader range of applications (Reaven et al. 2012b). For those who have difficulty with transitions to new settings, clinic-to-home telehealth delivery may be particularly appealing, both to persons with ASD and to their caregivers, who must assist in these transitions. Given that psychosocial interventions require active, consistent engagement of the participant and his/her caregiver (Kazdin et al. 1990), any modification that reduces treatment resistance and promotes interest and adherence is important to consider (Hollon et al. 2002).

Dissemination of Anxiety Interventions for Youth with ASD

Extending FYF to Clinical Settings

Efforts are underway in our own university clinic to bridge the research-to-practice gap. In an effort to enhance the portability of efficacious CBT treatments beyond the clinical research setting, we are training outpatient clinicians to fidelity on the FYF intervention for 8–14-year-old children with high-functioning ASD and anxiety (Facing Your Fears: Group Therapy for Managing Anxiety in Children with High-Functioning Autism Spectrum Disorders; Reaven et al. 2011). The study has three primary aims: (1) to train outpatient clinicians outside of our university clinic to deliver FYF, (2) to obtain direct feedback from all study participants regarding the acceptability of the intervention and incorporate feedback into future revisions of FYF, intervention (manual only, workshop only, workshop plus twice monthly phone consultation).

Our work on this project has included the development of a 2-day workshop and accompanying training materials, three versions of a conceptual knowledge test of CBT for group facilitators, intervention fidelity checklists, and intervention acceptability measures for facilitators, parents, and children. In an attempt to include best practice training principles, the workshop was designed to include training on the conceptual framework that underlies the intervention, session-by-session review of the intervention material, and active participation via behavioral rehearsal, role-plays and exposure hierarchy creation. The project has two phases: (1) training clinicians at the IWK Health Centre in Halifax, Nova Scotia, to fidelity on the intervention and incorporating feedback on the FYF facilitator training workshop and FYF program and (2) randomizing three outpatient clinics serving youth with ASD to one of the three instructional conditions referenced above for 3 years.

During the initial phase of this project, psychology graduate students and/or Ph.D. level psychologists with the IWK Health Centre conducted four treatment groups delivering the FYF intervention to children aged 8–14 with high-functioning ASD and anxiety. Biweekly phone conferencing occurred between the treatment developers and group facilitators for the duration of phase one. Results indicated very high adherence to the FYF protocol (all groups exceeded the 80% minimum threshold for treatment fidelity) and significant reductions in anxiety for child participants (Reaven et al. 2014). Reductions in anxiety symptoms were very similar to those obtained in our randomized clinical trial (53% of the Halifax sample met criteria for a clinically meaningful improvement in anxiety symptoms, compared with 50% in the previously conducted RCT) (Reaven et al. 2012a). Phase two of this project is ongoing.

Extending FYF to School Settings

Our research group recently conducted a small pilot study to determine whether FYF could be delivered in public school settings by a cross-disciplinary team of facilitators. The pilot study was an attempt to introduce a school-based version of FYF into schools early in the development process so that feedback from key stakeholders could inform the school treatment program. Eleven school providers enrolled as group leaders, along with 13 students aged 8–13 with ASD and anxiety and their parents. These students represented three elementary schools and one middle school. School providers included mental health professionals, educators, and school personnel from other disciplines. School providers took part in a 2-day training workshop. The workshop was similar in structure to the training in the implementation study described above (i.e., conceptual training, behavioral rehearsal, roleplay etc.), but specifically tailored to the needs of a cross-disciplinary school team. Similar to the feedback solicited in our previous study (Reaven et al. 2014), bidirectional feedback was requested on both the training workshop and intervention content. The providers indicated positive views of the both the training and the FYF curriculum, as reflected in their post evaluations. A larger scale school-based FYF project is currently in the planning stages. Based on feedback from the pilot study, a school-based version of FYF is anticipated to account for a shift in emphasis of child goals (e.g., address school-based fears) and further shifts from parents as coaches to educators as coaches.

Delivering FYF via Telehealth

When considering a novel dissemination strategy that involves a substantial change in the interpersonal context of the therapeutic encounter, one must consider how this novel way of relating impacts rapport, collaboration, and trust. Our team recently completed a study of the feasibility and potential efficacy of delivering a manualized CBT intervention (Facing Your Fears; Reaven et al. 2011) to youth with ASD and their parents through clinic-to-home videoconferencing (Hepburn, Blakeley-Smith, & Reaven, under review). We were primarily interested in how clinicians can establish and maintain a productive working alliance with dually diagnosed youth with ASD and their parents in this novel modality. Some "lessons learned" by therapists trying to promote a productive therapeutic alliance with youth with ASD and their parents included speaking slowly and deliberately, prolonging and exaggerating gesture use and facial expression to compensate for "lag time," e-mailing the family a few days prior to group, and attaching a session outline and any activity sheets to be used in the session. In our feasibility study, school-aged children (ages 8–14 years) and their mothers almost universally reported strong ratings of the quality of alliance with their therapist in both 1:1 and multifamily telehealth sessions. Overall, telehealth delivery of a manualized, family-focused intervention for anxious youth with ASD was found to be feasible and potentially efficacious in our pilot work (Hepburn et al., under review).

Telehealth delivery of psychosocial mental health interventions has the potential to improve access to care for persons with ASD and their families. In addition to providing direct intervention for individuals with ASD as described above, parent-to-parent support and peer-to-peer connections may be accessed through small group videoconferencing, helping families feel less isolated. Future studies will need to incorporate rigorous experimental designs that are developmentally appropriate for a broad range of persons with ASD in order to inform best practice parameters for the use of telehealth for people with ASD.

Conclusions

The development of evidence-based programs for individuals with ASD has accelerated over the past decade. However, the *dissemination and implementation* of evidence-based programs for ASD has only recently begun, and the implementation of treatments to address co-occurring psychiatric symptoms (e.g., anxiety) to "real-world" clinical settings is in its infancy. The increased prevalence of autism in recent years is indicative of a public health crisis, signaling the critical import of translating efficacious and evidence-based interventions from research to community settings. A bidirectional model of implementation may be essential not only in bridging the research to practice gap (Brookman-Frazee et al. 2012a, 2012b; Dingfelder and Mandell 2011) but also in developing meaningful, feasible, and cost-effective treatment programs. Once organizations view evidence-based programs as compatible with their values and as advantageous to deliver, individual practitioners stationed at the "front lines" will be better positioned to support individuals with ASD.

References

AACAP Official Action. (2008). Practice parameter for telepsychiatry with children and adolescents. *Journal of the American Academy of Child and Adolescent Psychiatry, 47,* 1468–1483. doi:10.1097/CHI.0b013e31818b4e13.

Abeles, P., Verduyn, C., Robinson, A., Smith, P., Yule, W., & Proudfoot, J. (2009). Computerized CBT for adolescent depression ("Stressbusters") and its initial evaluation through an extended case series. *Behavioural and Cognitive Psychotherapy, 37,* 151–165. doi:10.1017/S1352465808005067.

Baggett, K. M., Davis, B., Feil, E. G., Sheeber, L. L., Landry, S. H., Carta, J. J., & Leve, C. (2010). Technologies for expanding the reach of evidence-based interventions: Preliminary results for promoting social-emotional development in early childhood. *Topics in Early Childhood Special Education, 29,* 226–238. doi:10.1177/0271121409354782.

Baharav, E., & Reiser, C. (2010). Using telepractice in parent training in early autism. *Telemedicine Journal and e-Health: The Official Journal of the American Telemedicine Association, 16,* 727–731. doi:10.1089/tmj.2010.0029.

Baker, J. (2003). The social skills picture book: Teaching play, emotion, and communication to children with autism. *Arlington, TX: Future Horizons.*

Barrett, P., & Turner, C. (2001). Prevention of anxiety symptoms in primary school children: Preliminary results from a universal school-based trial. *The British Journal of Clinical Psychology, 40,* 399–410. doi:10.1348/014466501163887.

Barrett, P., Duffy, A., Dadds, M., & Rapee, R. (2001). Cognitive-behavioral treatment of anxiety disorders in children: Long term (6-year) follow up. *Journal of Consulting and Clinical Psychology, 69,* 135–141. doi:10.1037/0022-006X.69.1.135.

Barretto, A., Wacker, D. P., Harding, J., Lee, J., & Berg, W. K. (2006). Using telemedicine to conduct behavioral assessments. *Journal of Applied Behavior Analysis, 39,* 333–340. doi:10.1901/jaba.2006.173-04.

Bauminger, N. (2007). Brief report: Group social-multimodal intervention for HFASD. *Journal of Autism and Developmental Disorders, 37*(8), 1605–1615.

Beidas, R. S., Koerner, K., Weingardt, K. R., & Kendall, P. C. (2011). Training research: Practical recommendations for maximum impact. *Administration and Policy in Mental Health and Mental Health Services Research, 38,* 223–237. doi:10.1007/s10488-011-0338-z.

Bernard-Opitz, V., Sriram, N., & Nakhoda-Sapuan, S. (2001). Enhancing social problem solving in children with autism and normal children through computer-assisted instruction. *Journal of Autism and Developmental Disorders, 31,* 377–384. doi:10.1023/A:1010660502130.

Boisvert, M., Lang, R., Andrianopoulos, M., & Boscardin, M. L. (2010). Telepractice in the assessment and treatment of individuals with autism spectrum disorders: A systematic review. *Developmental Neurorehabilitation, 13,* 423–432. doi:10.3109/17518423.2010.499889.

Bölte, S., Golan, O., Goodwin, M. S., & Zwaigenbaum, L. (2010). What can innovative technologies do for autism spectrum disorders? *Autism, 14,* 155–159. doi:10.1177/1362361310365028.

Bouchard, S., Paquin, B., Payeur, R., Allard, M., Rivard, V., Fournier, T., et al. (2004). Delivering cognitive-behavior therapy for panic disorder with agoraphobia in videoconference. *Telemedicine Journal and e-Health, 10,* 13–25. doi:10.1089/153056204773644535.

Brannan, A. M., Heflinger, C. A., & Foster, E. M. (2003). The role of caregiver strain and other family variables in determining children's use of mental health services. *Journal of Emotional and Behavioral Disorders, 11,* 77–91. doi:10.1177/106342660301100202.

Brookman-Frazee, L. I., Drahota, A., & Stadnick, N. (2012a). Training community mental health therapists to deliver a package of evidence-based practice strategies for school-age children with autism spectrum disorders: A pilot study. *Journal of Autism and Developmental Disorders, 42,* 1651–1661. doi:10.1007/s10803-011-1406-7.

Brookman-Frazee, L., Stahmer, A. C., Lewis, K., Feder, J. D., & Reed, S. (2012b). Building a research-community collaborative to improve community care for infants and toddlers at-risk for autism spectrum disorders. *Journal of Community Psychology, 40*, 715–734. doi:10.1002/jcop.21501.

Bryson, S. E., Koegel, L. K., Koegel, R. L., Openden, D., Smith, I. M., & Nefdt, N. (2007). Large scale dissemination and community implementation of pivotal response treatment: Program description and preliminary data. *Research and Practice for Persons with Severe Disabilities (RPSD), 32*, 142–153. doi:10.2511/rpsd.32.2.142.

Cannon, L., Kenworthy, L., Alexander, K. C., Werner, M. A., & Anthony, L. (2011). *Unstuck and on Target! An Executive Function Curriculum to Improve Flexibility for Children with Autism Spectrum Disorders.* Baltimore, MD: Brookes Publishing.

Carroll, K. M. (2013). Treatment integrity and dissemination: Rethinking fidelity via the stage model. *Clinical Psychology: Science and Practice, 20*, 99–106. doi:10.1111/cpsp.12025.

Chalfant, A. M., Rapee, R., & Carroll, L. (2007). Treating anxiety disorders in children with high functioning autism spectrum disorders: A controlled trial. *Journal of Autism and Developmental Disorders, 37*, 1842–1857. doi:10.1007/s10803-006-0318-4.

Chen, C. Y., Liu, C. Y., Su, W. C., Huang, S. L., & Lin, K. M. (2008). Urbanicity-related variation in help-seeking and services utilization among preschool-age children with autism in Taiwan. *Journal of Autism and Developmental Disorders, 38*, 489–497. doi:10.1007/s10803-007-0416-y.

Cowain, T. (2001). Cognitive-behavioural therapy via videoconferencing to a rural area. *Australasian Psychiatry, 35*, 62–64. doi:10.1046/j.1440-1614.2001.00853.x.

Cunningham, M., Rapee, R., & Lyneham, H. (2006). The Cool Teens CD-ROM: A multimedia self-help program for adolescents with anxiety. *Youth Studies Australia, 25*, 50–56. doi:10.1007/s00787-008-0703-y.

Cunningham, M. J., Wuthrich, V. M., Rapee, R. M., Lyneham, H. J., Schniering, C. A., & Hudson, J. L. (2009). The cool teens CD-ROM for anxiety disorders in adolescents: A pilot case series. *European Child & Adolescent Psychiatry, 18*, 125–129. doi:10.1007/s00787-008-0703-y.

Dávalos, M. E., French, M. T., Burdick, A. E., & Simmons, S. C. (2009). Economic evaluation of telemedicine: Review of the literature and research guidelines for benefit-cost analysis. *Telemedicine and e-Health, 15*, 933–948. doi:10.1089/tmj.2009.0067.

Day, S. X., & Schneider, P. L. (2002). Psychotherapy using distance technology: A comparison of face-to-face, video, and audio treatment. *Journal of Counseling Psychology, 49*, 499–503. doi:10.1037/0022-0167.49.4.499.

Denis, J. L., & Lomas, J. (2003). Convergent evolution: The academic and policy roots of collaborative research. *Journal of Health Services Research & Policy, 8*, 1–6. doi:10.1258/135581903322405108.

Dingfelder, H. E., & Mandell, D. S. (2011). Bridging the research-to-practice gap in autism intervention: An application of diffusion of innovation theory. *Journal of Autism and Developmental Disorders, 41*, 597–609. doi:10.1007/s10803-010-1081-0.

Ehrenreich-May, J., & Bilek, E. L. (2011). Universal prevention of anxiety and depression in a recreational camp setting: An initial open trial. *Child & Youth Care Forum, 40*, 435–455. doi:10.1007/s10566-011-9148-4.

Elford, R., White, H., Bowering, R., Ghandi, A., Maddiggan, B., & St John, K. (2000). A randomized, controlled trial of child psychiatric assessments conducted using videoconferencing. *Journal of Telemedicine and Telecare, 6*, 73–82. doi:10.1258/135763300193506.

Elkins, M. R., McHugh, K. R., Santucci, L. C., & Barlow, D. H. (2011). Improving the transportability of CBT for internalizing disorders in children. *Clinical Child and Family Psychology Review, 14*, 161–173. doi:10.1007/s10567-011-0085-4.

Ferdig, R. E., Amberg, H. G., Elder, J. H., Valcante, G., Donaldson, S. A., & Bendixen, R. (2009). Autism and family interventions through technology: A description of a web-based tool to educate fathers of children with autism. *International Journal of Web-Based Learning and Teaching Technologies (IJWLTT), 4*, 55–69. doi:10.4018/jwbltt.2009090804.

Gibson, J. L., Pennington, R. C., Stenhoff, D. M., & Hopper, J. S. (2010). Using desktop videoconferencing to deliver interventions to a preschool student with autism. *Topics in Early Childhood Special Education, 29*, 214–225. doi:10.1177/0271121409352873.

Goldfield, G. S., & Boachie, A. (2003). Case report: Delivery of family therapy in the treatment of anorexia nervosa using telehealth. *Telemedicine Journal and E-Health, 9*, 111–114. doi:10.1089/153056203763317729.

Goodwin, M. S. (2008). Enhancing and accelerating the pace of autism research and treatment. *Focus on Autism and Other Developmental Disabilities, 23*(2), 125–128. doi:10.1177/1088357608316678.

Griffiths, L., Blignault, I., & Yellowlees, P. (2006). Telemedicine as a means of delivering cognitive-behavioural therapy to rural and remote mental health clients. *Journal of Telemedicine and Telecare, 12*(3), 136–140. doi:10.1258/135763306776738567.

Gunter, R. W., & Whittal, M. L. (2010). Dissemination of cognitive-behavioral treatments for anxiety disorders: Overcoming barriers and improving patient access. *Clinical Psychology Review, 30*, 194–202. doi:10.1016/j.cpr.2009.11.001.

Gutstein, S., Burgess, A., & Montfort, K. (2007). Evaluation of the relationship development intervention program. *Autism, 11*, 397–411. doi:10.1177/1362361307079603.

Henggeler, S. (2011). Efficacy studies to large-scale transport: The development and validation of multisystemic programs. *Annual Review of Clinical Psychology, 7*, 351–381. doi:10.1146/annurev-clinpsy-032210-104615.

Hepburn, S. L., Blakeley-Smith, A., & Reaven, J. A. (under review). Feasibility of a telehealth anxiety intervention for youth with ASD.

Herschell, A. D., Kolko, D. J., Baumann, B. L., & Davis, A. C. (2010). The role of therapist training in the implementation of psychosocial treatments: A review and critique with recommendations. *Clinical Psychology Review, 30,* 448–466. doi:10.1016/j.cpr.2010.02.005.

Hollon, S. D., Muñoz, R. F., Barlow, D. H., Beardslee, W. R., Bell, C. C., Bernal, G., et al. (2002). Psychosocial intervention development for the prevention and treatment of depression: Promoting innovation and increasing access. *Biological Psychiatry, 52,* 610–630. doi:10.1016/S0006-3223(02)01384-7.

Kazdin, A. E., & Weisz, J. R. (1998). Identifying and developing empirically supported child and adolescent treatments. *Journal of Consulting and Clinical Psychology, 66,* 19. doi:10.1037/0022-006X.66.1.19.

Kazdin, A. E., Siegel, T. C., & Bass, D. (1990). Drawing on clinical practice to inform research on child and adolescent psychotherapy: Survey of practitioners. *Professional Psychology: Research and Practice, 21,* 189–198. doi:10.1037/0735-7028.21.3.189.

Keehn, R. H. M., Lincoln, A. J., Brown, M. Z., & Chavira, D. A. (2013). The coping cat program for children with anxiety and autism spectrum disorder: A pilot randomized controlled trial. *Journal of Autism and Developmental Disorders, 43,* 57–67. doi:10.1007/s10803-012-1541-9.

Kelso, G., Fiechtl, B., Olsen, S., & Rule, S. (2009). The feasibility of virtual home visits to provide early intervention: A pilot study. *Infants & Young Children, 22,* 332–340. doi:10.1097/IYC.0b013e3181b9873c.

Kendall, P. C. (1994). Treating anxiety disorders in children: Results of a randomized clinical trial. *Journal of Consulting and Clinical Psychology, 62,* 100–110. doi:10.1037/0022-006X.62.1.100.

Kendall, P. C., & Beidas, R. S. (2007). Smoothing the trail for dissemination of evidence-based practices for youth: Flexibility within fidelity. *Professional Psychology Research and Practice, 38,* 13. doi:10.1037/0735-7028.38.1.13.

Kendall, P. C., Settipani, C. A., & Cummings, C. M. (2012). No need to worry: The promising future of child anxiety research. *Journal of Clinical Child & Adolescent Psychology, 41,* 103–115. doi:10.1080/15374416.2012.632352.

Kenworthy, L., Anthony, L. G., Naiman, D. Q., Cannon, L., Wills, M. C., Luong-Tran, C., & Wallace, G. L. (2013). Randomized controlled effectiveness trial of executive function intervention for children on the autism spectrum. *Journal of Child Psychology and Psychiatry, 55*(4), 374–383.

Khanna, M. S., & Kendall, P. C. (2010). Computer-assisted cognitive behavioral therapy for child anxiety: Results of a randomized clinical trial. *Journal of Consulting and Clinical Psychology, 78,* 737. doi:10.1037/a0019739.

Laugeson, E. A., Frankel, F., Gantman, A., Dillon, A. R., & Mogil, C. (2012). Evidence-based social skills training for adolescents with autism spectrum disorders: The UCLA PEERS program. *Journal of Autism and Developmental Disorders, 42,* 1025–1036. doi:10.1007/s10803-011-1339-1.

Liptak, G., Benzoni, L., Mruzek, D., Nolan, K., Thingvoll, M., Wade, C., & Fryer, G. E. (2008). Disparities in diagnosis and access to health services for children with autism: Data from the national survey of children's health. *Journal of Developmental Pediatrics, 29,* 152–160. doi:10.1097/DBP.0b013e318165c7a0.

Lord, C., Wagner, A., Rogers, S., Szatmari, P., Aman, M., Charman, T., et al. (2005). Challenges in evaluating psychosocial interventions for autistic spectrum disorders. *Journal of Autism and Developmental Disorders, 35,* 695–708. doi:10.1007/s10803-005-0017-6.

Machalicek, W. A. (2008). The use of video tele-conferencing to train teachers to assess the challenging behaviors of children with autism spectrum disorders. *Dissertation Abstracts International, Section A: Humanities and Social Sciences, 69,* 2221.

Machalicek, W., O'Reilly, M., Chan, J. M., Rispoli, M., Lang, R., Davis, T., et al. (2009). Using videoconferencing to support teachers to conduct preference assessments with students with autism and developmental disabilities. *Research in Spectrum Disorders, 3,* 32–41. doi:10.1016/j.rasd.2008.03.004.

Maheu, M. M., Pulier, M. L., Wilhelm, F. H., McMenamin, J. P., & Brown-Connolly, N. E. (2005). *The mental health professional and the new technologies: A handbook for practice today.* Mahwah: Erlbaum. doi:10.1192/bjp.186.6.545.

March, S., Spence, S. H., & Donovan, C. L. (2009). The efficacy of an internet-based cognitive-behavioral therapy intervention for child anxiety disorders. *Journal of Pediatric Psychology, 34,* 474–487. doi:10.1093/jpepsy/jsn099.

Marcin, J. P., Ellis, J., Mawis, R., Nagrampa, E., Nesbitt, T. S., & Dimand, R. J. (2004). Using telemedicine to provide pediatric subspecialty care to children with special health care needs in an underserved rural community. *Pediatrics, 113,* 1–6. doi:10.1542/peds.113.1.1.

Massatti, R. R., Sweeney, H. A., Panzano, P. C., & Roth, D. (2007). The de-adoption of innovative mental health practices (IMHP): Why organizations choose not to sustain an IMHP. *Administration and Policy in Mental Health, 35,* 50–65. doi:10.1007/s10488-007-0141-z.

McHugh, R., & Barlow, D. (2010). The dissemination and implementation of evidence-based psychological treatments: A review of current efforts. *American Psychologist, 65,* 73–84. doi:10.1037/a0018121.

McHugh, R. K., Murray, H. W., & Barlow, D. H. (2009). Balancing fidelity and adaptation in the dissemination of empirically-supported treatments: The promise of transdiagnostic interventions. *Behaviour Research and Therapy, 47,* 946–953. doi:10.1016/j.brat.2009.07.005.

McIntyre, L. L., Blacher, J., & Baker, B. L. (2002). Behaviour/mental health problems in young adults with intellectual disability: The impact on families.

Journal of Intellectual Disability Research, 46, 239–249. doi:10.1046/j.1365-2788.2002.00371.x.

Myers, S. M., & Johnson, C. P. (2007). Management of children with autism spectrum disorders. *Pediatrics, 120,* 1162–1182. doi:10.1542/peds.2007-2362, doi:10.1542/peds.2010-2549.

Myers, K. M., Valentine, J. M., & Melzer, S. M. (2008). Child and adolescent telepsychiatry: Utilization and satisfaction. *Telemedicine Journal and e-Health: The Official Journal of the American Telemedicine Association, 14,* 131–137. doi:10.1089/tmj.2007.0035.

Nelson, E. L., & Palsbo, S. (2006). Challenges in telemedicine equivalence studies. *Evaluation and Program Planning, 29,* 419–425. doi:10.1016/j.evalprogplan.2006.02.001.

Nelson, E. L., Barnard, M., & Cain, S. (2003). Treating childhood depression over videoconferencing. *Telemedicine Journal and e-Health, 9,* 49–55. doi:10.1089/153056203763317648.

Nesbitt, T. S., Rogers, S. J., Rich, B. A., Anders, T. F., Yellowlees, P. M., Brown, J. R., & Keast, P. R. (2006). *Enhancing mental health services to children with autism in rural areas: Guidelines for using telehealth to extend autism outreach.* Sacramento: MIND Institute, UC Davis.

O'Fallon, L. R., & Dearry, A. (2002). Community-based participatory research as a tool to advance environmental health sciences. *Environmental Health Perspectives, 110,* 155. doi:10.1289/ehp.02110s2155.

Pelham, W. E. Jr., & Hoza, B. (1996). Intensive treatment: A summer treatment program for children with ADHD. In E. D. Hibbs & P. S. Jensen (Eds.), *Psychosocial treatments for child and adolescent disorders: Empirically based strategies for clinical practice* (pp. 311–340). Washington, DC: American Psychological Association. doi:10.1037/10196-013.

Pesämaa, L., Ebeling, H., Kuusimäki, M. L., Winblad, I., Isohanni, M., & Moilanen, I. (2004). Videoconferencing in child and adolescent telepsychiatry: A systematic review of the literature. *Journal of Telemedicine and Telecare, 10,* 187–192.

PEW Internet and American Life Project. (2000, May 10). Tracking online life: How women use the Internet to cultivate relationships with family and friends. *Online Internet Life Report.*

Reaven, J., Blakeley-Smith, A., Beattie, T., Sullivan, A. Moody, E., Stern, J., Hepburn, S., & Smith, I. (2014). Improving transportability of a CBT intervention for anxiety in youth with ASD: Results from a US-Canada collaboration. *Autism, 2014.* Advance online publication.

Reaven, J., Blakeley-Smith, A., Nichols, S., & Hepburn, S. (2011). *Facing your fears: Group therapy for managing anxiety in children with high-functioning autism spectrum disorders.* Baltimore: Paul Brookes.

Reaven, J., Blakeley-Smith, A., Culhane-Shelburne, K., & Hepburn, S. (2012a). Group cognitive behavior therapy for children with high-functioning, autism spectrum disorders and anxiety: A randomized trial. *Journal of Child Psychology and Psychiatry, 53,* 410–419. doi:10.1111/j.1469-7610.2011.02486.x.

Reaven, J., Blakeley-Smith, A., Leuthe, E., Moody, E., & Hepburn, S. (2012b). Facing your fears in adolescence: Cognitive-behavioral therapy for high-functioning autism spectrum disorders and anxiety. *Autism Research and Treatment, 2012,* 1–13. doi:10.1155/2012/423905.

Reed, G. M., McLaughlin, C. J., & Milholland, K. (2000). Ten interdisciplinary principles for professional practice in telehealth: Implications for psychology. *Professional Psychology: Research and Practice, 31,* 170–178. doi:10.1037/0735-7028.31.2.170.

Reichow, B. (2011). Development, procedures, and application of the evaluative method for determining evidence-based practices in autism. In B. Reichow, P. Doehring, D. V. Cicchetti, & F. R. Volkmar (Eds.), *Evidence-based practices and treatments for children with autism* (pp. 25–39). New York: Springer. doi:10.1007/978-1-4419-6975-0_2.

Reivich, K., Gillham, J. E., Chaplin, T. M., & Seligman, M. E. P. (2005). From helplessness to optimism: The role of resilience in treating and preventing depression in youth. In S. Goldstein & R. B. Brooks (Eds.), *Handbook of resilience in children* (pp. 223–237). New York: Kluwer Academic/Plenum Publishers. doi:10.1007/978-1-4614-3661-4_12.

Rogers, E. M. (2003). *Diffusion of innovations* (5th ed.). New York: Free Press.

Rogers, S., & Dawson, G. (2010). *Early start Denver model for young children with autism. Promoting language, learning, and engagement.* New York: Guilford Press.

Rule, S., Salzberg, C., Higbee, T., Menlove, R., & Smith, J. (2006). Technology-mediated consultation to assist rural students: A case study. *Rural Special Education Quarterly, 25,* 3–8.

Santucci, L. C., Ehrenreich, J. T., Trosper, S. E., Bennett, S. M., & Pincus, D. B. (2009). Development and preliminary evaluation of a one-week summer treatment program for separation anxiety disorder. *Cognitive and Behavioral Practice, 16,* 317–331. doi:10.1016/j.cbpra.2008.12.005.

Schmidt, F., & Taylor, T. (2002). Putting empirically supported treatments into practice: Lessons learned in a children's mental health center. *Professional Psychology: Research and Practice, 33,* 483–489. doi:10.1037/0735-7028.33.5.483.

Schoenwald, S. K., & Hoagwood, K. (2001). Effectiveness, transportability, and dissemination of interventions: What matters when? *Psychiatric Services, 52,* 1190–1197. doi:10.1176/appi.ps.52.9.1190.

Seltzer, M. M., Greenberg, J. S., Krauss, M. W., & Hong, J. (1997). Predictors and outcomes of the end of co-resident caregiving in aging families of adults with mental retardation or mental illness. *Family Relations, 46*(1), 13–22. doi:10.2307/585602.

Sholomskas, D. E., Syracuse-Siewert, G., Rounsaville, B. J., Ball, S. A., Nuro, K. F., & Carroll, K. M. (2005). We don't train in vain: A dissemination trial of three strategies of training clinicians in cognitive-behavioral therapy. *Journal of Consulting and Clinical Psychology, 73*, 106. doi:10.1037/0022.006X.73.1.106.

Shortt, A., Barrett, P., Fox, T. (2001). Evaluating the FRIENDS program: A cognitive-behavioural group treatment of childhood anxiety disorders. *Journal of Clinical Child Psychology, 30*, 525–535. doi:10.1207/S15374424JCCP3004_09.

Slone, N. C., Reese, R. J., & McClellan, M. J. (2012). Telepsychology outcome research with children and adolescents: A review of the literature. *Psychological Services, 9*, 272–292. doi:10.1037/a0027607.

Smith, H. A., Allison, R. A., & Rockville, M. D. (1998). *Telemental health: Delivering mental health care at a distance*. Unpublished summary report, US Department of Health and Human Services, Office for the Advancement of Telehealth, Rockville, MD, USA.

Smith, T., Scahill, L., Dawson, G., Guthrie, D., Lord, C., Odom, S., et al. (2007). Designing research studies on psychosocial interventions in autism. *Journal of Autism and Developmental Disorders, 37*, 354–366. doi:10.1007/s10803-006-0173-3.

Sofronoff, K., Attwood, T., & Hinton, S. (2005). A randomised controlled trial of a CBT intervention for anxiety in children with Asperger syndrome. *Journal of Child Psychology and Psychiatry, 46*, 1152–1160. doi:10.1111/j.1469-7610.2005.00411.x.

Spence, S. H., Holmes, J. M., March, S., & Lipp, O. V. (2006). The feasibility and outcome of clinic plus internet delivery of cognitive-behavior therapy for childhood anxiety. *Journal of Consulting and Clinical Psychology, 74*, 614–621. doi:10.1037/0022-006X.74.3.614.

Stahmer, A. C., & Aarons, G. (2009). Attitudes toward adoption of evidence-based practices: A comparison of autism early intervention providers and children's mental health providers. *Psychological Services, 6*, 223. doi:10.1037/a0010738.

Storch, E. A., & Crisp, H. L. (2004). Taking it to the schools—transporting empirically supported treatments for childhood psychopathology to the school setting. *Clinical Child and Family Psychology Review, 7*, 191–193. doi:10.1007/s10567-004-6084-y.

Storch, E. A., Murphy, T. K., Arnold, E. B., Lewin, A. B., Nadeau, J. M., Jones, A. M., et al. (2013). The effect of cognitive-behavioral therapy versus treatment as usual for anxiety in children with autism spectrum disorders: A randomized, controlled trial. *Journal of the American Academy of Child & Adolescent Psychiatry, 52*, 132–142. doi:10.1016/j.jaac.2012.11.007.

Stout, K. A., & Martinez, K. (2011). Telehealth forging ahead: Overcoming barriers in licensure to improve access to care for service members. *International Journal of Telerehabilitation, 3*, 23–26. doi:10.5195/ijt.2011.6081.

Sung, M., Ooi, Y. P., Goh, T. J., Pathy, P., Fung, D. S., Ang, R. P., & Lam, C. M. (2011). Effects of cognitive-behavioral therapy on anxiety in children with autism spectrum disorders: A randomized controlled trial. *Child Psychiatry & Human Development, 42*, 634–649. doi:10.1007/s10578-011-0238-1.

Symon, J. B. (2001). Parent education for autism issues in providing services at a distance. *Journal of Positive Behavior Interventions, 3*, 160–174. doi:10.1177/109830070100300304.

Teachman, B. A., Drabick, D. A., Hershenberg, R., Vivian, D., Wolfe, B. E., & Goldfried, M. R. (2012). Bridging the gap between clinical research and clinical practice: Introduction to the special section. *Psychotherapy, 49*, 97. doi:10.1037/a0027346.

Vismara, L. A., Young, G. S., Stahmer, A. C., Griffith, E. M., & Rogers, S. J. (2009). Dissemination of evidence-based practice: Can we train therapists from a distance? *Journal of Autism and Developmental Disorders, 39*, 1636–1651. doi:10.1007/s10803-009-0796-2.

Vismara, L. A., Young, G. S., & Rogers, S. J. (2013). Community dissemination of the Early Start Denver Model: Implications for science and practice. *Topics in Early Childhood Special Education, 32*, 223–233. doi:10.1177/0271121411409250.

Volkmar, F. R., Reichow, B., & Doehring, P. (2011). Evidence-based practices in autism: Where we are now and where we need to go. In B. Reichow, P. Doehring, D. V. Cicchetti & F. R. Volkmar (Eds.), *Evidence-based practices and treatments for children with autism* (pp. 365–391). New York: Springer. doi:10.1007/978-1-4419-6975-0_14.

Walker, A. N., Barry, T. D., & Bader, S. H. (2010). Therapist and parent ratings of changes in adaptive social skills following a summer treatment camp for children with autism spectrum disorders: A preliminary study. *Child & Youth Care Forum, 39*, 305–322. doi:10.1007/s10566-010-9110-x.

Webb, C. A., DeRubeis, R. J., & Barber, J. P. (2010). Therapist adherence/competence and treatment outcome: A meta-analytic review. *Journal of Consulting and Clinical Psychology, 78*, 200–211. doi:10.1037/a0018912.supp.

Weisz, J. R., Chu, B. C., & Polo, A. J. (2004). Treatment dissemination and evidence-based practice: Strengthening intervention through clinician-researcher collaboration. *Clinical Psychology: Science and Practice, 11*, 300–307. doi:10.1093/clipsy/bph085.

White, S. W., Ollendick, T., Albano, A. M., Oswald, D., Johnson, C., Southam-Gerow, M. A., et al. (2013). Randomized controlled trial: Multimodal anxiety and social skill intervention for adolescents with autism spectrum disorder. *Journal of Autism and Developmental Disorders, 43*, 382–394. doi:10.1007/s10803-012-1577-x.

Wood, J. J., Drahota, A., Sze, K., Har, K., Chiu, A., & Langer, D. A. (2009). Cognitive behavioral therapy for anxiety in children with autism spectrum disorders: A randomized, controlled trial. *Journal of Child Psychology and Psychiatry, 50*, 224–234. doi:10.1111/j.1469-7610.2008.01948.x.

Christopher Lopata and Marcus L. Thomeer

Autism and Anxiety in School

Given the legal requirement of compulsory education, schools play a seminal role in the development of children and adolescents with autism spectrum disorder (ASD). Schools are required to assess the academic, social, management, and physical needs of students with ASD and provide appropriate programming as operationalized in their individualized education plan (IEP). The multiple domains addressed within each IEP represent a scope of functional areas that extends beyond academic achievement. Critical to the effectiveness of educational programming for students with ASD is an understanding of the clinical symptoms, techniques for assessing the presence and impact of these symptoms, and strategies for ameliorating symptoms and increasing adaptive functioning. Although these students are diagnosed and classified based on their ASD features, a substantial number also experience a range of co-occurring psychiatric symptoms and conditions including anxiety. Anxiety is of interest to educators as it is problematic on its own and can interfere with learning and effect the manifestation of ASD

symptoms (American Psychiatric Association [APA] 2013; Morgan 2006).

To date, there has been limited research examining problems with and interventions for anxiety in students with ASD in school settings. Studies involving clinically referred samples and nonschool settings have, however, yielded valuable insights into anxiety and treatments for anxiety in ASD. Several authors have proposed assessment strategies as well as ways to adapt anxiety-reducing treatments for use in schools. Given the limited research specifically in school settings, the following chapter was informed by the broader research involving anxiety in ASD. Particular attention was directed toward factors that may affect anxiety in students with ASD, assessment strategies, and anxiety interventions for ASD in school settings.

Comorbidity in Children and Adolescents with ASD

Students (children and adolescents) with ASD exhibit core diagnostic features involving social–communicative impairments and restricted and repetitive behaviors and interests (APA 2013). Recent changes in the diagnostic criteria reflect the perspective that individuals with ASD share a common set of symptoms, yet also exist along a continuum characterized by heterogeneity in symptom presentation and intensity. This framework also recognizes the broad variability in functional levels and degree of impairments

C. Lopata (✉) · M. L. Thomeer
Institute for Autism Research, Canisius College, 2001
Main Street, Buffalo, NY 14208, USA
e-mail: lopatac@canisius.edu

M. L. Thomeer
e-mail: thomeerm@canisius.edu

T. E. Davis III et al. (eds.), *Handbook of Autism and Anxiety,* Autism and Child Psychopathology Series,
DOI 10.1007/978-3-319-06796-4_14, © Springer International Publishing Switzerland 2014

that characterize ASD, including substantial differences in cognitive and language abilities along this continuum (APA 2013; see Chaps. 15–17 of this volume for in-depth discussion on the changes to ASD).

Another perspective that has evolved involves greater recognition of comorbid psychiatric symptoms and conditions in this population, as exemplified in the preceding chapters. According to Romanczyk and Gillis (2006), historically, ASD was considered orthogonal to other disorders. This perspective ran counter to empirical findings and clinical observations, suggesting that individuals with ASD experience a range of comorbid symptoms and disorders, and it likely contributed to the under-identification of co-occurring problems in this population (Tsai 2006; White et al. 2009). Despite the potential problem of under-identification of co-occurring problems, the APA (2013) reported that approximately 70 % of individuals with ASD have at least one comorbid psychiatric disorder.

One of the most common comorbid psychiatric symptoms among individuals with ASD is anxiety (White et al. 2009). Many studies of ASD and co-occurring problems, including anxiety, have examined the presence of comorbid or co-occurring psychiatric symptoms, with fewer reports based on formal diagnosis of the co-occurring condition (Gjevik et al. 2011). This is not meant to imply that studies of symptoms would not have yielded comparable rates of diagnoses, but to simply acknowledge the common use of symptoms or severity levels when characterizing anxiety in ASD. Before proceeding, a quick note on comorbidity is warranted. According to Szatmari and McConnell (2011), the identification of comorbid anxiety is based on the determination that the symptoms are independent of the ASD and result in impairment beyond the ASD diagnosis. The discussion of anxiety in this chapter is based on the perspective that anxiety symptoms occur in addition to the primary ASD diagnosis (but can effect and be affected by the core features of ASD). For the purpose of this chapter, the term *anxiety* will be used to refer to anxiety symptoms.

Anxiety in Children and Adolescents with ASD

The purpose of this chapter is to provide information on anxiety in students with ASD in schools. At present, research on anxiety in students with ASD in schools is very limited relative to studies involving clinically referred samples (Gjevik et al. 2011; see also earlier chapters in this volume). This section was included to provide a broader context for the limited findings from school samples. Results from the clinically derived samples provide some direction for school-based assessment and intervention, and a context for the current chapter.

A substantial body of research over the last decade has documented both a high prevalence of anxiety-related problems and elevated symptom levels/severity in children, adolescents, and adults with ASD relative to typically developing and clinical samples. A review by White et al. (2009) yielded prevalence estimates of anxiety problems in ASD samples ranging from 11 to 84 %. In a similar review of anxiety studies based on diagnostic interviews, Szatmari and McConnell (2011) reported prevalence estimates from 10 to 50 % in ASD samples. While prevalence estimates vary as a result of the heterogeneity of samples and measurement techniques used across studies, the data indicate that anxiety problems are common in the ASD population.

As noted, investigators have often examined anxiety-related problems in children and adolescents with ASD by assessing symptom levels. Studies by Lopata et al. (2010) and Gadow et al. (2005) on clinically referred samples with ASD illustrate this approach. Lopata et al. found significantly elevated parent-rated anxiety symptoms for high-functioning youth with ASD compared to typically developing youth, with 33 % of the ASD group having scores in the at-risk or clinical ranges. Gadow and colleagues also found significantly higher parent-rated anxiety severity for school-age youth with ASD compared to typical youth.

To better understand anxiety in ASD, researchers have considered its association with

ASD symptoms and other features. For example, Groden et al. (2006) noted that ASD features such as communication and social deficits can lead to stress in everyday social situations, and sensory sensitivities can lead to significant stress and anxiety when exposed to certain stimuli (e.g., sounds, light, etc.). Restricted and repetitive tendencies have also been linked to anxiety in ASD. Sukhodolsky et al. (2008) found greater stereotypic behavior as well as social impairment, which were associated with increased anxiety in youth with ASD. Similarly, Rodgers et al. (2012) found a strong positive association between repetitive behaviors and anxiety in children and adolescents with ASD. In a related large-scale study of youth with ASD, Gotham et al. (2013) found that anxiety was significantly associated with repetitive behaviors but only minimally related to the need for sameness.

Evidence has also indicated that anxiety problems occur across age and functional levels, but age, IQ, and language trends suggest that younger and lower-functioning (IQ and language) youth with ASD experience less anxiety than older and higher-functioning youth with ASD (Davis et al. 2011a; Szatmari and McConnell 2011; White et al. 2009). The reason for this is unknown, but potential explanations include increased self-awareness of impairments among higher-functioning youth (Szatmari and McConnell 2011), increased social and environmental demands and complexity during adolescents (White et al. 2009), and/or more impaired ability to label and express anxiety in youth with significant cognitive and language deficits (Davis et al. 2011b, 2012; Gjevik et al. 2011). While a number of factors have been associated with anxiety in ASD, the directionality of the relationships is not clear. It is possible that ASD symptoms and deficits increase anxiety symptoms, anxiety symptoms exacerbate ASD symptoms, and/or a bidirectional relationship exists (White et al. 2009). Regardless of the reasons, results of numerous investigations suggest that anxiety is a common but complex problem in school-age youth with ASD.

Anxiety in Students with ASD in School Settings

As mentioned, children and adolescents spend a considerable amount of time in school settings, and educational professionals assume significant responsibility for insuring that the students' needs are clearly understood and that effective interventions are delivered. Despite the critical role of teachers and school clinicians, parents and the students themselves have served as the main sources of information on anxiety in ASD, with few studies examining anxiety in ASD in school settings. While students with ASD and their parents are critical sources of information, school professionals (teachers, school psychologists, speech/language pathologists, etc.) represent an underutilized source of data on anxiety in ASD. School professionals may offer a number of advantages over other sources including advanced training and experience in typical development, learning, and behavior, as well as emotional, behavioral, and developmental disabilities. The lack of information derived from these sources and school populations led White et al. (2009) to call for studies of anxiety in ASD using school samples.

Although limited, some data have been generated on anxiety in students with ASD using teacher informants and/or school samples. Ashburner et al. (2010) collected teacher ratings of anxiety as part of a study of emotional/behavioral regulation skills in a school sample of 6–10-year-olds with ASD ($n=28$) compared to typical students ($n=51$). Students with ASD were in mainstream classrooms and the age- and gender-matched controls were drawn from the same classrooms. Results indicated significantly higher teacher ratings of anxiety in students with ASD compared to controls. Students with ASD were also rated as having significantly greater problems with perfectionism, emotional lability, and academic skills. Ashburner et al. suggested that, despite the availability of support services, the students with ASD were having significant problems coping with classroom and academic demands.

In another school-based study, Gjevik et al. (2011) assessed the prevalence of comorbidity in students attending a special school for students with ASD in Norway. Seventy-one students, 6–17 years of age, with ASD of various cognitive ability levels were rated by parents using a diagnostic interview. Results revealed that 72 % met criteria for at least one comorbid disorder. Anxiety disorders were most common, with 42 % meeting criteria for at least one anxiety disorder. This study was unique in that it assessed anxiety in a school sample; however, the setting was a specialized school for ASD which may have influenced the findings. Gjevik et al. suggested that the prevalence of comorbidity may have been higher in their sample than population-based samples of students with ASD. Unfortunately, the study did not include teacher ratings.

In the only identified study that assessed anxiety in a large school-based sample and included teachers as informants, Lecavalier (2006) examined the prevalence of anxiety problems (and other emotional and behavioral problems) in students with ASD drawn from 37 school districts in Ohio. Students were 3–21 years of age, of variable ability levels, and receiving special education services for ASD. From each of the 37 districts, 5–20 students were included in the study. Teachers provided ratings for 437 students and parents provided ratings for 353 students. Teacher results indicated that 18 % of the sample had moderate or severe problems being nervous/tense, 14 % had moderate or severe problems being worried, and 11 % had moderate or severe problems being fearful/anxious. Parent ratings in the moderate and severe problems ranges were generally similar to those of teachers (nervous/tense 21 %, worried 14 %, and fearful/anxious 17 %). Additional analyses based on teacher and parent ratings were consistent and indicated that younger students had significantly lower overall anxiety scores when compared with older students, and lower-ability students had lower overall anxiety scores when compared with higher-ability students.

Results of these investigations using school samples indicated that anxiety problems are present in a sizable number of students with ASD in school settings. The studies by Gjevik et al. (2011) and Lecavalier (2006) suggest that anxiety severity may differ based on the school setting, with

special schools specifically serving students with ASD being more likely to see a greater number of students with more severe anxiety symptoms. Similar to clinically referred samples, students needing a more restrictive specialized setting/school placement may have more complex psychiatric needs and comorbid symptoms. Despite these apparent patterns, anxiety has been reported across age and functional levels (White et al. 2009). Teachers and/or school clinicians should not assume an absence of anxiety in any student with ASD. Instead, teachers and school clinicians may benefit from a perspective that recognizes some of the communicative barriers of lower-ability and younger students with ASD and remain aware that anxiety may be manifested differently based on cognitive, language, and age levels.

Anxiety is of particular importance to educational professionals, as it can underlie and contribute to declines in school performance and interpersonal relationships, and it has been associated with increased problem behaviors among students with ASD (Kim et al. 2000; Reaven 2009). Anxiety results from stressful experiences and encounters (Morgan 2006), and many such stressors, can and do occur daily in school environments. During these events, students with ASD are expected to interpret, understand, cope with, and adapt to the circumstances. Many students with ASD have deficits that interfere with their self-regulation and ability to respond appropriately. This mismatch between environmental demands and the coping skills of students with ASD can lead to anxiety in the school environment. Teachers and school clinicians need to consider the array of factors that may be contributing to anxiety because chronic and sustained exposure to elevated anxiety can result in long-term negative effects on memory, learning, and brain functioning (Morgan 2006).

Student and School Factors Implicated in Anxiety in ASD

Research has suggested that younger and lower-ability students with ASD have lower anxiety symptoms compared to older and higher-ability students; this finding was replicated in the Lecavalier (2006) study which used a large school-derived sample of students with ASD. Although careful attention is warranted for all students with ASD, older and higher-ability students may be more susceptible to problems with anxiety. This suggestion is tempered, however, with the recognition that younger and lower-ability students with ASD also experience problems with anxiety and they may manifest the symptoms differently due to communication impairments.

Potential contributors to anxiety are often discussed in relation to the core diagnostic features of ASD and environmental factors that intersect with these features. Poor understanding of the social environment can present chronic and diverse challenges for students with ASD in school settings. The effort needed to interpret and respond during social exchanges can lead to stress and anxiety (APA 2013; Portway and Johnson 2005). Further, students with ASD often experience repeated social failures and social rejection, which can contribute to anxiety (Church et al. 2000). The increase in anxiety can further inhibit social functioning (Chang et al. 2012) and social overtures (Bellini 2004), and contribute to social fears (Evans et al. 2005). In this way, anxiety can result from and contribute to the characteristic social difficulties of students with ASD.

Research has also suggested that teasing and bullying at school may be especially influential in precipitating anxiety in students with ASD (Szatmari and McConnell 2011). A qualitative study of young adults with ASD revealed that being a victim of bullying was a nearly universal experience during childhood (Portway and Johnson 2005). These anxiety-producing interactions can contribute to further isolation and feelings of being *different* (Church et al. 2000; Portway and Johnson 2005). School environments also expose students with ASD to a number of familiar and unfamiliar adults and peers. Some evidence has suggested that exposure to unfamiliar peers can trigger anxiety and stress in high-functioning students with ASD. Lopata et al. (2008) found that unanticipated exposure to a play situation with an unfamiliar peer resulted in increased anxiety in contrast to a play situation with a familiar peer.

Results of that study suggested that social interactions can produce anxiety, particularly when they involve an unanticipated interaction with an unfamiliar individual. Lastly, the social–communicative impairments and anxiety in students with ASD need to be considered to understand their effect on classroom learning. Because learning is a social–communicative event, deficits in this area can interfere with everyday classroom learning and increase stress. Given the many demands of the school environment that involve social and communicative exchanges and the characteristic deficits in this area for students with ASD, school environments likely present a continual series of anxiety-producing stressors.

Another ASD feature commonly discussed in relation to anxiety is the students' need for predictable routines, as well as repetitive and ritualized behaviors. Church et al. (2000) documented a high need for rules and predictable routines in preschool through high school students with ASD. The broad array of school content, settings, and schedules is complex for students with ASD, and their routines and environments are often subject to change (Ashburner et al. 2010). This can be problematic as novel and unstructured situations and lack of predictability in school environments can increase anxiety (APA 2013; White et al. 2009). In addition, unanticipated disruptions in routines and ritualized behaviors can trigger and increase stress and anxiety in ASD (Groden et al. 2006; Portway and Johnson 2005; Tsai 2006) and negatively affect learning and academic performance (APA 2013; Morgan 2006). Church et al. (2000) found that repetitive behaviors emerged and were exacerbated during episodes of increased anxiety among students with ASD. The assertion that disruptions may increase anxiety appears to be consistent with several studies that have found anxiety to be significantly associated with repetitive behaviors (e.g., Rodgers et al. 2012; Sukhodolsky et al. 2008). While the directionality of this relationship is not certain, repetitive behaviors may serve a soothing function for students with ASD (Gjevik et al. 2011; Morgan 2006). Furthermore, a note on predictability and transitions is warranted (APA 2013). Educational staff should be mindful that the beginning of the school year constitutes a transition period which can increase anxiety (Tsai 2006). The transition to secondary school settings is also a period characterized by stress and anxiety, owing to more complex curriculum and organizational demands, as well as exposure to multiple teachers across the school day (Ashburner et al. 2010).

A final consideration involves the characteristic sensory sensitivities of some students with ASD. While the specific sensitivities often differ across students, exposure to certain sensory stimuli such as sounds, textures, and/or lighting can be distressing and can increase anxiety (Ashburner et al. 2010; Groden et al. 2006). School settings are characterized by environments that differ substantially in terms of these stimuli. Places such as loud cafeterias and gymnasiums, harshly and brightly lit rooms, and small spaces crowded with students and staff may be problematic for some students with ASD. Given the highly idiosyncratic nature of the sensitivities, school staff will need to assess the potential contribution of various stimuli to the anxiety symptoms of students with ASD.

The information in this section was not intended to be a comprehensive review of all factors that may contribute to or are affected by anxiety. Instead, it represents a framework from which to consider potential factors associated with anxiety in students with ASD. The student and school factors described in this section provide the educational team with a range of variables to consider when assessing and treating anxiety in students with ASD.

Assessment of Anxiety in ASD in School Settings

The key to determining the presence of anxiety, as well as appropriate intervention, is a systematic and structured assessment. School clinicians and teachers may be particularly suited for this, given their training and observations of the students in a variety of structured and unstructured settings. Anxiety is a complex construct that involves interrelated components including cogni-

tion, physiology, and behavior (Romanczyk and Gillis 2006). Assessing its presence is a challenge, given the significant heterogeneity of symptoms and functional levels that characterize ASD. Accessing information on some facets of anxiety (e.g., self-reported thoughts and internalized states) may not be possible for some with language and cognitive impairments, and its validity may be questionable even in higher-functioning students with ASD (Ollendick and White 2012; Reaven 2009; Tsai 2006; White et al. 2009). Compounding the problem is the lack of evidence or direction on how to best assess anxiety in students with ASD (White et al. 2009). The following is an overview of considerations that may inform the assessment practices of school assessment teams when evaluating anxiety in students with ASD.

Team Composition and Assessment Framework

Given the likelihood of anxiety in students with ASD, initial and routine assessments should include a screening for anxiety (Szatmari and McConnell 2011). The process of screening and assessment for anxiety is complex and warrants an interdisciplinary team that includes caregivers and service providers such as parents, teachers, school psychologists, speech/language pathologists, occupational and physical therapists, and physicians (Tsai 2006). With the exception of an external physician, this composition of parents and service providers is common in school-based assessment teams. Because the process of assessing anxiety is complex for students with ASD, some education may be necessary for team members (Tsai 2006) to operationally define and establish a common understanding of the construct of anxiety (Romanczyk and Gillis 2006).

Differentiating anxiety symptoms from the core features of ASD is a fundamental challenge (Kerns and Kendall 2012; White et al. 2009). In order to constitute comorbidity, the anxiety symptoms/disorder should be independent of and result in additional impairment beyond the ASD diagnosis (Szatmari and McConnell 2011). For example, the team may have to determine whether avoidance of social interactions or repetitive behavior is a reflection of the ASD or a symptom of anxiety (Gjevik et al. 2011). Another consideration is whether the student is experiencing state anxiety (situation specific) or trait anxiety (which may vary in intensity but is chronic; Romanczyk and Gillis 2006). This determination will help direct treatments so that the anxiety-inducing source is targeted. Although state and trait anxieties are characterized as distinct, Romanczyk and Gillis (2006) cautioned that environmental events that are linked to state anxiety can produce chronic anxiety if the events yield frequent and persistent anxious reactions.

Lastly, because anxiety is composed of several components (i.e., physiological, behavioral, cognitive, and affective; see Chaps. 3 and 6 for more details) and may be affected by a range of student and environmental factors, it should be assessed using multiple methods, measures, and sources (Groden et al. 2006; White et al. 2009). Data gathered in natural settings will likely yield more clinically useful information as it provides insights into setting factors and the relationship between environmental events and the student's physiological status and behavior (Romanczyk and Gillis 2006; Tsai 2006). It will also be essential to consider student-level variables when considering risk factors and the manner in which anxiety may be manifested. Because age, IQ, and severity of ASD symptoms will be important in selecting anxiety measures, a comprehensive assessment should include cognitive and language testing and assessment of ASD symptom severity. Academic achievement testing will also provide valuable information as many students with ASD underperform academically (Ashburner et al. 2010). Based on these basic student-level variables, the assessment team can select sources and measures that will help assess anxiety in students with ASD.

Source Considerations

The identification of appropriate informants is essential in the assessment of anxiety in students with ASD. Parents and teachers constitute critical

sources of information as they have longitudinal insights into the students' symptoms and behaviors in day-to-day settings (Lopata et al. 2010; Rodgers et al. 2012). This perspective may be particularly useful in determining whether a new or reemerging behavior is a symptom of anxiety or part of the student's baseline ASD symptoms. Several studies have found both teachers and parents reporting elevated symptoms in students with ASD (e.g., Lecavalier 2006); however, some informant differences may occur in the severity of symptoms (Weisbrot et al. 2005). In their review, White et al. (2009) noted a tendency for higher teacher-reported anxiety in students with ASD, which they suggested may have been associated with greater social and academic demands in school settings. While some differences may be observed in the severity or type of anxiety symptoms, the studies suggest that teachers and parents are capable of detecting anxiety in students with ASD and should continue to be a critical source of assessment information.

The other important source of information on anxiety is the student with ASD. For those with significant cognitive and language impairments, self-report information may not be possible (Gjevik et al. 2011; Groden et al. 2006); however, this should not preclude them from being a significant source of information. In such circumstances, the student's behaviors may signal the presence of anxiety (Szatmari and McConnell 2011). For higher-functioning (IQ and language) students with ASD, information can be collected on their behaviors and self-perceived anxiety. This self-reported information must be considered relative to other information, as students with ASD have characteristic self-report problems (APA 2013; Romanczyk and Gillis 2006). Although some have found high-functioning students with ASD reporting high levels of anxiety symptoms (e.g., Bellini 2004), others have found parents reporting higher levels of symptoms when compared with the students (e.g., Lopata et al. 2010). In a separate study, Lopata et al. (2008) compared a physiological indicator of anxiety/stress with self-reported anxiety among high-functioning students with ASD in different social situations. The overall correlation was moderate;

however, a complex relationship was observed. Specifically, low, self-reported anxiety did not yield useful data on the student's physiological status, whereas high self-reported anxiety was associated with elevated physiological anxiety. The complexity of the self-report capabilities and the sometimes observed tendency for students with ASD to underestimate symptoms may suggest that parents or teachers be given greater deference as a preferred source (Lopata et al. 2010).

Data Collection Methods and Considerations

Anxiety assessments in ASD should involve multiple measures such as rating scales, interviews, behavioral observations, and/or physiological measures (Groden et al. 2006; White et al. 2009). These measures yield important information on anxiety symptoms and arousal levels (Mazurek et al. 2013). A brief description of these types of measures and their use in the assessment of anxiety in students with ASD is provided. Caution is warranted, however, as there is a lack of psychometrically sound measures for assessing anxiety in ASD and the validity of existing scales for this population is unknown (Mazurek et al. 2013; Szatmari and McConnell 2011; White et al. 2009).

Rating scales and interviews are commonly used and have detected elevated anxiety symptoms in ASD (Sukhodolsky et al. 2008; Szatmari and McConnell 2011). Rating scales may offer a number of advantages. They can be done quickly, are simple to administer (Gosch et al. 2012), and can capture information across settings (e.g., home and school). They can also provide information not gathered in categorical measurement systems (Lecavalier 2006), specifically, information on the degree to which a symptom is exhibited or the severity of a symptom (Gadow et al. 2006). This may be important when anxiety symptoms are subthreshold for a diagnosis but still warrant intervention (Gosch et al. 2012). Despite these advantages, rating scales may be less sensitive in differentiating symptoms of anxiety from ASD. Clinical interviews have also been used to assess anxiety in ASD and may allow clinicians to make distinctions between ASD features and symptoms of anxiety (Gjevik et al. 2011; Reaven 2009). Clinical interviews are more flexible and allow evaluators to ask probing questions that help distinguish symptoms of anxiety and establish whether they are causing additional impairment (Chang et al. 2012; Szatmari and McConnell 2011). Interviews may also yield information on the thoughts and perceptions of students with ASD regarding objects, situations, and settings that may provoke anxiety. In schools, clinical interviews may be less feasible due to time constraints (Gosch et al. 2012). Both rating scales and interviews can be administered to parents and teachers and some students with ASD, allowing for data from multiple sources across settings: although problems with agreement and disagreement across reporters and environments may be an issue and should be treated carefully (Davis 2012).

Behavioral observations are another useful measurement technique for assessing anxiety in all students with ASD, but may be especially important for nonverbal and/or cognitively impaired students (Sukhodolsky et al. 2008; Szatmari and McConnell 2011). When using observations, it is essential that the anxiety symptoms are operationalized to be observable and measurable (Tsai 2006). Anxiety may be manifested in new behaviors and/or in increases in anxiety-related behavior compared to base rates (APA 2013). Behaviors such as tantrums, clinginess, crying, withdrawal and agitation, changes in eating and sleep patterns, and/or increases in repetitive behaviors may reflect increased anxiety (APA 2013; Tsai 2006; White et al. 2009). Observations of social functioning may also reveal anxiety-related problems (Chang et al. 2012). While these constitute potential indicators of anxiety, behavioral manifestations of anxiety can be highly idiosyncratic. Once behavioral indicators are identified, educational teams should conduct a functional behavioral assessment to document base rates, antecedents, and consequences (Tsai 2006). This information will inform subsequent interventions.

A final set of measurement options involves physiological indicators of anxiety. Given the self-report and cognitive and/or language deficits, anxiety may be more accurately measured using physiological indices (Evans et al. 2005). While physiological symptoms can vary significantly among students with ASD, measurements of heart rate, skin temperature and conductance, and cortisol can be used to detect anxiety and stress in these students (Mazurek et al. 2013; Romanczyk and Gillis 2006). If using a physiological measure, the least intrusive and most tolerable technique should be selected, as the technique itself may be stressful for some students with ASD (e.g., Putnam et al. (2012) reported on the acceptability of saliva collection methods in students with ASD). While physiological indices are a potentially important contributor, there is significant variability in the physiological levels of anxiety across individuals with ASD (Romanczyk and Gillis 2006), and normative comparisons are typically not feasible. As a result, physiological measures are perhaps most useful in terms of assessing the student's anxiety level relative to baseline (Groden et al. 2006) or when exposed to various stimuli (e.g., social situations; Lopata et al. 2008). Physiological indices may provide valuable information when assessing anxiety in ASD; however, their feasibility in schools will be influenced by factors such as cost, time requirements, and expertise (Romanczyk and Gillis 2006).

School Interventions for Anxiety in Students with ASD

Effective school interventions to reduce anxiety of students with ASD are needed, as mental health problems such as anxiety can negatively affect long-term outcomes (APA 2013). Despite this need, there is a paucity of school-based interventions that target anxiety in students with ASD. Emerging evidence from clinical studies has, however, yielded a number of techniques that appear applicable to school settings (Rotheram-Fuller and MacMullen 2011). The following was developed to provide school professionals with a framework for anxiety-reducing interventions for students with ASD. Given the lack of evidence

for a school-based model, the following should be viewed as guidelines and factors to consider for school professionals.

Intervention Team and Framework

A multimodal approach to intervention for anxiety in students with ASD is needed (Reaven 2009; White et al. 2009), and this requires an interdisciplinary team (Mazurek et al. 2013). Intervention teams in schools are comprised of professionals from diverse areas of expertise (special educators, school psychologists, counselors, speech/language pathologists, nurses, occupational and physical therapists, etc.) and they typically include parents. This may make them particularly suited for such interventions. Although not typically a part of the school intervention team, physicians often prescribe psychotropics and school staff is accustomed to providing feedback on medication responsiveness. As such, physicians may play a role in school interventions for many with ASD and will likely have their decisions informed by school staff and parents (Tsai 2006). Although there are diverse disciplines represented in school teams, each member's expertise and training related to anxiety and ASD should be assessed prior to intervention (Rotheram-Fuller and MacMullen 2011). This will help determine roles within the intervention and the extent of training needed by the team members. Sound training in anxiety, ASD, and treatment strategies is considered essential for school staff (Gosch et al. 2012; Szatmari and McConnell 2011).

Another factor to consider is the extent to which multicomponent interventions are feasible in schools. This is critical as anxiety treatments for students with ASD are comprised of several therapeutic elements. Multicomponent interventions require considerable coordination and staffing, and their exportability is unknown (White et al. 2013). Further, the typical responsibilities of teachers and other school clinicians may limit their time available to implement such treatments (Rotheram-Fuller and MacMullen 2011). Despite these challenges, recent comprehensive school-based intervention studies for students with ASD suggested that school staff found the multicomponent programs feasible and were capable of implementing them with a high degree of fidelity (e.g., Lopata et al. 2012). The authors suggested that feasibility was enhanced by having different members of the team assume responsibility for different treatment components, thus avoiding overburdening any individual. Although the program targeted social and communication skills and ASD symptoms, the distribution of roles may be important for multicomponent anxiety treatments for students with ASD.

A final note involves the fact that schools may be ideal for treating anxiety as they constitute a setting that is often problematic for students with ASD. Interventions in this setting can exploit building-level resources, make use of concrete examples, and take advantage of practice opportunities in natural environments that foster generalization (Bolton et al. 2012; Gosch et al. 2012). Outpatient programs generally do not afford practice opportunities in authentic environments which may hinder generalization (Rotheram-Fuller and MacMullen 2011). Schools also offer a unique opportunity to coordinate the multiple components as intervention teams have regular access to and contact with one another. They can also coordinate the targets of the intervention so that the student's IEP goals are integrated. Interventions for anxiety in students with ASD often target social proficiencies which can overlap with social and communication goals.

Intervention Components

A multimodal approach to intervention allows for targeting of the multiple components that comprise anxiety (i.e., cognition, physiology, and behavior), as well as skills to improve social performance. Most commonly, anxiety in students with ASD has been treated using cognitive and behavioral techniques, as well as medication (Romanczyk and Gillis 2006). For school teams, development of the intervention is based on results of the assessment which should have included information on IQ and language levels, as well as anxiety and ASD symptoms. Understanding the student's cognitive and language abilities

is imperative as the intervention techniques will be adopted based on these factors (Davis 2012).

To date, the preponderance of treatment research on anxiety in ASD has examined the use of cognitive–behavioral (CB) interventions. Because CB interventions utilize cognitive elements and require relatively intact cognitive and language abilities, they are most appropriate for high-functioning students with ASD. For students with ASD and cognitive and language impairments, less is known about how to reduce anxiety (White et al. 2009). For these students, interventions may have to rely more exclusively on behavioral techniques (Bolton et al. 2012; Chang et al. 2012). While studies of CB interventions in ASD have generally included students with an IQ > 70, clinicians in schools will have to decide which elements are appropriate for a specific child and the extent to which the intervention employs CB elements or relies more exclusively on behavioral strategies. The following is an overview of elements commonly used in anxiety interventions for students with ASD that appear applicable to school environments.

Based on the existing research, school staff should develop interventions that target the cognitive, physiological, and behavioral aspects of anxiety. Although researchers have developed different treatment packages, the interventions share common elements (e.g., Reaven et al. 2012; White et al. 2013; Wood et al. 2009), and different members of the intervention team can assume responsibility for one or more of the elements (based on expertise and time). Initially, students and parents are taught about anxiety, symptoms, how thoughts and behaviors trigger and sustain symptoms, and treatment strategies. For students, it may be necessary to discuss anxiety in terms of physiological symptoms as emotions can be abstract (Romanczyk and Gillis 2006; Rotheram-Fuller and MacMullen 2011). Students can then be taught relaxation techniques to reduce physiological aspects of anxiety and arousal. Techniques such as progressive muscle relaxation and controlled breathing can be used in response to a triggering event or preventively (i.e., practiced daily to decrease general anxiety; Groden et al. 2006). To address automatic and negative thoughts associated with anxiety, cognitive restructuring is used. Students are taught to recognize automatic thoughts and distortions, and these are challenged and replaced with more adaptive thoughts and self-statements (Reaven et al. 2012; Rotheram-Fuller and MacMullen 2011). In addition to cognitive restructuring, students are taught problem-solving skills to increase their ability to cope with different circumstances. Problem-solving skills can be taught verbally or using visual techniques involving behavioral sequences that depict adaptive coping (Groden et al. 2006). Modeling and behavioral rehearsal can also be used to teach and practice problem solving (Bolton et al. 2012; Reaven 2009). Team members including school psychologists, counselors, and social workers have training consistent with these therapeutic techniques and may be appropriate for implementing one or more of these elements.

Once students with ASD have learned anxiety-reducing techniques and adaptive cognitive and coping strategies, exposure exercises are used. Anxiety-provoking situations are systematically confronted in a hierarchical manner using graded exposures (Gosch et al. 2012; Reaven 2009). Schools offer a wide range of in vivo exposure opportunities that can be selected based on the student's problem area. Students can rehearse their responses prior to exposure but should have daily exposure activities (Reaven 2009). During these exercises, the student should use her/his coping and relaxation strategies (Romanczyk and Gillis 2006) but remain in the situation until the anxiety subsides (Wood et al. 2009). For students with cognitive and language impairments, exposure exercises may constitute a more behaviorally oriented approach to anxiety reduction. In vivo exposure exercises can be facilitated by a number of members of the intervention team. Direct teaching and support staff (e.g., aides) may be able to integrate these practice opportunities across the school day. Clear communication among the team members will be essential in supporting effective exposure exercises. The coping skills and relaxation strategies the student has learned should be understood by the team so that planned exposure activities, as well as unanticipated exposures, can be supported.

Another important intervention element, familiar to school intervention teams, for anxiety reduction in students with ASD involves contingency management. Contingency management is used to systematically reinforce desired behaviors and coping skills (Rotheram-Fuller and MacMullen 2011), and it has been effectively used in anxiety treatment studies for youth with ASD (e.g., Reaven et al. 2012; Wood et al. 2009). School staff should reinforce attempts to cope with anxiety-provoking situations (Reaven 2009) including engagement and approach behaviors (Gosch et al. 2012). Although contingency management is important for all students with ASD, it may be even more essential for those with significant cognitive and language impairments who may be confronting stressors without the cognitive strategies of higher-functioning students. In school settings, a contingency management system can be instituted across the school day to support learning during planned exposures and unplanned naturalistic situations and promote generalization. The utility and feasibility of contingency management systems used across the school day has been demonstrated in a multicomponent psychosocial intervention for students with ASD (Lopata et al. 2012) and as a component of an anxiety program for students with ASD (Wood et al. 2009). Though teachers and aides are in the best position to implement this system across the day, other members of the team should provide reinforcement when target skills are observed. Parents should also be involved to insure practice and reinforcement across settings (Bolton et al. 2012).

A number of anxiety treatments for youth with ASD that have yielded positive effects have incorporated social skills training (e.g., Reaven et al. 2012; White et al. 2013; Wood et al. 2009). This was based on the notion that social impairments of students with ASD can contribute to anxiety, which in turn can negatively affect social performance and engagement. As such, social skills instruction may increase social skills and reduce anxiety (Szatmari and McConnell 2011). Social skills can be taught using direct instruction, modeling, role-play, rehearsal, and feedback (Bolton et al. 2012). Members of the intervention team including school psychologists and speech/language pathologists have been effective in conducting these groups in school-based psychosocial interventions for students with ASD (Lopata et al. 2012). Across these therapeutic elements, instructional adjustments may need to be made to help students with ASD learn the range of cognitive and coping skills. Modifications such as the use of visual supports and cues, concrete examples and lessons, and hands-on activities can be useful. High levels of consistency, predictability, and structure are also recommended (Groden et al. 2006; Reaven 2009; Rotheram-Fuller and MacMullen 2011; White et al. 2009).

An additional component to be included is parent education and involvement (White et al. 2009). Parent education should include instruction about anxiety and ASD symptoms and treatment strategies, and parents should contribute to development of the intervention. Parents are also required to insure that students practice coping skills and are reinforced outside the school setting (i.e., generalization; Bolton et al. 2012). Parents should also learn to model courageous behavior, as well as titrate exposures, so that the student has the skills to successfully cope with the given situation (Reaven 2011).

A final note on medication treatment is warranted. School staffs do not make determinations about psychotropic treatments for anxiety in students with ASD; however, they are an important source of information on efficacy and side effects for physicians (Tsai 2006). Psychotropic medications can offer symptom reduction, which may help with other intervention efforts.

Progress Monitoring

School intervention staff must be proficient in monitoring progress (Bolton et al. 2012). Progress monitoring for anxiety in students with ASD is complicated by a number of factors including the complexity of anxiety, overlap of anxiety and ASD features, and significant cognitive and language heterogeneity. Despite these challenges, a few factors may help inform the monitoring techniques and outcome determinations. Given the various settings in which anxiety occurs,

data from multiple sources using various methods should be obtained (Rotheram-Fuller and MacMullen 2011). An important consideration in selecting an assessment technique involves the degree to which it taps the targeted skill or reaction. The closer the measure aligns with the treatment target and the more focused the goals, the greater the likelihood that gains will be detected (Bolton et al. 2012; Wood et al. 2009).

Given the critical roles of teachers and parents, information should be attained from these sources on an ongoing basis. These sources have extensive knowledge of the student's symptom levels and behaviors (Lopata et al. 2010; Rodgers et al. 2012), including during the baseline phase against which gains will be determined. Progress monitoring data from these sources can be gathered using rating scales (Reaven 2009). These scales can be particularly useful as they assess symptoms at both clinical and subclinical levels (Lecavalier 2006) and can be used to track progress on a continuous scale. It is important that the same scales used to establish baseline levels be used for monitoring change. Diagnostic anxiety scales designed for categorical determinations may be less useful in tracking treatment responsiveness (Bolton et al. 2012). When appropriate, data can also be gathered from the student via self-reports. Although this may or may not be useful given some of the self-report challenges previously described, a simple numerical rating of anxiety or stress may provide some indication of the student's self-perceived stress (e.g., Lopata et al. 2008).

Another useful technique for monitoring outcomes involves direct behavioral observations (Bolton et al. 2012). This focuses on operationally defined behaviors that have been attributed to and/or associated with anxiety and that were tracked during the baseline assessment. Changes in behavior attributed to anxiety can be useful in tracking anxiety levels in all students with ASD (APA 2013), but may be especially useful for those with cognitive and language impairments who are unable to or have difficulty describing their anxiety levels (Szatmari and McConnell 2011; Tsai 2006). Using operationally defined behavioral indicators of anxiety, classroom staff can track changes in behaviors resulting from the intervention.

A final strategy for monitoring progress involves physiological measures. These may not be readily available in many schools but, if available, can serve as a way to overcome some of the shortcomings of other measures (Evans et al. 2005). Physiological indices can be used to measure students' anxiety in response to different situations and help determine whether their coping skills are effective in reducing anxiety (Romanczyk and Gillis 2006). Physiological measures may be especially useful for monitoring the progress of students with significant cognitive and language impairments (Reaven 2011). Although these measures require training and practice, they may prove to be very useful as part of a multi-method monitoring system.

Together, these measures provide school teams with an extensive array of progress-monitoring options. Teams will have to decide on tracking techniques that are appropriate, given the characteristics of the student and targeted symptoms, and that are also feasible within the school. Whichever measures are selected, data should be reviewed regularly and used to inform decisions about intervention effectiveness and modifications. Regular and open communication and shared responsibility among the members of the school team and parents will be essential in insuring effective and integrated assessment, treatment, and progress monitoring.

References

American Psychiatric Association. (2013). *Diagnostic and statistical manual of mental disorders* (5th ed.). Arlington: American Psychiatric Association.

Ashburner, J., Ziviani, J., & Rodger, S. (2010). Surviving in the mainstream: Capacity of children with autism spectrum disorders to perform academically and regulate their emotions and behavior at school. *Research in Autism Spectrum Disorders, 4*, 18–27.

Bellini, S. (2004). Social skill deficits and anxiety in high-functioning adolescents with autism spectrum disorders. *Focus on Autism and Other Developmental Disorders, 19*(2), 78–86.

Bolton, J. B., McPoyle-Callahan, J. E., & Christner, R. W. (2012). Autism: School-based cognitive-behavioral interventions. In R. B. Mennuti, R. W. Christner, & A. Freeman (Eds.), Cognitive-behavioral interventions in educational settings: A handbook for practice (2nd ed., pp. 469–501). New York: Routledge.

Chang, Y., Quan, J., & Wood, J. J. (2012). Effects of anxiety disorder severity on social functioning in children with autism spectrum disorders. Journal of Developmental and Physical Disabilities, 24, 235–245.

Church, C., Alisanski, S., & Amanullah, S. (2000). The social, behavioral, and academic experiences of children with Asperger syndrome. Focus on Autism and Other Developmental Disabilities, 15(1), 12–20.

Davis III, T. E. (2012). Where to from here for ASD and anxiety? Lessons learned from child anxiety and the issue of DSM-5. Clinical Psychology: Science and Practice, 19, 358–363.

Davis III, T. E., Hess, J. A., Moree, B. N., Fodstad, J. C., Dempsey, T., Jenkins, W., & Matson, J. L. (2011a). Anxiety symptoms across the lifespan in people with autistic disorder. Research in Autism Spectrum Disorders, 5, 112–118.

Davis III, T. E., Moree, B., Dempsey, T., Reuther, E., Fodstad, J., Hess, J., Jenkins, W., Matson, J. L. (2011b). The relationship between autism spectrum disorders and anxiety: The moderating effect of communication. Research in Autism Spectrum Disorders, 5, 324–329.

Davis III, T. E., Moree, B., Dempsey, T., Hess, J., Jenkins, W., Fodstad, J., & Matson, J. L. (2012). The effects of communication deficits on anxiety symptoms in infants and toddlers with autism spectrum disorders. Behavior Therapy, 43, 142–152.

Evans, D. W., Canavera, K., Kleinpeter, F. L., Maccubbin, E., & Taga, K. (2005). The fears, phobias, and anxieties of children with autism spectrum disorders and Down syndrome: Comparison with developmentally and chronologically age matched children. Child Psychiatry and Human Development, 36(1), 3–26.

Gadow, K. D., DeVincent, C. J., Pomeroy, J., & Azizian, A. (2005). Comparison of DSM-IV symptoms in elementary school-age children with PDD versus clinic and community samples. Autism, 9(4), 392–415.

Gadow, K. D., DeVincent, C. J., & Pomeroy, J. (2006). ADHD symptom subtypes in children with pervasive developmental disorder. Journal of Autism and Developmental Disorders, 36(2), 271–283.

Gjevik, E., Eldevik, S., Fjaeran-Granum, T., & Sponheim, E. (2011). Kiddie-SADS reveals high rates of DSM-IV disorders in children and adolescents with autism spectrum disorders. Journal of Autism and Developmental Disorders, 41, 761–769.

Gosch, E. A., Flannery-Schroeder, E., & Brecher, R. J. (2012). Anxiety disorders: School-based cognitive-behavioral interventions. In R. B. Mennuti, R. W. Christner, & A. Freeman (Eds.), Cognitive-behavioral interventions in educational settings: A handbook for practice (2nd ed., pp. 117–160). New York: Routledge.

Gotham, K., Bishop, S. L., Hus, V., Huerta, M., Lund, S., Buja, A., Krieger, A., Lord, C. (2013). Exploring the relationship between anxiety and insistence on sameness in autism spectrum disorders. Autism Research, 6, 33–41.

Groden, J., Baron, M. G., & Groden, G. (2006). Assessment and coping strategies. In M. G. Baron, J. Groden, G. Groden, & L. P. Lipsitt (Eds.), Stress and coping in autism (pp. 15–41). New York: Oxford University Press.

Kerns, C. M., & Kendall, P. C. (2012). The presentation and classification of anxiety in autism spectrum disorder. Clinical Psychology: Science & Practice, 19, 323–347.

Kim, J. A., Szatmari, P., Bryson, S. E., Streiner, D. L., & Wilson, F. J. (2000). The prevalence of anxiety and mood problems among children with autism and Asperger syndrome. Autism, 4(2), 117–132.

Lecavalier, L. (2006). Behavioral and emotional problems in young people with pervasive developmental disorders: Relative prevalence, effect of subject characteristics, and empirical classification. Journal of Autism and Developmental Disorders, 36, 1101–1114.

Lopata, C., Volker, M. A., Putnam, S. K., Thomeer, M. L., & Nida, R. E. (2008). Effect of social familiarity on salivary cortisol and self-reports of social anxiety and stress in children with high functioning autism spectrum disorders. Journal of Autism and Developmental Disorders, 38, 1866–1877.

Lopata, C., Toomey, J. A., Fox, J. D., Volker, M. A., Chow, S. Y., Thomeer, M. L., Lee, G. K., Rodgers, J. D., McDonald, C. A., Smerbeck, A. M. (2010). Anxiety and depression in children with HFASD: Symptom levels and source differences. Journal of Abnormal Child Psychology, 38(6), 765–776.

Lopata, C., Thomeer, M. L., Volker, M. A., Lee, G. K., Smith, T. H., Smith, R. A., McDonald, C. A., Rodgers, J. D., Lipinski, A. M., Toomey, J. A. (2012). Feasibility and initial efficacy of a comprehensive school-based intervention for high-functioning autism spectrum disorders. Psychology in the Schools, 49(10), 963–974.

Mazurek, M. O., Vasa, R. A., Kalb, L. G., Kanne, S. M., Rosenberg, D., Keefer, A., Murray, D. S., Freedman, B., Lowery, L. A. (2013). Anxiety, sensory overresponsivity, and gastrointestinal problems in children with autism spectrum disorders. Journal of Abnormal Child Psychology, 41, 165–176.

Morgan, K. (2006). Is autism a stress disorder? What studies of nonautistic populations can tell us. In M. G. Baron, J. Groden, G. Groden, & L. P. Lipsitt (Eds.), Stress and coping in autism (pp. 129–182). New York: Oxford University Press.

Ollendick, T. H., & White, S. W. (2012). The presentation and classification of anxiety in autism spectrum disorder: Where to from here? Clinical Psychology: Science and Practice, 19, 352–355.

Portway, S. M., & Johnson, B. (2005). Do you know I have Asperger's syndrome? Risks of a non-obvious disability. Health, Risk and Society, 7(1), 73–83.

Putnam, S. K., Lopata, C., Fox, J. D., Thomeer, M. L., Rodgers, J. D., Volker, M. A., Lee, G. K., Neilans, E. G., Werth, J. (2012). Comparison of saliva collection methods in children with high-functioning autism spectrum disorders: Acceptability and recovery of cortisol. Child Psychiatry and Human Development, 43(4), 560–573.

Reaven, J. A. (2009). Children with high-functioning autism spectrum disorders and co-occurring anxiety symptoms: Implications for assessment and treatment. Journal for Specialists in Pediatric Nursing, 14, 192–199.

Reaven, J. (2011). The treatment of anxiety symptoms in youth with high-functioning autism spectrum disorders: Developmental considerations for parents. Brain Research, 1380, 255–263.

Reaven, J., Blakely-Smith, A., Culhane-Shelburne, K., & Hepburn, S. (2012). Group cognitive behavior therapy for children with high-functioning autism spectrum disorders and anxiety: A randomized trial. Journal of Child Psychology and Psychiatry, 53(4), 410–419.

Rodgers, J., Riby, D. M., Janes, E., Connolly, B., & McConachie, H. (2012). Anxiety and repetitive behaviours in autism spectrum disorders and Williams syndrome: A cross-syndrome comparison. Journal of Autism and Developmental Disorders, 42, 175–180.

Romanczyk, R. G., & Gillis, J. M. (2006). Autism and the physiology of stress and anxiety. In M. G. Baron, J. Groden, G. Groden, & L. P. Lipsitt (Eds.), Stress and coping in autism (pp. 183–204). New York: Oxford University Press.

Rotheram-Fuller, E., & MacMullen, L. (2011). Cognitive-behavioral therapy for children with autism spectrum disorders. Psychology in the Schools, 48(3), 263–271.

Sukhodolsky, D. G., Scahill, L., Gadow, K. D., Arnold, E., Aman, M. G., McDougle, C. J., McCracken, J. T., Tierney, E., White, S. W., Lecavalier, L., Vitiello, B. (2008). Parent-rated anxiety symptoms in children with pervasive developmental disorders: Frequency and association with core autism symptoms and cognitive functioning. Journal of Abnormal Child Psychology, 36, 117–128.

Szatmari, P., & McConnell, B. (2011). Anxiety and mood disorders in individuals with autism spectrum disorder. In D. G. Amaral, G. Dawson, & D. H. Geschwind (Eds.), Autism spectrum disorders (pp. 330–338). New York: Oxford University Press.

Tsai, L. Y. (2006). Diagnosis and treatment of anxiety disorders in individuals with autism spectrum disorder. In M. G. Baron, J. Groden, G. Groden, & L. P. Lipsitt (Eds.), Stress and coping in autism (pp. 388–440). New York: Oxford University Press.

Weisbrot, D. M., Gadow, K. D., DeVincent, C. J., & Pomeroy, J. (2005). The presentation of anxiety in children with pervasive developmental disorders. Journal of Child and Adolescent Psychopharmacology, 15(3), 477–496.

White, S. W., Oswald, D., Ollendick, T., & Scahill, L. (2009). Anxiety in children and adolescents with autism spectrum disorders. Clinical Psychology Review, 29, 216–229.

White, S. W., Ollendick, T., Albano, A. M., Oswald, D., Johnson, C., Southam-Gerow, M. A., Kim, I., Scahill, L. (2013). Randomized controlled trial: Multimodal anxiety and social skill intervention for adolescents with autism spectrum disorder. Journal of Autism and Developmental Disorders, 43, 382–394.

Wood, J. J., Drahota, A., Sze, K., Har, K., Chiu, A., & Langer, D. A. (2009). Cognitive behavioral therapy for anxiety in children with autism spectrum disorders: A randomized, controlled trial. Journal of Child Psychology and Psychiatry, 53(3), 224–234.

Part IV
Implications and Future Directions

The Evolution of Autism
as a Diagnostic Concept: From
Kanner to *DSM-5*: A commentary

15

Fred R. Volkmar and Brian Reichow

The growth of research in the field, particularly over the past two decades has been remarkable. For example, in the two decades following Kanner's 1943 report there were, on average, about 2.5 scientific papers a *year*. Between 2003 and 2012, well over 10,000 papers were published—i.e., about 1,000 papers per year or 2.5 papers *per day* (Reichow and Volkmar 2011)! This dramatic rise in research productivity reflects greater awareness of the condition and, in particular, its official recognition (first provided in *Diagnostic and Statistical Manual-III* (*DSM-III*); APA 1980). The growth of research has been particularly dramatic over the past decade reflecting, in part, a stability of diagnostic approach and the convergence (in *DSM-IV*, APA 1994) of the American (*DSM*) and international (*International Classification of Disease*, ICD) diagnostic approaches. This convergence, unique in some ways to autism, has also encouraged cross-national collaborations both in research and clinical work and service.

The explosion of interest and knowledge has not been an unmixed blessing. A recent search on one of the standard Internet search engines for "autism" yielded more than 70 million hits. Research on website information has shown a convergence of search engines in their yield of the most popular sites although, unfortunately, a substantial number are either pushing a "cure" or providing questionable information (Reichow et al. 2012). A new study (Reichow et al. 2013) showed that websites that provide references or were from government agencies (e.g., NIMH, CDC) were more likely to be of high quality with reliable information to have a higher quality rating score than websites without references or websites with a .com top-level domain. Happily, good sources of information are increasingly available—including some with a degree of quality control either through peer review or some other such mechanism. Although historically oriented in many respects, the present review does not provide a comprehensive history of autism (please see Chap. 1 for a comprehensive review). Fortunately, some good resources that provide a detailed background are available (e.g., Feinstein 2010; Volkmar et al. 2014). In this chapter, we provide a concise and selective summary of these issues. It is appropriate that we begin with Kanner's initial description of infantile autism.

F. R. Volkmar (✉)
Child Study Center, Yale University, PO Box 207900,
New Haven, CT 06520, USA
e-mail: Fred.Volkmar@yale.edu

B. Reichow
A.J. Pappanikou Center for Excellence in Developmental
Disabilities, University of Connecticut, Storrs,
CT 06269, USA

Kanner's Description of Infantile Autism

Kanner's work remains remarkably accurate and worth review. His approach was ahead of its time in that he "stuck to the facts" and was more phenomenologically oriented than many of his contemporaries who often adopted particular theoretical notions or approaches. In this way, he was anticipating developments more generally in psychiatric diagnosis (e.g., the research diagnostic criteria approach, see Spitzer and Williams 1988).

The first child psychiatrist in the USA, Kanner, an émigré from Nazi Germany, had written the first textbook of Child Psychiatry in 1935. His report, in 1943, of 11 children with an "inborn" disturbance of affective contact (autism) noted two aspects of the condition that Kanner felt were central to the definition—(1) autism—or being cut off from the world of people and (2) an over-engagement in the nonsocial world, e.g., not tolerating change, insisting on routines, or otherwise engaging in a search for sameness. The child's lack of interest in the social world contrasted markedly from his intense interest in the nonsocial world; this has become an area of great research interest—i.e., in understanding what it is about social interaction difficulties that are unique and might lead to an engagement in the nonsocial world (Klin et al. 2003).

Kanner, a careful clinical observer, used developmental data to guide his observations, building upon and citing the work of Arnold Gesell at Yale who had emphasized that typical babies were clearly socially engaged within the first weeks of life (Gesell 1934). We now know that this engagement is typically present from the moment of birth if not before (Klin et al. 2003; Volkmar and Wiesner 2009).

In his report, Kanner noted many of the features still viewed as frequent prominent characteristics of autism spectrum disorder (ASD) in autism (e.g., echolalia, difficulties with pronoun use and idiosyncratic language, unusual responses to the environment, apparently incredible feats of memory, or problem solving). Other aspects of his original description served to mislead early work on the condition. For example, his use of the word "autism" was taken from Bleuler's (1911) use of the term for self-centered thinking in schizophrenia. Given broad views of schizophrenia then widely held, this raised the issue of whether autism was the earliest manifestation of schizophrenia—a question not answered satisfactorily for nearly three decades. Somewhat paradoxically, we now believe that childhood onset schizophrenia is quite rare and certainly much less common than autism (Volkmar and Wiesner 2009).

Some other aspects of his original report were also misleading. For example, his original impression of normal intellectual levels in autism was based on the observation that certain (nonverbal) abilities were preserved and, although children did poorly on other parts of IQ tests, the presumption was that if they did as well on the rest of the test they would have normal IQ. It took several decades to realize that unusual patterns of ability, often with great scatter, were present and that many children did function in the intellectual disability range if overall scores were examined (Goldstein et al. 2009).

Kanner was also careful to note that other medical conditions or syndromes were not obviously present and that the children appeared to be physically normal (e.g., in contrast to Trisomy 21). Over time, it became clear that was not the case and that as many as 20% of children would go on to develop seizures while in a smaller proportion of cases there were associations with genetic conditions like fragile X and tuberous sclerosis (Rutter et al. 1994). Finally, he noted that in his original cases a parent was, in 10 of 11 cases, remarkably successful. This led to an impression that autism was strongly related to educational and social status and, in part, lent to an impression that parental factors might be involved in syndrome pathogenesis. As a result, in the 1950s, parents were referred for psychotherapy along with their child—traumatizing a generation of parents who felt responsible for their child's difficulties. We now know that autism is seen in all social classes and that factors that bias case detection (e.g., greater parent education and sophisticate) may skew the demographics of clinic samples (Wing 1980). At the same time, children with autism in lower-income families may be less likely to receive a diagnosis (Mandell et al. 2002). Much of the work done on autism in the 1950s and 1960s is difficult to understand given the ambiguities of diagnosis and the various confusions about it. During the 1970s, a body of work began to emerge that clarified these issues and led to the official recognition of autism in *DSM-III* in 1980.

Before turning our attention to *DSM-III*, it is reasonable to ask were there cases of autism before Kanner. The short answer is that of course there must have been, but if so how were they viewed?

Although children with intellectual impairment had been known since antiquity, it was only with the enlightenment and a focus on providing an educated citizenry and electorate that broader interest in child development and education began to increase (Hunt 1961). This also corresponded, roughly, with a gradual decrease in infant mortality. Reports began to appear of "wild" or so-called feral (reared by animals) children. These reports (Candland 1995) may have in fact been the first recorded cases of autism. For example, the description of Victor the "wild boy" described by Itard (Wolff 2004) includes many features suggestive of autism. By the mid-1800s, the great British psychiatrist Maudsley noted that he felt children were not immune (as had been believed previously) to insanity and that, like adults, they could have severe psychiatric illness. The description of dementia praecox (or what now would be recognized as schizophrenia in young adults) was quickly followed by a description of the condition, dementia praecossisima, in children (de Sanctis 1906) setting the stage for much of the early confusion about autism. At around this time, other clinicians (e.g., Heller 1908) also described children with unusual patterns of development and behavior (Heller's concept known as childhood disintegrative disorder was included in *DSM-IV*).

DSM-III and the Official Recognition of Autism

Several lines of work in the 1970s began to suggest that autism was a unique and distinctive condition. For example, the work of Kolvin (1972) and Rutter (1972) suggested that childhood

schizophrenia differed from autism in many ways including onset, clinical features, and family history. As children with autism were followed over time, it became apparent that they were at risk for developing recurrent seizures (Volkmar and Nelson 1990) and in the late 1970s the first studies of twins (Folstein and Rutter 1978) suggested a strong genetic basis for the condition. Other work (Rutter and Bartak 1973) also suggested the importance of recognizing autism relative to the provision of structured special educational and behavioral interventions rather than the psychotherapy that was favored in the 1950s and 1960s. Rimland's highly influential book on autism (Rimland 1964) also focused on neurobiological mechanisms and provided an initial, if now seen as somewhat dated, instrument to help objectively make the diagnosis. It began an entire body of work which has now come to include screening instruments (for infants and older individuals), diagnostic instruments (parent or teacher interviews and direct observational procedures), and measures of severity that might be followed in a study of intervention (see Volkmar and Wiesner 2009).

By the late 1970s, several important developments impacted the recognition of autism in *DSM-III*. For autism in particular several approaches to updating Kanner's "definition" into a more formal set of diagnostic guidelines were completed. For example, Rutter (1978) provided a definition that profoundly influenced *DSM-III*. Rutter's approach extended Kanner's description by noting three areas of difficulties that must be present from early in life: social difficulties (not just due to intellectual delay), language problems (also not just due to cognitive problems), and unusual behaviors consistent with Kanner's notion of "resistance to change/insistence on sameness." As with Kanner's original description, this approach "stuck to the facts," was theoretical, and phenomenological in nature. At the same time another approach, the National Society for Autistic Children (NSAC) definition (NSAC 1978) emphasized other aspects of the condition that were slightly harder to conceptualize and/or that relied heavily on parental report (e.g., unusual rates or sequences of development, hyper/hyposensitivity to the environment). For child psychiatry, the development of multiracial approaches to diagnosis also attracted interest and for general psychiatry the development of the Research Diagnostic Criteria approach at Washington University in St. Louis (Spitzer et al. 1978) had a major impact.

The growing body of research led to a decision to include autism (as "infantile autism") in the landmark 3rd edition of the *DSM* (*DSM-III*; APA 1980). A new term, "pervasive developmental disorder" (PDD), was also coined to denote the class of disorder to which autism was assigned. The definition of autism provided was indeed more of the "infantile form" (e.g., with "pervasive lack" of social interest). Given that many older individuals would not meet such a criteria, a category for "residual infantile autism" was included as well as a poorly described (but well operationalized) condition of childhood onset PDD (COPDD) and its "residual" counterpart (the latter two conditions reflected an awareness that children rarely developed autism after 30 months of age).

Clearly, the inclusion of autism as a diagnostic category was a major advance. On the other hand, some parts of the approach were clearly problematic. The "residual" idea seemed to minimize the many difficulties older children, adolescents, and adults exhibited (i.e., the difficulties were different but in no way "residual"). Also, the lack of a developmental orientation was problematic as with the overall "monothetic" approach (i.e., all criteria had to be present); this left little flexibility to clinicians (see Volkmar and Klin 2005). Accordingly, changes were planned for the revision of *DSM-III* for which planning quickly began.

DSM-III-R

Work on a revision of *DSM-III* began shortly after it appeared. Although initially started as just minor revisions, the scope of the project quickly expanded into a major redo—in part to address problems arising with *DSM-III*. Major changes were introduced for autism as it evolved from "infantile autism" to "autistic disorder" (Siegel et al. 1989; Spitzer and Siegel 1990; Waterhouse

et al. 1993). As may now be true again with *DSM-5,* a rapid change posed some challenges for clinicians and researchers alike.

The definition of autistic disorder in *DSM-III-R* was strongly influenced by the somewhat broader views of Lorna Wing on the diagnosis of autism (Wing and Gould 1979). Consistent with *DSM-III,* the three major domains of dysfunction were included, with specific criteria provided for each domain: qualitative impairment in reciprocal social interaction, qualitative impairment in verbal and nonverbal communication and in imagination, and restricted repertoire of activities and interests. The criteria were more developmentally oriented and detailed and, in some cases, included practical examples.

The final *DSM-III-R* definition rested on a national field trial (Spitzer and Siegel 1990) and, in its final version, 16 criteria for autistic disorder were grouped into three broad categories. Several problems with this field trial were evident. Cases could be rated based on chart review (i.e., rather than current exam) and the comparison group included cases that were essentially wildly inappropriate (conduct disorder cases). A diagnosis of autism required that an individual, regardless of age (child or adult), had to exhibit at least eight of the 16 criteria. These criteria had to include two symptoms from the social domain and one each from the communication and restricted activities categories. In *DSM III-R,* the onset by 30 months was dropped as an essential feature; however, the diagnostician could specify onset before or after age 3 years. Essentially, the various changes in the definition meant that the diagnosis of autism could be made on the basis of current exam only (i.e., knowledge of early history was not required).

Several of the *DSM-III-R* changes were positive. These changes included attention to an awareness of the broader range of expression as well as to changes expressed over age and developmental level (Volkmar et al. 1992a). Given the stronger emphasis on developmental factors and the more flexible, polythetic, diagnostic approach of the *DSM-III,* the concept of "residual autism" was dropped. The name change—infantile autism to autistic disorder—rightly emphasized the persistence of the condition.

Other changes included dropping the older COPDD category although this then left the (rare) child who developed autism after age 3 in a diagnostic limbo. The *DSM-III* "atypical" (i.e., subthreshold) categories were changed to "not otherwise specified," because, in part, this reflected an awareness of the earlier history of atypical personality development as a diagnostic concept (Rank 1949).

In some ways, *DSM III-R* was a conceptual advance over *DSM-III*. The description itself was more detailed and developmentally oriented (Volkmar et al. 1992a). However, it expanded the concept and included more cases as autistic than either the *DSM-III* or most experienced clinicians likely would (Factor et al. 1989; Hertzig et al. 1990; Volkmar et al. 1992a, b). The rate of "false positive" cases (using clinician judgment as the standard) was nearly 40 % (see Rutter and Schopler 1992; Spitzer and Siegel 1990 for a discussion of some of these issues).

Other problems were identified. Given the focus on a broader spectrum (over age and developmental level), it was clear that the diagnostic criteria set was more complex and detailed, thus requiring more from the diagnostician. Although understandable in some ways, the inclusion of specific examples within the actual criteria was problematic in that it tended to reify the examples rather than the broader criterion concept. Elimination of age of onset was a source of controversy. A final complication was the apparent major difference with the pending approach to classification of autism and similar conditions in the 10th edition of the *ICD* (*ICD-10*; WHO 1990). In essence, it appeared that *DSM-III-R* markedly over diagnosed autism relative to the draft *ICD-10* definition (Volkmar et al. 1992b)

DSM-IV and ICD-10

Concerns about *DSM-III-R* and awareness of the pending major changes presented in *the ICD-10* prompted the move towards a major revision of *DSM*. Although the international (*ICD*) and American (*DSM*) systems are fundamentally related and must share diagnostic coding, there

are, however, some major differences between the systems. *DSM* has traditionally been used for both clinical work and research, whereas *ICD-10* had one set of research diagnostic criteria and an entirely different set of clinical descriptions. Other differences exist as well (e.g., relative to an emphasis on history vs. current examination and approaches to comorbidity; Volkmar et al. 2002). The provision of research definitions meant that *ICD-10* could be much more detailed than would like be the case for *DSM-IV*. Another potential difference was the provisional decision to include additional disorders within the PDDs. As a result, there was clearly potential for major differences in the *ICD* and *DSM* approaches to autism that would presumably complicate both research and clinical work. Early studies of the *ICD-10* system for autism (e.g., Volkmar et al. 1992b) suggested that it did not correspond well with *DSM-III-R* but did with *DSM-III* (in the "lifetime" sense of infantile autism) and with diagnoses of experienced clinicians.

Substantial groundwork was done as part of the *DSM-IV* process. Work groups were charged with reviewing the existing research and identifying areas of both consensus and controversy. Issues of clinical utility, reliability, and descriptive validity of categories and criteria were considered. Changes from *DSM-III-R* had to be well justified and given due consideration given to potential differences in *ICD-10* (Volkmar et al. 2002).

A series of literature reviews were commissioned for each of the potential diagnostic categories. These reviews focused on aspects of diagnostic validity, definition, and noted areas where research was lacking. For autism, the reviews were published well before *DSM-IV* appeared (*Journal of Autism and Developmental Disorders,* December, 1992 issue). It was noted that the absence of "official" or other generally agreed upon definitions for Asperger's syndrome had contributed to markedly different uses of the term in clinical and research work (Sharma et al. 2012; Szatmari 1991). With Rett's syndrome, the issues had less to do with the validity of the diagnostic concept itself and more to do with whether it was best included as a PDD (otherwise it would not have been included at all; Gillberg 1994; Rutter 1994; Tsai 1992). At that time, the consensus was that additional categories might well be included in the PDD category in *DSM-IV* and there was general agreement that, for autism, there be substantive compatibility of *DSM-IV* and ICD-10 (Rutter and Schopler 1992).

A number of data reanalyses were undertaken to address issues related to the definition of autism. These reanalyses generally suggested that the *DSM-III-R* definition of autistic disorder was overly broad (Volkmar et al. 1992b) although also clearly more developmentally oriented than its predecessor (Volkmar et al. 1992b). Issues identified for *DSM-IV* included the nature of discrepancies between *DSM-III-R* and other approaches, how to provide a developmentally oriented approach without sacrificing specificity, the need to include history (e.g., early onset) as an essential feature, patterns of similarity and difference with *ICD-10*, and justification for including other conditions in the PDD class. Given the large number of issues, a field trial was undertaken to see how well current, and potential new, criteria actually worked in clinical and research settings.

The *DSM-IV* field trial for autism (Volkmar et al. 1994) was undertaken in collaboration with *ICD-10* with a goal, if possible, of having, diagnostic convergence across nosologies for autism. The field trial included 21 sites, and 125 raters participated from the USA and around the world who provided ratings of nearly 1000 cases. Raters had a range of experience in the diagnosis of autism and various professional backgrounds. Nearly half reported that they had evaluated more than 25 patients with autism; other raters were less experienced, providing an opportunity to assess possible moderators of both rater and item reliability (Klin et al. 2000). Most cases were rated based on current examination although in some cases (for low-frequency disorders) case records were used. To be included, a case had to present features that would suggest autism as a reasonable part of the differential diagnosis (i.e., unlike the *DSM-III-R* field trial where conduct disorder cases were part of the comparison group).

Typically, multiple sources of information were available to the raters who judged the equality of the information to be excellent or good in about 75 % of cases. A standard system of coding was created and included basic information on the individual and rater as well as the rater's clinical diagnosis and explicit ratings of *DSM-III, DSM III-R, ICD-10,* and potential new *DSM-IV* diagnostic criteria. The coding form also provided criteria for Asperger's syndrome, Rett's syndrome, and childhood disintegrative disorder, based on the draft *ICD-10* definitions (Klin et al. 2000).

The results of this extensive trial can be briefly summarized. The *DSM-III* diagnoses of infantile autism and residual autism (taken together) had a reasonable balance of sensitivity and specificity although clearly residual autism was problematic. *DSM-III-R* criteria had a higher sensitivity but lower specificity and a relatively high rate of false positive cases; this was particularly true in individuals with significant intellectual disability where the false positive rate reached 60 % (Volkmar et al. 1994). As expected, the *ICD-10* research definition had higher specificity. Consistent with Kanner's report and subsequent work, the onset of autism was noted to be typically within the first 18 months of life and almost invariably by age 3 years.

Inter-rater reliability of individual criteria was assessed using chance-corrected statistics such as kappa and was generally in the good to excellent range. The more detailed *ICD-10* criteria had greater reliability. The experienced evaluators usually had excellent agreement among themselves and were more likely to agree with each other than with less experienced raters. Among the experienced raters, disagreements were more common over "fine-grained" distinctions between autism and other disorders in the PDD class, although even with this disagreement reliability remained good. Less experienced raters had the same pattern, albeit with lower overall levels of reliability. A series of additional analyses were undertaken. For example, signal detection procedures confirmed (consistent with Kanner) that the domain of social difficulties was the single most powerful discriminating feature. Factor analysis yielded several potential solutions underlying symptom structures, with the traditional three-category approach (social, communication, and restricted interests) as well as a two- and five-factor solution. In the two-factor solution, social-communication items grouped together while, in the five-factor solution, the restricted interests items formed three different groups. Other analyses looked at temporal diagnostic stability, coverage relative to age and IQ level, and so forth.

Data collected as part of the field trial provided some justification for including conditions other than autism in the PDD class (see Szatmari 1992; Tsai 1992; Volkmar 1992). For example, the series of cases with clinical diagnoses of Asperger's disorder differed both from those with PDD-not otherwise specified (PDD-NOS) and higher functioning autism in significant ways: e.g., Asperger's cases had greater levels of social severity than those with PDD-NOS and had different profiles of cognitive ability as compared to those with autism.

The collaboration with *ICD-10* provided an opportunity for convergence with *DSM-IV*. A number of scenarios were considered. In the end, it appeared that possible, data-based, modifications in the draft *ICD-10* provided a reasonably robust definition also suitable for *DSM-IV*. This definition balanced clinical and research needs, was reasonably concise, and provided reasonable coverage over the range of syndrome expression in autism from early childhood through adulthood.

Dimensional Approaches to Diagnosis

Rimland provided one of the first checklists to use in screening for autism many years ago (Rimland 1964). Over time, a number of instruments have been developed—some for screening and others for purposes of diagnosis (see Lord 2014; Stone et al. 2014, for comprehensive reviews). Some of these focus on infants and younger children, other older individuals, or the more cognitively able. Some instruments are based on parent or teacher reports, others on direct observation. As one might imagine, issues of standardization and development of these instruments are complex as

are issues with intended levels of coverage, relevance to the broader "autism phenotype," and so forth (see Volkmar and Wiesner 2009 for a discussion). As a practical matter, particularly since *DSM-IV* and *ICD-10* were published, there has been a strong movement towards convergence of these instruments with categorical approaches (e.g., the Autism Diagnostic Interview Revised, Lord et al. 1994; and the Autism Diagnostic Observation Schedule, de Bildt et al. 2004). Many of the same challenges exist for dimensional instruments as for categorical ones, the broad range of syndrome expression, age- and IQ-related issues in syndrome expression, the relevance of historical information versus current examination, evaluation of important but low frequency behaviors such as self-injury along with issues of reliability, and so forth (see Lord et al. 2014). Issues of how items are administered and scored can be problematic, not to mention the issue of relevance, or lack thereof, to normative functioning. Not surprisingly, a range of different diagnostic approaches have been undertaken.

The issue of quantifying symptoms has significant research interest in that it might help us improve the validity of subgrouping, particularly if these could be related to biological or other markers in some way. Another major result of the convergence of *ICD-10* and *DSM-IV* has been the ability to use these measures to ensure consistency of diagnostic approaches (e.g., for genetic studies). However, such instruments may be impractical for general clinical use and thus clinicians might opt not to use standardized instruments for diagnosing autism in their practice.

These approaches have had important uses, but also possess limitations. On balance, they have seemed to work the best with school-aged children who have mild to moderate cognitive disability with some spoken language. They become more challenging, on balance, as one moves to individuals with greater cognitive impairment or individuals with gifted levels of cognition and to older and younger ages. Screening instruments (see Barton et al. 2012; Stone et al. In press) have a different set of concerns. Given the overall decision in *DSM-5* to rely heavily on data from such instruments (i.e., rather than field trials as in *DSM-IV*), they have assumed a major role in development of the new *DSM-5* approach to diagnosis.

DSM-5

The most recent revision of *DSM* (*DSM-5*, APA 2013) has just appeared. This new version of the manual sought to address a number of concerns with the prior DSM including the many advances made in our understanding of disorders in the two decades since *DSM-IV* appeared (APA 1994; see Rutter 2011). Several important overarching decisions clearly impacted the final product. These included the decision to eliminate all subthreshold categories and the plan to use diagnostic instruments rather than data reanalyses or true field trials as a major source of information for diagnostic criteria (see Regier et al. 2010). In comparison to its various predecessors, the *DSM-5* autism definition aroused much controversy before it even officially appeared (Baron-Cohen 2009; Carey 2012; Ritvo 2012; Singer 2012, Wing et al. 2011).

For autism, a decision was made to change both the overall approach conceptually with a move to a single overarching category of "ASD" and to use a rather different set of diagnostic criteria (Lord and Jones 2012). The *DSM-IV* model of distinct PDD (i.e., autistic disorder, Asperger's disorder, childhood disintegrative disorder, and PDD-NOS) was replaced by an overarching category of ASD. Rett's disorder is included in *DSM-5* as a specifier for ASD rather than a distinctive category (e.g., a child who meets diagnostic criteria for ASD and has Rett's disorder would be indicated as a child with ASD with associated Rett syndrome). More importantly, the traditional (since Rutter 1978) triadic symptom grouping of social, communication, and restrictive and repetitive features has been collapsed into a dyad with social-communication features and restricted interests features; this decision, based on factor analytic work on Autism Diagnostic Interview/ Autism Diagnostic Observation Schedule (ADI/ ADOS) data (Huerta et al. 2012) has some important practical implications.

For example, it greatly reduced the number of criteria combinations that can produce a diagnosis from more than 2000 in *DSM-IV* to 11 in *DSM-5*. Factor analysis is, of course, always somewhat complicated to interpret given the inherent difficulties introduced by any constraints chosen for the analysis—not to mention what is entered in the first place (Gould 1996); other factor analytic approaches have found the traditional three factors as well as other solutions (Sipes and Matson In press). As mentioned earlier, the factor analysis of the *DSM-IV* field trial data yielded either three-, two-, or five-factor solutions (in the five-factor solution, the "restricted interests" items formed three different factors). As a practical matter, the return, in part, to the monothetic approach last employed in *DSM-III* (1980) does intrinsically pose some obstacles for flexible diagnosis. Similarly, the new approach also increases the number of restricted interests/repetitive behaviors that have to be met, increasing from one of four for DSM-IV autistic disorder to two of four for DSM-5 ASD—likely tending to "pull" for individuals with greater cognitive difficulty given the strong association of such behaviors with intellectual disability (Burbidge et al. 2010). The new criterion of hyper- or hyporeactivity had been evaluated in *DSM-IV* and found to be unsatisfactory given its strong association with intellectual disability (Volkmar et al. 1994). One additional change is the explicit note that criteria can be rated on either current behavior or past history (in *DSM-IV,* previously the emphasis was generally on current functioning but with problems of early onset); this presumably reflects the use of both parent report and observational diagnostic instruments used to generate criteria (although as noted below, there is strong suggestion that BOTH need to be used for the best results). It should also be noted that *DSM-5* introduces a "grandfathering" clause suggesting that previous *DSM-IV* diagnoses of autistic disorder, Asperger's disorder, or PDD-NOS should continue to apply in *DSM-5* (i.e., regardless of the actual changes in criteria or current symptom presentation). Although undoubtedly well intentioned, this becomes highly problematic since, if it is honored in practice, we will now have two different groups of individuals with ASD diagnoses. *DSM-5* also provides specifiers relative to functional severity level (i.e., requiring support, requiring substantial support, and requiring very substantial support). These also can be used in relation to intellectual disability, language impairment, as well as associations with other conditions (e.g., other neurodevelopmental, behavioral, genetic, or medical conditions), including a specific mention of catatonia.

Difficulties with *DSM-5* conceptually came from several decisions made early in the *DSM-5* process. For autism, the overarching decision is to eliminate sources. Eliminating subthreshold categories and an almost exclusive reliance on data from research instruments (rather than a field trial) has resulted in changes that effectively increase the stringency of the ASD diagnosis; put another way, the "spectrum" becomes, in essence, something more like autism as first conceptualized in *DSM-III* or as first described by Kanner in 1943. There will also be important issues both for clinical work and research.

On the clinical side, individuals with very significant social impairment who do not meet criteria for ASD will presumably lose eligibility for services (the somewhat backhanded acknowledgement of this in *DSM-5* may or may not eliminate this problem but certainly will not for the future). Individuals with Asperger's disorder have significantly impaired social skills that merit intervention (Baron-Cohen 2009; Ghaziuddin 2010; Kaland 2011) and although the merits of this category and its connection to (or identity with) high-functioning autism have been debated (Lord et al. 2012; Sharma et al. 2012), studies using reasonably stringent criteria do suggest significant differences, for example, in neuropsychological profile (Klin et al. 1996; Mayes et al. 2001; Ozonoff and Griffith 2000) and family history (DeLong and Dwyer 1988; Ghaziuddin 2005; Gillberg 1991; Klin et al. 2005). Thus, even for individuals who currently have the diagnosis (and presumably may not lose it if "grandfathered in") the broader ASD label has potential for important clinical differences that may have important treatment implications. The new social

(pragmatic) communication disorder (SCD) remains confusing in that its relation to ASD is unclear and as proposed the concept seems to have a rather considerable overlap with PDD-NOS and maybe Asperger's syndrome. In *DSM-5,* it appears that SCD is ASD without restricted and repetitive behaviors (one cannot have any such symptoms to receive a diagnosis of SCD). This does leave a gap, however, of children presenting with all of the social criteria of ASD and only one repetitive and restricted behavior; they would not qualify for ASD or SCD. Further confusion lies in that although ASD must be ruled out to receive a diagnosis of SCD, it has been lumped with ASD in prevalence estimates of ASD in the *DSM-5* field trial reports to show ASD prevalence was equal across *DSM-IV* and *DSM-5* (Regier et al. 2012). It remains unclear whether the *ICD* will adopt a similar model; in *DSM-5,* the actual code number of SCD is one consistent with a communication disorder.

The move away from Rutter's (1978) triad of difficulties (social difficulties, communication problems, resistance to change) to a two-cluster groupings (social-communication, restrictive behaviors) model is justified based on results of a factor analysis (Huerta et al. 2012). Of course, one of the problems with factor analysis is that the results are dependent on the data entered in the first place and also on the constraints used to guide the analysis. For example, in *DSM-IV* a factor analysis of all the potential criteria showed that three-, two-, or five-factor solutions could be derived (in the five-factor approach, the resistance to change criteria split into three subgroups).

One, probably unintended, result of this move to a "two-factor" model is there is less flexibility than in *DSM-IV* for clinicians to combine diagnoses. Put another way, there are now many fewer (11) ways to combine criteria to achieve ASD while in *DSM-IV* the situation was very different (more than 2000 combinations at the minimum of six of 12 criteria). By design in *DSM-IV,* social factors were more heavily weighted since other analyses confirmed their centrality to the definition of autism (e.g., signal detection analysis, Siegel et al. 1989; Volkmar et al. 1994). Yet another practical problem is returning, for the social-communication criteria, to a monothetic approach—the same model employed in *DSM-III* (i.e., all criteria must be present). Again, this speaks to a lack of diagnostic flexibility. As noted above, this lack of flexibility is seen in several groups—including the higher-functioning cases as well as in toddlers (the latter is somewhat paradoxical since a stated concern with *DSM-IV* was its failure to adequately capture toddlers' difficulties!).

Although *DSM-5* has literally just appeared, a number of studies have already focused on the new approach to autism. Consistent with the *DSM-5* emphasis on the use of diagnostic instruments a large body of data were used including siblings (some with and others without ASD). In this sample of 2- to 18-year-olds, Frazier et al. (2012) suggest that the sensitivity of *DSM-5* was higher than *DSM-IV* although with slightly lower specificity, which they noted could be improved by relaxing diagnostic threshold. The major study used to evaluate the proposed change used a large data set of extremely well-characterized individuals with ADI-revised (ADI-R) and ADOS results (Huerta et al. 2012); if both instruments were available to use in generating diagnosis, the authors suggested that only a few cases diagnosed under *DSM-IV* would not meet new *DSM-5* criteria. Unfortunately, specificity fell if only one instrument was available and as the authors rightly noted this large data analysis (the major support of the new approach) was not a field trial. In this study, results were obtained in research settings and as Tsai (2012) noted the actual sensitivity and specificity in "real-world" settings remain unclear.

A number of other studies have already appeared and questioned aspects of the *DSM-5* approach. Mazefsky et al. (2012), in a study comparing *DSM-IV* and *DSM-5* using the ADOS and ADI-R, found minimal differences between *DSM-IV* and *5* if BOTH instruments were used, but a lower sensitivity if only parent report were available, and even lower if only the ADOS was available. In a study of reliability of the new diagnostic criteria (Regier et al. 2012), there was

good sensitivity but questionable specificity (although see Frances 2012; Jones 2012 for other views of this study); in addition, only a small number of cases of ASD were actually seen so that, as Tsai has pointed out (Tsai 2012), the actual sensitivity and specificity remain unclear.

Mattila et al. (2011) studied an epidemiological sample of 8-year-olds in Finland and found *DSM-5* to be less sensitive than *DSM-IV* particularly for the higher IQ cases. Similarly, and using a subsequent iteration of the *DSM-5* criteria, McPartland et al. (2012) reanalyzed data from the *DSM-IV* field trial (Volkmar et al. 1994) "cross-walking" the many criteria evaluated in the field trial to the new *DSM-5* criteria. Specificity of *DSM-5* was high but sensitivity varied dramatically by clinical group. For autism, this was at acceptable levels but was very poor for both Asperger's disorder and PDD-NOS. Furthermore, McPartland et al. found moderate levels of sensitivity for individuals with IQ < 70 and poor levels of sensitivity for individuals with IQ ≥ 70.

Similarly, Worley and Matson (2012) reported on a large sample of cases and found children who met *DSM-IV* but not *DSM-5* criteria. In a subsequent study focused on toddlers, they found similar results (Matson et al. 2012). A similar result has been noted by Barton et al. (2013) raising serious concerns about the applicability of *DSM-5* in both higher functioning cases and toddlers.

Difficulties in the use of the new criteria for cases of children who had received previous *DSM-IV* diagnoses of PDD-NOS have been noted by Gibbs et al. (2012) as well as Taheri and Perry (2012). In another study of adults who were more cognitively able, Wilson et al. (In press) compared *DSM-IV, ICD-10,* and *DSM-5* in a large sample of adults. In their study, they also addressed the issue of what proportion of cases might fail *DSM-5* for ASD but achieve a diagnosis of SCD. In their sample, more than half of the cases with an *ICD-10* PDD diagnosis also met *DSM-5* criteria for ASD. Nearly 20 % of those not meeting criteria for ASD would meet *DSM-5* criteria for SCD. Several of the studies just mentioned had addressed potential "fixes" for *DSM-5* (mostly in terms of adjustment of scoring rules).

Summary and Issues for the Future

From a researcher's point of view, all of these studies highlight the potential for significant change in the composition of research samples. Some ongoing research projects may face significant challenges in this regard. Clearly, epidemiological work and similar work with significance for program planning may be impacted. From the research side, it would appear that we will now be in the position (as in the 1970s) of having a number of different diagnostic approaches in operation—i.e., *DSM-IV/ICD-10*, new *DSM-5* cases, *DSM-5* cases "grandfathered in," and *ICD-11* (presuming it is different from any of the previously mentioned criteria that are currently in practice). This appears to be most unfortunate with negative implications for a range of studies: epidemiological studies may be disrupted, samples from longitudinal studies might be affected, and comparisons across multiple studies at different time points combined in meta-analyses might be difficult to interpret. This is of great concern given how the field has increased its research and moved closer to identifying biomarkers and underlying etiologies of the distinctive disorders, like has been done for the genetic cause of Rett's syndrome. Finally, some studies have suggested that a small percentage of individuals no longer meet diagnostic criteria later in life. With the "grandfather clause," it is unclear how this research will be impacted (taken literally, no one with a *DSM-IV* diagnosis of autistic disorder, Asperger's disorder, or PDD-NOS would receive the ASD diagnosis), which is unfortunate given these are best outcome cases and learning how this best outcome was achieved could greatly advance treatment for all individuals with autism.

The changes in *DSM-5* also present great challenges for practice. It is still not known how the diagnostic criteria will be used in practice. Moreover, the two "gold standard" diagnostic tools, the ADOS and ADI-R will need to be modified to match the new criteria (this has already been done for the ADOS, which is now in its second edition, the ADOS-2; see Lord et al. 2014). Changing these tools and others will require re-training clinicians on the new instruments, not to mention the new criteria. It is also unclear how school systems will be impacted by the changes; although the *DSM* is not meant to be directly tied to education eligibility in the USA, some states use the *DSM* definition verbatim for eligibility criteria and most other states have criteria that are closely related. Further complicating the issues in education would be what, if any, services a child with SCD might be entitled to.

In essence, it appears that if taken at face value without the special "grandfathering" rule, the spectrum in ASD as defined in *DSM-5* is rather a misnomer, in some ways it seems much closer to the narrower view of "classic" autism as first described by Kanner (i.e., with lower-functioning individuals).

References

American Psychiatric Association. (1980). *Diagnostic and statitical manual of mental disorders* (3rd ed.). Washington, DC: American Psychiatric Association.

American Psychiatric Association. (1987). *Diagnostic and statitical manual of mental disorders* (3rd revised ed.). Washington, DC: American Psychiatric Association.

American Psychiatric Association. (1994). *Diagnostic and statitical manual of mental disorders* (4th ed.). Washington, DC: American Psychiatric Association.

American Psychiatric Association. (2000). *Diagnostic and statitical manual of mental disorders* (4th ed.—text revision). Washington, DC: American Psychiatric Association.

American Psychiatric Association. (2005). *Diagnostic and statitical manual of mental disorders* (5th ed.). Washington, DC: American Psychiatric Association.

American Psychiatric Association. (2013). DSM 5. Washington, DC: American Psychiatric Association.

Baron-Cohen, S. (9 Nov 2009). The short life of a diagnosis. *New York Times*.

Barton, M. L., Dumont-Mathieu, T., & Fein, D. (2012). Screening young children for autism spectrum disorders in primary practice. *Journal of Autism and Developmental Disorders, 42*(6), 1165–1174.

Barton, M. D., Robins, D., Jashar, D., Brennan, L., & Fein, D. (2013). Sensitivity and specificity of proposed DSM-5 criteria for autism spectrum disorder in toddlers. *Journal of Autism and Developmental Disorders, 43*(5),1184–1195.

Bleuler, E. (1911). *Dementia praecox oder Gruppe der Schizophrenien* (trans: J. Zinkin). New York: International Universities Press.

Burbidge, C., Oliver, C., Moss, J., Arron, K., Berg, K., Furniss, F., Hill, L., et al. (2010). The association between repetitive behaviours, impulsivity and hyperactivity in people with intellectual disability. *Journal of intellectual Disability Research, 54*(12), 1078–1092.

Candland, D. C. (1995). *Feral children and cleber animals: Reflections on human nature*. New York: Oxford University Press.

Carey, B. (19 Jan 2012). New denfinition of autism may exclude many, study suggests. *New York Times*.

de Bildt, A., Sytema, S., Ketelaars, C., Kraijer, D., Mulder, E., Volkmar, F., et al. (2004). Interrelationship between Autism Diagnostic Observation Schedule-Generic (ADOS-G), Autism Diagnostic Interview-Revised (ADI-R), and the Diagnostic and Statistical Manual of Mental Disorders (DSM-IV-TR) classification in children and adolescents with mental retardation. *Journal of Autism and Developmental Disorders, 34*(2), 129–137.

de Sanctis, S. (1906). On some variations of dementia praecox. *Revista Sperimentali di Frenciatria, 32,* 141–165.

DeLong, G. R., & Dwyer, J. T. (1988). Correlation of family history with specific autistic subgroups: Asperger's syndrome and bipolar affective disease. *Journal of Autism and Developmental Disorders, 18*(4), 593–600.

Factor, D. C., Freeman, N. L., & Kardash, A. (1989). A comparison of DSM-III and DSM-III-R criteria for autism. Clarke institute of psychiatry conference: Challenge and change in childhood psychopathology (1988, Toronto, Canada). *Journal of Autism and Developmental Disorders, 19*(4), 637–640.

Feinstein, A. (2010). A history of autism conversations with the pioneers. *A history of autism conversations with the pioneers*. Chichester: Wiley Blackwell.

Folstein, S., & Rutter, M. (1978). Genetic influences and infantile autism. *Annual Progress in Child Psychiatry and Child Development, 1978,* 437–441.

Frances, A. (2012). Better safe than sorry. *Australian and New Zealand Journal of Psychiatry, 46*(8), 695–696.

Frazier, T. W., Youngstrom, E. A., Speer, L., Embacher, R., Law, P., Constantino, J., et al. (2012). Validation of proposed DSM-5 criteria for autism spectrum disorder. *Journal of the American Academy of Child and Adolescent Psychiatry, 51*(1), 28–40.e3.

Gesell, A. (1934). *Atlas of infant behavior*. New Haven: Yale University Press.

Ghaziuddin, M. (2005). A family history study of Asperger syndrome. *Journal of Autism and Developmental Disorders, 35*(2), 177–182.

Ghaziuddin, M. (2010). Should the DSM V drop Asperger syndrome? *Journal of Autism and Developmental Disords, 40*(9), 1146–1148.

Gibbs, V., Aldridge, F., Chandler, F., Witzlsperger, E., & Smith, K. (2012). An exploratory study comparing diagnostic outcomes for autism spectrum disorders under DSM-IV-TR with the proposed DSM-5 revision. *Journal of Autism and Developmental Disorders, 42*(8), 1750–1756.

Gillberg, C. (1991). Clinical and neurobiological aspects of Asperger syndrome in six family studies. In U. Frith (Ed.), *Autism and Asperger syndrome* (pp. 122–146). x, 247 pp. Cambridge: Cambridge University Press.

Gillberg, C. (1994). Debate and argument: Having Rett syndrome in the ICD-10 PDD category does not make sense.[comment]. *Journal of Child Psychology, Psychiatry and Allied Disciplines, 35*(2), 377–378.

Goldstein, S., Naglieri, J. A., & Ozonoff, S. (2009). *Assessment of autism spectrum disorders* (pp. xiv, 384). New York: Guilford.

Gould, S. J. (1996) *The mismeasure of man*. NY: Norton.

Heller, T. (1908). Dementia infantilis. *Zeitschrift fur die Erforschung und Behandlung des Jugenlichen, Schwachsinns, 2,* 141–165.

Hertzig, M. E., Snow, M. E., New, E., & Shapiro, T. (1990). DSM-III and DSM-III-R diagnosis of autism and pervasive developmental disorder in nursery school children. *Journal of the American Academy of Child and Adolescent Psychiatry, 29*(1), 123–126.

Huerta, M., Bishop, S. L., Duncan, A., Hus, V., & Lord, C. (2012). Application of DSM-5 criteria for autism spectrum disorder to three samples of children with DSM-IV diagnoses of pervasive developmental disorders. *American Journal of Child Psychiatry, 169*(10), 1056–1064.

Hunt, J. M. (1961). *Intelligence and experience*. New York: Roland.

Jones, K. D. (2012). A critique of the DSM-5 field trials. *Journal of Nervous and Mental Disease, 200*(6), 517–519.

Kaland, N. (2011). Brief report: Should Asperger syndrome be excluded from the forthcoming DSM-V? *Research in Autism Spectrum Disorders, 5*(3), 984–989.

Kanner, L. (1943). Autistic disturbances of affective contact. *Nervous Child, 2,* 217–250.

Klin, A., Volkmar, F. R., Sparrow, S. S., Cicchetti, D. V., & Rourke, B. P. (1996). Validity and neuropsychological characterization of asperger syndrome: Convergence with nonverbal learning disabilities syndrome. *Annual Progress in Child Psychiatry & Child Development,* 241–259.

Klin, A., Lang, J., Cicchetti, D. V., & Volkmar, F. R. (2000). Brief report: Interrater reliability of clinical diagnosis and DSM-IV criteria for autistic disorder: results of the DSM-IV autism field trial. *Journal of Autism and Developmental Disorders, 30*(2), 163–167.

Klin, A., Jones, W., Schultz, R., & Volkmar, F. (2003). The enactive mind, or from actions to cognition: lessons from autism. *Philosophical Transactions of the Royal Society of London-Series B: Biological Sciences, 358*(1430), 345–360.

Klin, A., Pauls, D., Schultz, R., & Volkmar, F.R. (2005). Three diagnostic approaches to asperger syndrome: Implications for research. *Journal of Autism and Developmental Disorders, 35*(2), 221–234.

Kolvin, I. (1972). Infantile autism or infantile psychoses. *British Medical Journal, 3*(829), 753–755.

Lord, C., & Jones, R. M. (2012). Annual research review: Re-thinking the classification of autism spectrum disorders. *Journal of Child Psychology and Psychiatry, 53*(5), 490–509.

Lord, C., Corsello, C., & Grzadzinski, R. (2014). Diagnostic Instruments in autistic spectrum disorders. Children. In F. Volkmar, R. Paul, K. Pelphrey, & S. Rogers (Eds.), *Handbook of autism* (4th ed., Vol. 2, pp. 609–660). Hoboken: Wiley.

Lord, C., Rutter, M., DiLavore, P. C., & Risi, S. (2000). Autism diagnostic observation schedule: ADOS. Torrance, CA: Western Psychological Services.

Lord, C., Rutter, M., & Le Couteur, A. (1994). Autism diagnostic interview-revised: A revised version of a diagnostic interview for caregivers of individuals with possible pervasive developmental disorders. *Journal of Autism and Developmental Disorders, 24*(5), 659–685.

Lord, C., Petkova, E., Hus, V., Gan, W., Lu, F., Martin, D. M., & Risi, S. (2012). A multisite study of the clinical diagnosis of different autism spectrum disorders. *Archives of General Psychiatry, 69*(3), 306–313.

Mandell, D. S., Listerud, J., Levy, S. E., & Pinto-Martin, J. A. (2002). Race differences in the age at diagnosis among Medicaid-eligible children with autism. *Journal of the American Academy of Child and Adolescent Psychiatry, 41*(12), 1447–1453.

Matson, J. L., Hattier, M. A., & Williams, L. W. (2012). How does relaxing the algorithm for autism affect DSM-V prevalence rates? *Journal of Autism and Developmental Disorders, 42*(8), 1549–1556.

Mattila, M. L., Kielinen, M., Linna, S. L., Jussila, K., Ebeling, H., Bloigu, R., et al. (2011). Autism spectrum disorders according to DSM-IV-TR and comparison with DSM-5 draft criteria: An epidemiological study. *Journal of the American Academy of Child and Adolescent Psychiatry, 50*(6), 583–592.e11.

Mayes, S. D., Calhoun, S. L., & Crites, D. L. (2001). Does DSM-IV Asperger's disorder exist? *Journal of Abnormal Child Psychology, 29*(3), 263–271.

Mazefsky, C. A., McPartland, J. C., Gastgeb, H. Z., & Minshew, N. J. (2012). Brief report: Comparability of DSM-IV and DSM-5 ASD research samples. *Journal of Autism and Developmental Disorders, 42*(5), 1236–1242.

McPartland, J. C., Reichow, B., & Volkmar, F. R. (2012). Sensitivity and specificity of proposed DSM-5 diagnostic criteria for autism spectrum disorder. *Journal of the American Academy of Child and Adolescent Psychiatry, 51*(4), 368–383.

NSAC. (1978). National Society for Autistic Children definition of the syndrome of autism. *Journal of Autism and Childhood Schizophrenia, 8*(2), 162–169.

Ozonoff, S., & Griffith, E. M. (2000). Neuropsychological function and the external validity of Asperger syndrome. In: A. Klin, & F. R. Volkmar (Eds.), *Asperger syndrome* (pp. 72–96). New York: Guilford.

Rank, B. (1949). Adaptation of the psychoanalytic technique for the treatment of young children with atypical development. *American Journal of Orthopsychiatry, 19,* 130–139. (American Psychological Assn/Educational Publishing Foundation, US).

Regier, D. A., Narrow, W. E., Kuhl, E. A., & Kupfer, D. J. (2010). *The conceptual evolution of DSM-5.* Arlington: American Psychiatric Publishing.

Regier, D. A., Narrow, W. E., Clarke, D. E., Kraemer, H. C., Kuramoto, S. J., Kuhl, E. A., & Kupfer, D. J. (2012). DSM-5 field trials in the United States and Canada, Part II: Test-retest reliability of selected categorical diagnoses. *American Journal of Psychiatry, 168,* 1122–1122.

Reichow, B., & Volkmar, F. R. (2011). Introduction to evidence-based practices in autism: Where we started. In B. Reichow, P. Doehring, D. V. Cicchetti, & F. R. Volkmar (Eds.), *Evidence-based practices and treatments for children with autism* (pp. 3–24). New York: Springer.

Reichow, B., Halpern, J., Steinhoff, T., Letsinger, N., Naples, A., & Volkmar, F. R. (2012). Characteristics and quality of autism websites. *Journal of Autism and Developmental Disorders, 42*(6), 1263–1274.

Reichow, B., Shefcyk, A., & Bruder, M. B. (2013). Quality comparison of websites related to developmental disabilities. *Research in Developmental Disabilities, 34,* 3077–3083.

Rimland, B. (1964). *Infantile autism: The syndrome and its implications for a neural theory of behavior.* New York: Appleton-Century-Crofts.

Ritvo, E. R. (2012). Postponing the proposed changes in DSM 5 for autistic spectrum disorder until new scientific evidence adequately supports them. *Journal of Autism and Developmental Disorders, 42*(9), 2021–2022.

Rutter, M. (1972). Childhood schizophrenia reconsidered. *Journal of Autism and Childhood Schizophrenia, 2*(4), 315–337.

Rutter, M. (1978). Diagnosis and definitions of childhood autism. *Journal of Autism and Developmental Disorders, 8*(2), 139–161.

Rutter, M. (1994). Debate and argument: There are connections between brain and mind and it is important that Rett syndrome be classified somewhere. *Journal of Child Psychology and Psychiatry and Allied Disciplines, 35*(2), 379–381.

Rutter, M. (2011). Research review: Child psychiatric diagnosis and classification: concepts, findings, challenges and potential. *Journal of Child Psychology & Psychiatry & Allied Disciplines, 52*(6), 647–60.

Rutter, M., & Bartak, L. (1973). Special educational treatment of autistic children: A comparative study. II. Follow-up findings and implications for services. *Journal of Child Psychology and Psychiatry and Allied Disciplines, 14*(4), 241–270.

Rutter, M., & Schopler, E. (1992). Classification of pervasive developmental disorders: Some concepts and practical considerations. Special Issue: Classification and diagnosis. *Journal of Autism and Developmental Disorders, 22*(4), 459–482.

Rutter, M., Bailey, A., Bolton, P., & Le Couteur, A. (1994). Autism and known medical conditions: Myth and substance. *Journal of Child Psychology and Psychiatry and Allied Disciplines, 35*(2), 311–322.

Sharma, S., Woolfson, L. M., & Hunter, S. C. (2012). Confusion and inconsistency in diagnosis of Asperger syndrome: A review of studies from 1981 to 2010. *Autism, 16*(5), 465–486.

Siegel, B., Vukicevic, J., Elliott, G. R., & Kraemer, H. C. (1989). The use of signal detection theory to assess DSM-III-R criteria for autistic disorder. *Journal of the American Academy of Child and Adolescent Psychiatry, 28*(4), 542–548.

Singer, E. (2012). Diagnosis: Redefining autism. *Nature, 491,* S12–S13.

Sipes, M., & Matson, J. (In press). Factor structure for autism spectrum disorders with toddlers using DSM-IV and DSM-5 criteria. *Journal of Autism and Developmental Disorders.*

Spitzer, R. L., & Siegel, B. (1990). The DSM-III-R field trial of pervasive developmental disorders. *Journal of the American Academy of Child & Adolescent Psychiatry, 29*(6), 855–862.

Spitzer, R. L., & Williams, J. B. (1988). Having a dream. A research strategy for DSM-IV [see comments]. *Archives of General Psychiatry, 45*(9), 871–874.

Spitzer, R. L., Endicott, J. E., & Robbins, E. (1978). Resarch diagnostic criteria. *Archives of General Psychiatry, 35,* 773–782.

Stone, W., Ibanez L., & Coonrod, E. E. (2014). Screening for autism in young children. In F. Volkmar, R. Paul, K. Pelphrey, & S. Rogers (Eds.), *Handbook of autism* (4th ed., Vol. 2, pp. 585–608). Hoboken: Wiley.

Szatmari, P. (1991). Asperger's syndrome: Diagnosis, treatment, and outcome. *Psychiatric Clinics of North America, 14*(1), 81–93.

Szatmari, P. (1992). The validity of autistic spectrum disorders: A literature review. *Journal of Autism & Developmental Disorders, 22*(4), 583–600.

Taheri, A., & Perry, A. (2012). Exploring the proposed DSM-5 criteria in a clinical sample. *Journal of Autism and Developmental Disorders, 42*(9), 1810–1817.

Tsai, L. (1992). Is rett syndrome a subtype of pervasive developmental disorder? *Journal of Autism and Developmental Disorders, 22,* 551–561.

Tsai, L. Y. (2012). Sensitivity and specificity: DSM-IV versus DSM-5 criteria for Autism spectrum disorder. *American Journal of Psychiatry, 169*(10), 1009–1011. doi:10.1176/appi.ajp.2012.12070922.

Volkmar, F. R. (1992). Childhood disintegrative disorder: Issues for DSM-IV. *Journal of Autism and Developmental Disorders, 22*(4), 625–642.

Volkmar, F. R., & Klin, A. (2005). Issues in the classification of autism and related conditions. In F. R. Volkmar, A. Klin, R. Paul, & D. J. Cohen (Eds.), *Handbook of autism and pervasive developmental disorders* (3rd ed., Vol. 1, pp. 5–41). Hoboken: Wiley.

Volkmar, F. R., & Nelson, D. S. (1990). Seizure disorders in autism. *Journal of the American Academy of Child and Adolescent Psychiatry, 29*(1), 127–129.

Volkmar, F., & Wiesner, L. (2009). *A practical guide to autism.* Hoboken: Wiley.

Volkmar, F. R., Reichow, B., Westphal, A., & Mandell, D. S. (2014). Autism and the autism spectrum: Diagnostic concepts. In F. R. Volkmar, S. Rogers, K. Pelphrey, & R. Paul (Eds.), *Handbook of autism and the pervasive developmental disorders* (4th ed., Vol. 1, pp. 3–27). Hoboken: Wiley.

Volkmar, F. R., Cicchetti, D. V., Bregman, J., & Cohen, D. J. (1992a). Three diagnostic dystems for Autism: DSM-III, DSM-III-R, and ICD-10. Special issue: Classification and diagnosis. *Journal of Autism and Developmental Disorders, 22*(4), 483–492.

Volkmar, F. R., Cicchetti, D. V., Cohen, D. J., & Bregman, J. (1992b). Brief eeport: Developmental aspects of DSM-III-R criteria for Autism. *Journal of Autism and Developmental Disorders, 22*(4), 657–662.

Volkmar, F. R., Klin, A., Siegel, B., Szatmari, P., Lord, C., Campbell, M., et al. (1994). Field trial for autistic disorder in DSM-IV. *American Journal of Psychiatry, 151*(9), 1361–1367.

Volkmar, F. R., Scwab-Stone, M., & First, M. (2002). Classification in child psychiatry: principles and issues. In M. Lewis (Ed.), *Child and adolescent psychiatry: A comprehensive textbook* (3rd ed., pp. 499–506). Baltimore: Williams & Wilkins.

Waterhouse, L., Wing, L., Spitzer, R. L., & Siegel, B. (1993). Diagnosis by DSM-III-R versus ICD-10 criteria. *Journal of Autism & Developmental Disorders, 23*(3), 572–573.

Wilson, C. E., Gillan, N., Spain, D., Robertson, D., Roberts, G., Murphy, C. M., et al. (In press). Comparison of ICD-10R, DSM-IV-TR and DSM-5 in an adult autism spectrum disorder diagnostic clinic. *Journal of Autism and Developmental Disorders.*

Wing, L. (1980). Childhood autism and social class: A question of selection? *British Journal of Psychiatry, 137,* 410–417.

Wing, L., & Gould, J. (1979). Severe impairments of social interaction and associated abnormalities in children: Epidemiology and classification. *Journal of Autism & Developmental Disorders, 9*(1), 11–29.

Wing, L., Gould, J., & Gillberg, C. (2011). Autism spectrum disorders in the DSM-V: Better or worse than the DSM-IV? *Research in Developmental Disabilities, 32,* 768–73.

Wolff, S. (2004). The history of autism. *European Child & Adolescent Psychiatry, 13*(4), 201–208.

World Health Organization. (1993). *The ICD-10 classification of mental and behavioural disorders: Diagnostic criteria for research* (10th ed.). Geneva: World Health Organization.

Worley, J. A., & Matson, J. L. (2012). Comparing symptoms of autism spectrum disorders using the current DSM-IV-TR diagnostic criteria and the proposed DSM-V diagnostic criteria. *Research in Autism Spectrum Disorders, 6*(2), 965–970.

James C. McPartland and Geraldine Dawson

In May 2013, the American Psychiatric Association published the fifth edition of the *Diagnostic and Statistical Manual of Mental Disorders* (*DSM-5*; American Psychiatric Association 2013). Substantive changes were made in the criteria of the *DSM-5* defining many of the psychiatric diagnoses it classifies. Included among these changes were major revisions to the structure and diagnostic criteria for autism and related disorders. With current prevalence estimated to be approximately 1 in 88 (CDC 2012), this class of neurodevelopmental disorders affects numerous children and families; for this reason, the revisions to prior criteria, contained in the *DSM: Fourth Edition—Text Revision* (*DSM-IV-TR*; American Psychiatric Association 2000), have been closely followed not only within the scientific and clinical literature but also by the popular media. In this commentary, we review the *DSM-5* diagnostic criteria, highlighting changes from the *DSM-IV-TR*. We next review several of the strengths of revised criteria. The final section outlines key issues related to implementing *DSM-5* criteria that have garnered discussion, focusing

on both the advantages of this revised approach to diagnosing autism and potential concerns that have been voiced regarding the new system. In closing, we provide our opinions about the future of diagnostic taxonomy for autism and anticipated challenges for both scientists and clinicians moving forward.

DSM-5 Diagnostic Criteria for Autism Spectrum Disorder

The most salient change to the new criteria for autism spectrum disorder (ASD) is a conceptualization of autism and related disorders as a continuum, per se, rather than a group of related but taxonomically distinct diagnoses. In the *DSM-IV-TR,* autism was included in a class of pervasive developmental disorders. This broad class included five different disorders: autistic disorder, Asperger's disorder, pervasive developmental disorder—not otherwise specified (PDD-NOS), Rett syndrome, and childhood disintegrative disorder (CDD). Over time, the first three of these disorders came to be colloquially and commonly recognized as ASD. In the *DSM-5,* this trend is rendered official, with the text describing ASD as the nominal diagnosis, subsuming preexisting subcategories of autistic disorder, Asperger's disorder, PDD-NOS, and CDD. The exclusion of Rett syndrome is described in the differential diagnosis section as based on the existence of only a constrained developmental period in which its clinical phenotype resembles ASD.

J. C. McPartland (✉)
Assistant Professor of Child Psychiatry and Psychology,
Director, Yale Developmental Disabilities Clinic,
Yale Child Study Center, 230 South Frontage Road,
New Haven, CT 06520, USA
e-mail: james.mcpartland@yale.edu

G. Dawson
Duke Center for Autism and Brain Development,
Duke University School of Medicine, Box 3454,
Durham, NC, USA

T. E. Davis III et al. (eds.), *Handbook of Autism and Anxiety,* Autism and Child Psychopathology Series,
DOI 10.1007/978-3-319-06796-4_16, © Springer International Publishing Switzerland 2014

A second major change reflected in the current diagnostic criteria is the collapsing of the traditional "triad of impairments" into two symptom domains. *DSM-IV-TR* grouped clusters of symptoms into three categories, comprised of social interaction, communication, and repetitive and restricted behaviors and interests (RRBs). The *DSM-5* structurally reorganizes symptoms into two domains. The first integrates the first two symptom domains of *DSM-IV-TR's* triad, reflecting enduring problems with social communication *and* social interaction. Within this domain, there are three broad symptom clusters, roughly approximating (1) verbal and nonverbal social–emotional reciprocity; (2) nonverbal communication; and (3) development, maintenance, and comprehension of social relationships. Language delay is now identified as an associated condition rather than a symptom of ASD. The second domain corresponds directly to *DSM-IV-TR's* RRB domain and describes four symptom clusters, corresponding to stereotyped or repetitive language or movement, insistence on sameness, circumscribed or unusual interest, and atypical interest in or reactivity to sensory information. This final symptom represents a meaningful revision to the *DSM-IV-TR* criteria, which did not reference sensory characteristics explicitly. Moreover, for a diagnosis of ASD, two symptoms in the RBB domain rather than one are required.

A potentially influential revision to the diagnostic criteria for ASD is a change from exclusively polythetic criteria to a combination of monothetic and polythetic criteria. *Monothetic* indicates a list of symptoms in which each individual feature must be present for endorsement of the overarching category. A *polythetic* criteria set, in contrast, presents a list of individual features or symptoms from which a subset may be endorsed to reach threshold for the overarching category. In *DSM-IV-TR,* each of the three symptom domains in the triad was polythetic, presenting four individual symptom clusters and requiring a person to meet zero, one, or two symptoms in each domain to qualify for a diagnosis of one of the Pervasive Developmental Disorders (PDDs). The reorganization in *DSM-5* preserves the polythetic structure for RBBs, requiring individuals

to manifest difficulty in two of the four symptom clusters. However, the *DSM-5* restructures the social-communication domain to be monothetic, requiring individuals to manifest a symptom in each cluster for endorsement of this portion of the *DSM-5* "dyad" of impairments. This restructuring entails reducing the number of clusters relating to social-communicative impairment to three (from eight), with these broader symptom descriptions encompassing the breadth of symptoms described across *DSM-IV-TR's* eight clusters. Within both the social and communicative domain and the RBB domain, *DSM-5* permits endorsement of symptom clusters by current presentation or by history.

Three additional features of the *DSM-5* ASD criteria inform context for evaluating the presence of the symptoms described above in terms of chronological development, relative functional level, and cognitive development. It is required that symptoms are present in childhood, although the text acknowledges that problems may not become evident until later in development due to limited developmental expectations (e.g., a verbally proficient child with ASD may not evince obvious social difficulties until school enrollment) and may become less evident in later development due to compensatory strategies. Consistent with *DSM-IV-TR,* the revised criteria clarify that symptoms must result in clinically significant impairment and must be manifest across contexts. The final caveat is that the difficulties experienced by the individual cannot be explained by intellectual disability or global developmental delay alone, i.e., that social and communicative difficulties exceed those predicted based on overall developmental level.

Reflecting a general effort of the *DSM-5* to introduce themes and descriptors that apply across multiple diagnoses, the criteria for ASD introduce a series of specifiers. These diagnostic corollaries provide a mechanism to convey additional relevant information about the current presentation of a person meeting criteria for ASD. A first specifier describes whether a known etiological factor (i.e., medical condition, genetic syndrome, or environmental exposure) is present. The second, a severity specifier, is implemented across diagnostic categories in the *DSM-5*. Severity is specified separately for each domain of symptoms (i.e., social communicative and RBB) and is intended to reflect required level of support and impact on a person's levels of functioning; the severity specifier is not intended to be a proxy for global functioning or severity of comorbid features. Severity levels range from Level 1–3, denoting requirement of support, substantial support, or very substantial support, respectively. It is made explicit that severity specifiers do not correspond directly to qualification for or need for services as they do not account for a person's profile of abilities or an individual hierarchy of intervention objectives. The third specifier indicates whether or not intellectual impairment is present. The fourth specifier indicates whether or not language impairment is present and is to be provided separately for receptive and expressive language along with a concise description of the actual language skills possessed by the individual. The fifth and final specifier is used to indicate whether catatonia is present.

In addition to these changes to the actual criteria for ASD, the *DSM-5* introduces a novel diagnosis relevant to individuals exhibiting social communication symptomatology. Social (pragmatic) communication disorder (SCD) has been included as a communication disorder within the overarching category of neurodevelopmental disorders (in which ASD also lies). This disorder is characterized by problems in the social application of both verbal and nonverbal communication in terms of: using communication socially, adapting communication to match contextual or individual factors, adhering to conventional guidelines for issuing a narrative or conversing, and understanding figurative language and implicit meanings. To qualify for a diagnosis of SCD, these challenges must lead to functional impairment and must not be explained by basic problems with language or other medical or neurological conditions. Consistent with ASD, the criteria specify early developmental onset. SCD is described as distinct from ASD (with ASD as a rule out), representing a separate disorder sharing common phenotypic characteristics with respect to vulnerabilities in pragmatic language.

Although SCD is a type of communication disorder, it is not considered a part of the autism spectrum. Notably, the SCD criteria describe symptoms that would not be expected to be present until approximately 4–5 years of age (or later). As noted in the *DSM-5* manual, diagnosis of SCD in children under age 4 would be rare.

The *DSM-5* criteria for ASD indicate carryover from *DSM-IV-TR* to the revised rubric. In the accompanying text, it is stated that patients with a "well-established" diagnosis of one of the *DSM-IV* ASD qualify for *DSM-5* ASD. It is recommended that individuals with social communication deficits who do not meet *DSM-5* criteria for ASD be evaluated for SCD.

Strengths of *DSM-5*

DSM-5 moves forward from previous criteria by explicitly addressing several factors that are poorly understood in ASD but hold great significance. The *DSM-5* text expounding upon the ASD diagnostic criteria introduces specific considerations related to individual characteristics, such as sex and cultural issues, which are not addressed in *DSM-IV-TR*. *DSM-5* highlights the importance of adaptive functioning and an estimation of actual impact on a person's life by introducing severity specifiers (described previously). *DSM-5* also alters the relationship of comorbidities to ASD by eliminating diagnostic rule outs for other common childhood disorders. Below, we explore these factors in the context of implementing *DSM-5*.

Sex and ASD Diagnosis

ASD is more common in males than females and this skewed sex ratio has remained constant as diagnostic criteria have evolved (Bryson et al. 1988; Fombonne 2003; Ritvo et al. 1989; Yeargin-Allsopp et al. 2003). The disproportionate prevalence in males has resulted in a corresponding skew in scientific research, with most studies focusing primarily or exclusively on males. Although research literature explicitly addressing sex differences is limited (Koenig and Tsatsanis 2005; Kreiser and White 2013), investigation of clinical, genetic, and etiologic factors in females is a recognized research priority, with suggestive evidence for distinct profiles and pathways across sex. Females with ASD tend to display reduced cognitive abilities (Lord et al. 1982; Volkmar et al. 1993) and a higher proportion of females is observed among those with IQs under 55 (Lord and Schopler 1985; Tsai and Beisler 1983; Wing 1981b). Among individuals with normative cognitive abilities, the gender ratio is even more pronounced (as high as 8:1; Scott et al. 2002). In the cognitively able segment of the spectrum, females show fewer social problems early in life but have more difficulties in adolescence (McLennan et al. 1993). Females are also noted to exhibit more associated (non-core) features, including sleep difficulties (Hartley and Sikora 2009), sensory issues (Lai et al. 2011), and motor impairment (Carter et al. 2007). Females have also been observed to display reduced RBBs relative to males (Mandy et al. 2012). The body of research on sex differences in ASD is limited in scope and complicated by methodological weaknesses, including wide variation in age range and cognitive function within studies.

The text accompanying *DSM-5* specifically acknowledges the importance of gender-related diagnostic issues. In a designated section, the manual warns evaluators that girls of average intellectual ability or greater are at risk for going undetected due to potentially less salient manifestation of impairments in social interaction and communication. By drawing attention to these factors, *DSM-5* may facilitate diagnosis of ASD among females. In this regard, the new criteria are likely to foster increased research on the topic.

Culture and ASD Diagnosis

DSM-5 also introduces issues related to culture. The manual acknowledges cultural variation in many of the behaviors encompassed in diagnostic criteria (e.g., eye contact) for ASD and other disorders. The text makes clear that the difficulties observed in ASD must be impaired with respect to the individual's cultural mores. For example, for children from cultures in which direct or sustained eye contact with an adult is considered inappropriate, their behavior should be gauged in the context of the family's cultural expectations rather than expectations or values held by the evaluator. Given recognized cultural variation in social customs related to ASD (Kang-Yi et al. 2013) and prevalence estimates that have varied by culture (Kim et al. 2011), this represents a significant advance in conceptualizing ASD. The text also describes a correspondence between cultural and socioeconomic factors, highlighting discrepancies in age at recognition. These changes, though peripheral to the actual diagnostic criteria, reflect an increasing awareness of factors in society and community that are essential for advancing clinical practice and research in ASD.

Adaptive Function

The importance of understanding adaptive function in ASD has long been acknowledged. Adaptive functioning refers to the application of one's aptitudes for daily functioning in practical areas, such as self-care, maintaining a household, and communicating with others. Irrespective of intellectual ability, individuals with ASD exhibit great difficulties functioning adaptively across contexts in real life. Even individuals with ASD with strong cognitive abilities tend to display a markedly weaker performance on measures of adaptive functioning (Klin et al. 2007), highlighting the dissociation between intellect and functional abilities in individuals on the spectrum. A noted problem with *DSM-IV-TR* was inappropriate application of diagnostic subcategories as proxies for functional levels. For example, an individual with a symptom profile consistent with autism but with fairly intact adaptive skills might be given a diagnosis of PDD-NOS to reflect his relatively high performance in daily life. By introducing severity specifiers, *DSM-5* emphasizes the importance of considering the functional impact of symptoms in an explicit and straightforward fashion. When applying diagnoses, clinicians are required to describe the level of support warranted by the individual's profile (i.e., requiring support, requiring substantial support, or requiring very substantial support). Taken together with specifiers characterizing language level and cognitive ability, this revised diagnostic protocol offers greater insight into the nuances of clinical presentation for individuals meeting criteria for ASD. Although *DSM-5* criteria have been criticized for the omission of diagnostic subcategories, if clinicians thoroughly complete the recommended profile of specifiers, it is likely that even more practically useful information will be available for understanding individuals affixed with the label of an extremely heterogeneous disorder.

Comorbidity and ASD

DSM-5 also addresses the relationship between ASD and comorbidity. For example, in *DSM-IV-TR,* a diagnosis of attention-deficit/hyperactivity disorder (ADHD) was ruled out in individuals meeting criteria for ASD. This reflected the presumably distinct etiology and developmental origins of problems with attention in ASD. In contrast to ADHD, in which attentional difficulties and hyperactivity are primary problems, for many individuals with ASD, these challenges are sequelae of social deficits in many instances. For example, a child in a classroom might be distractible because of problems with focus or, in the case of ASD, because the teacher at the front of the room is less salient than he is for other children. This dichotomy failed to acknowledge that, within the autism spectrum, there is great variability in attentional abilities; even among children on the spectrum, there are those who display severe attention problems and hyperactivity with respect to a cohort of individuals with ASD. Given the poorly understood brain basis of ASD, it is also likely that an individual child could possess neuropathology in distributed circuitry affecting both social-communicative behavior and attentional regulation. Despite the diagnostic rule out, these factors led to a high prevalence of "unofficial" diagnosis of ADHD among children with ASD, as well as treatment of children with ASD using

approaches recommended for ADHD children (Matson et al. 2013). In *DSM-5,* the elimination of this rule out acknowledges that ASD sometimes but not always has accompanying ADHD and, in so doing, provides a structure for organizing this already-recognized problem to help clinicians recognize attention problems in ASD and to support treatment. In addition to recognizing psychiatric comorbidities, such as ADHD and anxiety disorders, both intellectual and language disabilities are identified as common comorbidities. Furthermore, medical comorbidities such as seizures and gastrointestinal problems are coded as part of *DSM-5* ASD diagnoses.

Key Issues in the Transition to *DSM-5* Criteria

Scientists, clinicians, individuals with ASD, family members, and other stakeholders have debated planned changes to *DSM-5* criteria since well before their publication (Baron-Cohen 2009). Below we summarize key discussion points involved in the revision of the diagnostic criteria of ASD: (1) elimination of diagnostic subcategories, (2) potential impact on the prevalence and composition of ASD, (3) continuity of clinical and research samples over time and internationally, and (4) introduction of SCD as a novel diagnosis. Our review focuses, whenever possible, on published empirical data. In this way, we aim to provide a concrete, objective estimation of what is understood about potential changes thus far.

Elimination of Diagnostic Subcategories

As described above, *DSM-5* enacts a major change in the granularity of autism diagnosis. In *DSM-IV-TR,* ASD fell under a broad category of PDDs and included three distinct diagnoses: autistic disorder, Asperger's disorder, and PDD-NOS. These diagnoses utilized the same list of 12 diagnostic criteria and were differentiated based on the nature and severity of social, communicative, and RRB symptoms manifest, as well as the presence or absence of associated features, such as age of onset and cognitive ability. In general terms, autistic disorder represented significant difficulties spanning all three domains (social interaction, communication, and rigid and repetitive behaviors) with early onset. Asperger's disorder was characterized by the presence of problems with social interaction and repetitive behaviors in the context of relatively preserved language and normative intellectual ability. PDD-NOS was a residual category for individuals with social difficulties who did not meet criteria for another PDD due to insufficient breadth or severity of symptoms. In *DSM-5,* these sub-diagnostic categories are eliminated in lieu of an umbrella category of ASD.

The removal of these sub-diagnoses follows more than a decade of debate regarding the validity of these diagnostic constructs (Happe 2011). Given the vague definition of *DSM-IV-TR* PDD-NOS and the absence of formal operational diagnostic criteria, there has been less debate about its removal from the *DSM-5*; more productive research and discussion has focused specifically on Asperger's disorder. Introduced into the *DSM* subsequent to Lorna Wing's translation (Wing 1981a) of Hans Asperger's original account (Asperger 1944), the disorder is (like the rest of ASD) based primarily on nuanced clinical observations of differences in the behavioral phenotype. During the tenure of *DSM-IV-TR,* there has been inconsistent evidence establishing the disorder as a distinct taxonomic entity from autism; to do so, psychiatric disorders must differ meaningfully and usefully from extant diagnoses in clinically relevant respects, such as neuropsychological profiles, brain bases, or genetic etiology.

Patterns of performance in neuropsychological testing have been pursued as a means of validating Asperger's disorder as distinct from autistic disorder as it presents in higher-functioning individuals. Cognitively able individuals with autism tend to exhibit impairment in the areas of language and verbal abilities with strengths in nonverbal cognitive skills (Siegel et al. 1996). In contrast, studies have suggested that those with Asperger's disorder display an opposite profile of verbal strengths and weaknesses in nonverbal abilities, visual–spatial organization, and grapho-

motor skills (Ghaziuddin and Mountain-Kimchi 2004). Multiple studies have observed a learning profile described as nonverbal learning disability (NLD; Rourke 1989) in Asperger's disorder relative to ASD (Ehlers et al. 1997), though others have failed to detect this difference in neuropsychological function (Ozonoff et al. 2000). Others have suggested that, rather than indicating distinct etiology or brain basis, observed discrepancies between verbal and nonverbal ability may simply reflect different diagnostic criteria in that individuals with Asperger's disorder, by definition, have preserved language skills (Miller and Ozonoff 1997). There have also been few studies providing strong evidence for differential response to treatment or outcome in Asperger's disorder, when controlling for nondiagnostic associated features, such as cognitive ability (Mesibov 1992; Scahill and Martin 2005).

Direct measures of biological factors, such as genetics and brain structure and function, have also provided limited evidence of Asperger's disorder as a distinct diagnostic construct. Asperger's original report (Asperger 1944) observed similar characteristics in family members, particularly in fathers and grandfathers. Case report data have frequently reported high rates of social difficulties in family members of individuals with Asperger's disorder, especially among fathers (Bowman 1988; DeLong and Dwyer 1988; Volkmar et al. 1998). Several case reports have suggested genetic anomalies specific to Asperger's disorder (Anneren et al. 1995; Bartolucci and Szatmari 1987; Saliba and Griffiths 1990; Tentler et al. 2003), but no specific genetic etiology has consistently emerged. The preponderance of evidence suggests shared genetic liabilities between autism and Asperger's disorder, with no distinct or specific profile characterizing Asperger's disorder (Burgoine and Wing 1983). Several studies have provided some data regarding brain differences between individuals with Asperger's disorder and autism, including differences in brain structure (Berthier et al. 1993; Lotspeich et al. 2004), regional brain activity (McKelvey et al. 1995), and patterns of brain connectivity (Duffy et al. 2013). Despite this suggestive evidence, neither medical nor neurobiological

(Pina-Camacho et al. 2012) factors have been found to differ consistently between groups or to effectively validate as a distinct diagnosis (Macintosh and Dissanayake 2004).

In summary, the research described above in the areas of neuropsychology, developmental course, brain structure and function, and genetics provide limited support for the conceptualization of Asperger's disorder as a diagnostic construct distinct from autism. Nevertheless, a separate line of debate has focused on the validity of the diagnosis based on clinical observation alone. Although some research has suggested that, among highly experienced clinicians, diagnostic distinctions among subcategories of ASD are made reliably (Volkmar et al. 1994), most studies have not substantiated reliable distinctions based on clinical factors alone (Allen et al. 2001; Howlin 2003; Mordre et al. 2011). A recent study of an extremely large and thoroughly characterized sample collected across 12 university-based sites (Lord et al. 2011) revealed high reliability across sites at the level of distinction between ASD vs. non-ASD; however, even when controlling for cognitive and behavioral factors, subcategorical diagnoses were not reliably applied, suggesting that clinician-related factors, rather than phenotypic characteristics, were most influential in application of sub-diagnoses. This was consistent with most evidence to-date, which has indicated diagnostic reliability at the level of ASD versus non-ASD. There are now widely available standardized measures that are valid and reliable at determining this threshold, such as the Autism Diagnostic Observation Schedule-2 (ADOS-2; Lord et al. 2012) and the Autism Diagnostic Interview—Revised (ADI-R; Lord et al. 1994); there do not exist well-standardized instruments that reliably distinguish among *DSM-IV-TR* sub-diagnoses.

Debate commenced regarding the elimination of diagnostic subcategories years prior to publication of the *DSM-5,* immediately upon disclosure by the Neurodevelopmental Disorders Working Group that a transition to a spectrum category was likely. Despite weak evidence for the reliability of diagnostic subcategories during the tenure of *DSM-IV-TR,* much of the initial commentary was critical of the elimination of sub-diagnoses. One of the first public comments appeared in the New York Times, in which Baron-Cohen observed that, having been acknowledged in the *DSM* for merely a decade, scientists had been provided scant time to biologically validate the diagnostic construct (Baron-Cohen 2009). Ghaziuddin (2010) argued that, despite inconsistent application of the diagnosis and limited validation of the construct as a distinct etiology, the term was clinically beneficial, offering professionals information germane to case conceptualization and treatment; he recommended revising diagnostic criteria rather than eliminating the diagnosis entirely. Others expressed concern about the potential impact on individuals who benefited from a diagnosis of Asperger's disorder and had found the label pragmatically or socio-emotionally beneficial (Kaland 2011). Even among those who continued to qualify for a *DSM-5* diagnosis of ASD, elimination of the diagnosis could be a stressful or anxiety-producing event. Wing and colleagues suggested attaching descriptive diagnoses, such as a specifier for Asperger's disorder, to *DSM-5* criteria to avoid this possibility (Wing et al. 2011). While acknowledgment of the effects on individuals and on a "culture of autism" is clinically relevant, Vivanti and colleagues (Vivanti et al. 2013) emphasize that medical diagnoses must be distinguished from social and cultural factors and should rely on empirical foundations rather than issues related to personal identity. Given the specifiers appended to a diagnosis in *DSM-5,* Asperger's disorder endures as an implicit category when specifiers regarding intact language and cognitive ability and an early course that does not include substantial language delay are endorsed (Baron-Cohen 2013).

In summary, the transition to a spectrum category rather than individual sub-diagnoses promises several substantive benefits while introducing several risks. The official taxonomy now reflects the most consistent and reliable level of specificity among most professionals applying the diagnosis. Although individuals with great expertise or individuals practicing in specific locales may have applied sub-diagnoses appropriately, the bulk of evidence suggests that, even under

DSM-IV-TR, the only reliable diagnostic distinction has been ASD versus non-ASD, which will now correspond directly to *DSM-5* criteria. An added benefit of this change will be direct correspondence between diagnostic categories and gold-standard diagnostic instruments. This correspondence will support more widespread and reliable differentiation of ASD from typical development and other developmental and psychiatric disorders with reduced dependence on the amount and nature of experience of individual clinicians. As *DSM-5* is implemented in clinical and research settings, more information will be available about potential risks related to change in diagnostic label, such as whether individuals carrying a diagnosis of Asperger's disorder experience disenfranchisement. In many regards, the elimination of diagnostic subcategories is a semantic issue as long as the same group of individuals continues to meet threshold for ASD.

Potential Impact on the Prevalence and Composition of ASD

Whether or not the same group of individuals will continue to meet the threshold for ASD has been hotly contested. *DSM-5* diagnostic criteria alter the symptom profile required to meet diagnostic threshold for an ASD. They introduce sensory behavior as an official diagnostic criterion, and they require the endorsement of two symptom clusters within the RBB domain. These changes, along with a monothetic social-communication domain, have been interpreted as potentially more restrictive than *DSM-IV* criteria (Volkmar and Reichow 2013). Based on this concern, a number of studies have attempted to discern the correspondence between *DSM-IV-TR* samples and *DSM-5* samples, to ascertain whether or not the population of individuals meeting criteria for ASD could change according to the new criteria. A number of such studies have now been published and results have varied widely. An early report by the first author's research group suggested that individuals with milder forms of *DSM-IV ASD,* such as Asperger's disorder and PDD-NOS, and individuals with normative cog-

nitive abilities (McPartland et al. 2012) might be less likely to meet *DSM-5* criteria, findings consistent with a prior study that had utilized an earlier version of draft criteria (Mattila et al. 2011). Other studies have suggested that individuals meeting proposed *DSM-5* criteria evince more significant impairments than those meeting *DSM-IV-TR* criteria (Matson et al. 2012; Worley and Matson 2012). Some studies indicate that *DSM-5* criteria may exhibit reduced sensitivity for females (Frazier et al. 2012) or very young children (Barton et al. 2013), which could result in under-identification in these groups. In a study of several thousand cases assessed across several cites, Huerta and colleagues demonstrated excellent sensitivity (approximately 91%) for *DSM-5* criteria, suggesting a high level of correspondence between *DSM-IV-TR* and *DSM-5* criteria (Huerta et al. 2012). Although the strength of this study is its sample size, it relied on retrospective diagnostic data based on the previous diagnostic system that were adapted to correspond to the new criteria.

In the past several years, multiple studies have attempted to estimate the *DSM-5's* potential influence on ASD prevalence by retrospectively applying *DSM-5* criteria to existing datasets. As illustrated by the subset of studies described above, results have been extremely variable. Estimates have ranged from very low (e.g., 27% of individuals with a *DSM-IV-TR* diagnosis meeting *DSM-5* criteria for ASD in a sample of individuals with PDD-NOS; Mayes et al. 2013) to extremely high (e.g., 91% of individuals with a clinical *DSM-IV-TR* diagnosis; Huerta et al. 2012). These studies all have notable limitations, including reliance on older datasets, use of outdated versions of proposed *DSM-5* criteria, or exclusive reliance on clinician observation or parent report. There has been significant methodological variability among these studies in terms of data collection (e.g., reanalysis of historical data vs. prospective data collection using *DSM-5* criteria) and in terms of symptom endorsement (e.g., clinical observation vs. endorsement on one or more standardized assessment instruments). These factors are demonstrated to influence ascertainment; for example, observational measures alone may fail to detect some low-frequency behaviors and result in reduced symptom endorsement and consequently decreased proportion of individuals meeting criteria (Mazefsky et al. 2013). Most importantly, none of these studies compared diagnostic rubrics in a prospective manner, concurrently evaluating children on both criteria sets using the actual *DSM-5* criteria set (in lieu of an algorithm approximating the concepts but employing different symptom-specific wording); only with this information can any true change in prevalence associated with alteration in the diagnostic rubric be estimated. Such studies are now in progress and will provide critical information for the preparation of the next revision of *DSM-5*.

At present, very few studies have examined *DSM-5* criteria prospectively and they too have delivered heterogeneous results. The *DSM-5* field trials were designed to prioritize estimation of reliability, validity, clinical utility, and feasibility, with, compared to prior field trials, reduced prioritization of evaluating change in prevalence (Regier et al. 2013). In a small sample of 64 children assessed at two separate sites, diagnoses of ASD showed very good test–retest reliability (as measured by intraclass Kappa). *DSM-5* prevalence was similar to *DSM-IV* prevalence at one site (0.24 to 0.23, respectively) but slightly lower at a second site (0.26 to 0.19); the difference in prevalence at this second site primarily reflected a shift of some cases into the new diagnostic category, SCD (Regier et al. 2013). Young and colleagues (Young and Rodi 2013) evaluated 233 patients in a clinical setting, concurrently evaluating children and adults according to both *DSM-IV-TR* and *DSM-5* criteria. Results indicated that 57.1% of individuals meeting *DSM-IV-TR* criteria for an ASD met *DSM-5* criteria. Another study conducted a similar procedure internationally, evaluating 132 patients presenting to a specialty clinic in Australia (Gibbs et al. 2012). In this sample, 76.6% of those meeting *DSM-IV-TR* criteria also met *DSM-5* criteria, with the majority of individuals failing to reach threshold displaying a symptom profile consistent with *DSM-IV-TR* PDD-NOS. Each of these prospective studies included a modest sample size. Though larger-scale studies have com-

menced, results are not yet available. An important consideration is the impact of the diagnostic changes on the monitoring of prevalence of ASD over time by the Centers on Disease Control and Prevention (CDC). Studies are underway to examine the next cohort of children collected by the CDC's surveillance studies using both the *DSM-IV-TR* and *DSM-5* systems. A specific goal is to better understand how the diagnostic changes impact prevalence estimates across subpopulations based on race/ethnicity, socioeconomic status (SES), and gender. Another objective will be to determine whether the removal of an explicit onset rule (i.e., age 3 in *DSM-IV-TR*) impacts on prevalence estimates.

Taken together, the majority of studies suggest improved specificity (i.e., decrease in false positive diagnoses) with potentially reduced sensitivity (i.e., increased failure to detect true positive diagnoses). Many questions about the impact of *DSM-5* criteria on prevalence will not be answered conclusively until well into the period of implementation. Because most research conducted to date has taken place at major academic research centers, a key short-term objective will be to understand the application of new criteria in purely clinical and community-based settings and in contexts in which the diagnostic criteria set itself will be employed as a checklist without reliance on standardized assessment measures. More research is particularly needed to understand the effects of the new diagnostic criteria among younger, older, and more ethnically diverse individuals and in community-based settings, as well as their application to females.

Consistency of Past and Future Research

Any change in diagnostic criteria entails discontinuity in samples characterized before and after the shift in rubric. In the case of ASD, changes associated with *DSM-5* represent only one of several shifts in conceptualization and diagnostic criteria since its inclusion in the *DSM*. If, as some studies suggest, diagnoses issued according to *DSM-5* criteria would, in some cases, differ from those based on previous criteria, the comparability of future studies with prior research would be reduced, complicating the interpretation of research conducted before and after publication of the *DSM-5*. Longitudinal studies could also be impacted, with children diagnosed at one point in the study according to *DSM-IV-TR* being evaluated at subsequent time points according to discrepant criteria. This is not a novel challenge to ASD or to psychiatric diagnosis in general, but, given the large volume of research conducted on ASD in the past few years, loss of correspondence could represent a significant loss of information. By this metric, the transition from *DSM-IV* to *DSM-5* is more weighty than previous transitions in that more research is at stake. The elimination of diagnostic subcategories would preclude a straightforward mapping of historical samples to future samples, in studies relying on these clinical diagnoses alone. In addition to this chronological complexity, the transition also presents a challenge in terms of international consistency. The international community of researchers has benefited from common standards in the USA and other countries because of shared criteria in the *DSM,* used in the USA, and the International Classification of Diseases (ICD; World Health Organization 1993). *DSM-IV* and the tenth edition of the ICD (ICD-10) were developed in congruence, and, for the past 20 years, comparable diagnostic systems have been employed internationally. With the publication of the *DSM-5*, this is no longer the case. The eleventh edition of the ICD is currently in preparation and it is not yet known whether correspondence among international systems will be maintained. Obviously, for studies adhering to these criteria, inconsistency would complicate comparison of studies conducted internationally.

Although inconsistency in diagnostic systems undoubtedly complicates interpretation of research studies, several factors suggest that research consistency between historical and future samples may be preserved. Some studies indicate that there may be little alteration in the composition of research samples (Huerta et al. 2012). This improves confidence in comparability from sample to sample but does not provide a concrete means of determining degree of overlap or discrepancy. If, for example, even a small portion of individuals differ between samples, e.g., a subset shifting into SCD (Regier et al. 2013), comparison would be inexact. An alternative and more robust means of ensuring comparable samples capitalizes upon the field's increasing reliance on standardized diagnostic measures. Since the publication and popularization of the ADOS and ADI-R, nearly all rigorous scientific research, across disciplines, includes samples restricted to those meeting criteria on both instruments. As long as extant diagnostic algorithms for these instruments remain consistent, it is likely that the majority of high-quality scientific publications can be retrospectively compared to prior work. Looking forward from *DSM-5,* the monothetic criteria and specifiers may serve to reduce heterogeneity and enhance comparability of studies in the long term.

Social Communication Disorder

Social communication disorder is a new diagnosis included in the *DSM-5,* also in the category of neurodevelopmental disorders. Within this broad category, it is classified as a communication disorder and is not considered part of the autism spectrum. It reflects specific difficulties in the social application of verbal and nonverbal communication and in pragmatic language that are not accounted for by gross language impairment or other psychiatric or developmental disorders. Although specifically related to communication, SCD is described as potentially exerting more widespread impact on social functioning, such as leading to avoidance of social interactions. The *DSM-5* specifies that SCD must be present in early development, while noting that it is rarely detected prior to 4 years of age, when social communication becomes sufficiently complex to permit detection of specific impairment. SCD is distinct from ASD though ASD is described as a familial risk factor. *DSM-5* differentiates SCD from ASD based on the presence or absence of RRBs in current and historical presentation and in requiring deficits that would only be apparent in older children. In this way, SCD has been compared to PDD-NOS featuring only social and communicative symptoms, without evidence of RRBs, and it has been suggested that many individuals meeting *DSM-IV-TR* criteria for PDD-NOS would fall into the category of SCD (Skuse 2012). This notion was borne out in the *DSM-5* field trials in which a portion of individuals did not meet criteria for ASD and instead met criteria for SCD (Regier et al. 2013). Tanguay (Tanguay 2011) has commented that SCD may, rather than representing a distinct disorder, represent a mild form of ASD. Skuse (Skuse 2012) has expressed concern that SCD recreates a potentially problematic residual diagnostic category, akin to PDD-NOS. Because of limited assessment instruments to accurately measure pragmatic language function, it may also be difficult to reliably and validly quantify the impairments defining SCD as a diagnosis (Tager-Flusberg 2013). Aside from concerns about the validity of SCD as a diagnostic construct distinct from ASD, it is possible that it could alter service access. Tanguay (Tanguay 2011) cautioned about potentially disruptive effects of this inclusion on research, education, service delivery systems, and insurance. There is limited evidence to indicate specific courses of treatment for SCD versus ASD. For this reason, SCD's classification as a communication disorder might restrict educational service provision or reimbursement for care by insurance companies compared to ASD (Grant and Nozyce 2013). These points of debate will remain unresolved as service delivery systems adapt to incorporate new diagnostic criteria into their policies. The main concerns regarding the pragmatic effects of SCD rely on the presumption that it would be classified in such a fashion as to qualify individuals carrying the diagnosis for a more limited service package. Although classification as a communication disorder raises this possibility, it is not yet known how SCD will be treated by schools and other provider agencies. Many of the individuals diagnosed with SCD would likely benefit from interventions and other services that are designed to address the social communication and reciprocity deficits associated with ASD. Until treatment guidelines are created and empirically

validated for SCD, it will be important to assess the specific needs of each individual child and to match those needs to available services and therapeutic interventions, which may include treatments developed for ASD.

Summary and Remaining Questions

In May 2013, the field of autism experienced the first revision to diagnostic practice in nearly two decades. The revisions presented in *DSM-5* are significant. They advance clinical science by acknowledging critical issues, such as the role of sex and culture, which have been understudied thus far. They increase the level of detail included in diagnostic reports, adding important information about the impact of symptomatology on daily life and other factors, such as language and cognitive ability, which are focal in describing a person with ASD and planning intervention. Comorbidities associated with ASD are included in a manner that more accurately corresponds to clinical practice. Etiologies are described more precisely through the use of specifiers. Several changes have been particularly controversial, such as the elimination of diagnostic subcategories, the addition of a novel diagnosis of SCD, and the alteration of the diagnostic rubric and the risk of associated changes in the composition of individuals meeting diagnostic criteria for ASD.

Several concerns about *DSM-5* relate to changes in the composition of the spectrum. In the short term, these are rendered moot by the stipulation that a diagnosis of *DSM-5* ASD should be granted to individuals with well-established *DSM-IV* diagnoses on the autism spectrum. By prequalifying individuals with a *DSM-IV* diagnosis, this clause helps assuage worries about changes in research and practice associated with revised criteria. The existing population of individuals with ASD will maintain their diagnosis and access to clinical, medical, and educational services should remain unchanged. This clause also makes clear that reevaluations according to *DSM-5* criteria are not deemed obligatory, though the text suggests reevaluations in the case of individuals more closely resembling SCD than ASD.

A deeper understanding of any potential changes wrought by the revised criteria will emerge as the next generation of people, seeking evaluation for the first time, are assessed in the context of *DSM-5*. Of particular interest will be to understand the implications of the *DSM-5* for making first-time diagnoses in very young children. Children who have ASD may not manifest the full range of ASD symptoms before age 3. For example, a toddler who eventually qualifies for an ASD diagnosis based on *DSM-5* criteria may exhibit a significant impairment in social communication and only one symptom in the repetitive behavior domain early in life; for example, many typically developing children display repetitive motor movements during infancy or toddlerhood. Such children would not meet criteria for a diagnosis of ASD but would likely benefit from early intensive behavioral intervention. Understanding how the new criteria affect access to services is an important public health priority.

This state of affairs offers interesting challenges for clinicians to consider as *DSM-5* is implemented. Under *DSM-IV-TR,* individuals making marked progress might no longer meet criteria and lose their diagnosis. The transition period, in which preexisting diagnoses carry over, complicates the process of reevaluation. It will be necessary to set guidelines for the frequency of reevaluation of individuals, acknowledging that, in addition to change in diagnostic criteria, change in individuals may alter who meets or fails to meet criteria. The field now enters a period in which individuals may carry the same diagnosis based on different systems of classification. Though this presents a challenge for clinical research, the commonality of intervention protocols across the autism spectrum suggests that clinical practice will be robust to this heterogeneity. Even under *DSM-IV,* treatment recommendations related more directly to the individual features of a person rather than a specific sub-diagnosis.

The heated debate regarding *DSM-5's* impact on research may shift as new considerations emerge. The National Institute of Mental Health, a primary sponsor of autism research, has made explicit the objective to transition from research based on categorical diagnoses to research focused on transdiagnostic biological processes germane to multiple disorders. When diagnostic criteria are next revisited, the notion of autism research is likely to be less relevant than at present. The co-occurrence of major changes in diagnostic classification and reformulation of research priorities promises unprecedented opportunities for clinical practice and research advances in ASD.

References

Allen, D. A., Steinberg, M., Dunn, M., Fein, D., Feinstein, C., Waterhouse, L., & Rapin, I. (2001). Autistic disorder versus other pervasive developmental disorders in young children: same or different? *European Child & Adolescent Psychiatry,* 10(1), 67–78. doi: 10.1007/s007870170049.

American Psychiatric Association. (2000). *Diagnostic and statistical manual of mental disorders: DSM-IV-TR* (4th ed.). Washington, DC: American Psychiatric Association.

American Psychiatric Association. (2013). *Diagnostic and statistical manual of mental disorders: DSM-5* (5th ed.). Washington, DC: American Psychiatric Association.

Anneren, G., Dahl, N., Uddenfeldt, U., & Janols, L. (1995). Asperger syndrome in a boy with a balanced de novo translocation. *American Journal of Medical Genetics, 56,* 330–331.

Asperger, H. (1944). Die "autistichen Psychopathen" im Kindersalter. *Archive fur psychiatrie und Nerven-krankheiten, 117,* 76–136.

Baron-Cohen, S. (2009). The short life of a diagnosis. *New York Times.* http://www.nytimes.com/2009/2011/2010/opinion/2010baron-cohen.html. Accessed 9 Nov 2009.

Baron-Cohen, S. (2013). Despite fears, DSM-5 is a step forward. http://sfari.org/news-and-opinion/specials/2013/dsm-5-special-report/despite-fears-dsm-5-is-a-step-forward/. Accessed 24 Sept 2013.

Bartolucci, G., & Szatmari, P. (1987). Possible similarities between the fragile X and Asperger's syndromes. *American Journal of Diseases of Children, 141*(6), 601–602.

Barton, M. L., Robins, D., Jashar, D., Brennan, L., & Fein, D. (2013). Sensitivity and specificity of proposed DSM-5 criteria for autism spectrum disorder in toddlers. *Journal of Autism and Developmental disorders, 43*(5), 1184–1195. doi:10.1007/s10803-013-1817-8.

Berthier, M. L., Bayes, A., & Tolosa, E. S. (1993). Magnetic resonance imaging in patients with concurrent Tourette's disorder and Asperger's syndrome. *Journal of the American Academy of Child & Adolescent Psychiatry, 32*(3), 633–639.

Bowman, E. (1988). Asperger's syndrome and autism: The case for a connection. *British Journal of Psychiatry, 152,* 377–382.

Bryson, S. E., Clark, B. S., & Smith, I. M. (1988). First report of a Canadian epidemiological study of autistic syndromes. *Journal of Child Psychology and Psychiatry, 29*(4), 433–445.

Burgoine, E., & Wing, L. (1983). Identical triplets with Asperger's syndrome. *British Journal of Psychiatry, 143,* 261–265.

Carter, A. S., Black, D. O., Tewani, S., Connolly, C. E., Kadlec, M. B., & Tager-Flusberg, H. (2007). Sex differences in toddlers with autism spectrum disorders. *Journal of Autism and Developmental Disorders, 37*(1), 86–97. doi:10.1007/s10803-006-0331-7.

CDC. (2012). Prevalence of autism spectrum disorders-autism and developmental disabilities monitoring network, 14 Sites, United States, 2008. *MMWR Surveillance Summaries, 61*(SS-3), 1–19.

DeLong, G., & Dwyer, J. (1988). Correlation of family history with specific autistic subgroups: Asperger's syndrome and bipolar affective disease. *Journal of Autism & Developmental Disorders, 18*(4), 593–600.

Duffy, F. H., Shankardass, A., McAnulty, G. B., & Als, H. (2013). The relationship of Asperger's syndrome to autism: A preliminary EEG coherence study. *BMC Medicine, 11,* 175. doi:10.1186/1741-7015-11-175.

Ehlers, S., Nyden, A., Gillberg, C., Sandberg, A., Dahlgren, S., Hjelmquist, E., & Oden, A. (1997). Asperger syndrome, autism and attention disorders: A comparative study of the cognitive profiles of 120 children. *Journal of Child Psychology and Psychiatry, 38*(2), 207–217.

Fombonne, E. (2003). The prevalence of autism. *JAMA: Journal of the American Medical Association, 289*(1), 87–89.

Frazier, T. W., Youngstrom, E. A., Speer, L., Embacher, R., Law, P., Constantino, J., Eng, C., et al. (2012). Validation of proposed DSM-5 criteria for autism spectrum disorder. *Journal of the American Academy of Child & Adolescent Psychiatry, 51*(1), 28–40e23. doi:10.1016/j.jaac.2011.09.021.

Ghaziuddin, M. (2010). Should the DSM V drop Asperger syndrome? *Journal of Autism and Development Disorders, 40*(9), 1146–1148. doi:10.1007/s10803-010-0969-z.

Ghaziuddin, M., & Mountain-Kimchi, K. (2004). Defining the intellectual profile of Asperger syndrome: Comparison with high-functioning autism. *Journal of Autism and Developmental Disorders, 34*(3), 279–284.

Gibbs, V., Aldridge, F., Chandler, F., Witzlsperger, E., & Smith, K. (2012). Brief report: An exploratory study comparing diagnostic outcomes for autism spectrum disorders under DSM-IV-TR with the proposed DSM-5 revision. *Journal of Autism and Developmental Disorders.* doi:10.1007/s10803-012-1560-6.

Grant, R., & Nozyce, M. (2013). Proposed changes to the American Psychiatric Association diagnostic criteria for autism spectrum disorder: Implications for young children and their families. *Maternal and Child Health Journal, 17*(4), 586–592. doi:10.1007/s10995-013-1250-9.

Happe, F. (2011). Criteria, categories, and continua: Autism and related disorders in DSM-5. *Journal of the American Academy of Child & Adolescent Psychiatry, 50*(6), 540–542. doi:10.1016/j.jaac.2011.03.015.

Hartley, S. L., & Sikora, D. M. (2009). Sex differences in autism spectrum disorder: An examination of developmental functioning, autistic symptoms, and coexisting behavior problems in toddlers. *Journal of Autism and Developmental Disorders, 39*(12), 1715–1722. doi:10.1007/s10803-009-0810-8.

Howlin, P. (2003). Outcome in high-functioning adults with autism with and without early language delays: implications for the differentiation between autism and Asperger syndrome. *J Autism Dev Disord, 33*(1), 3–13.

Huerta, M., Bishop, S. L., Duncan, A., Hus, V., & Lord, C. (2012). Application of DSM-5 criteria for autism spectrum disorder to three samples of children with DSM-IV diagnoses of pervasive developmental disorders. *American Journal of Psychiatry, 169*(10), 1056–1064. doi:10.1176/appi.ajp.2012.12020276.

Kaland, N. (2011). Brief report: Should Asperger syndrome be excluded from the forthcoming DSM-V? *Research in Autism Spectrum Disorders, 5*(3), 984–989. doi:10.1016/j.rasd.2011.01.011.

Kang-Yi, C. D., Grinker, R. R., & Mandell, D. S. (2013). Korean culture and autism spectrum disorders. *Journal of Autism and Developmental Disorders, 43*(3), 503–520. doi:10.1007/s10803-012-1570-4.

Kim, Y. S., Leventhal, B. L., Koh, Y. J., Fombonne, E., Laska, E., Lim, E. C., Grinker, R. R., et al. (2011). Prevalence of autism spectrum disorders in a total population sample. *The American Journal of Psychiatry.* doi:10.1176/appi.ajp.2011.10101532.

Klin, A., Saulnier, C. A., Sparrow, S. S., Cicchetti, D. V., Volkmar, F. R., & Lord, C. (2007). Social and communication abilities and disabilities in higher functioning individuals with autism spectrum disorders: The Vineland and the ADOS. *Journal of Autism and Developmental Disorders, 37*(4), 748–759.

Koenig, K., & Tsatsanis, K. (2005). Pervasive developmental disorders in girls. In D. Bell-Dolan, S. L. Foster, & E. J. Mash (Eds.), *Behavioral and emotional problems in girls.* New York: Kluwer Academic/Plenum.

Kreiser, N. L., & White, S. W. (2013). ASD in females: Are we overstating the gender difference in diagnosis? *Clinical Child and Family Psychology Review.* doi:10.1007/s10567-013-0148-9.

Lai, M. C., Lombardo, M. V., Pasco, G., Ruigrok, A. N., Wheelwright, S. J., Sadek, S. A., Baron-Cohen, S., et al. (2011). A behavioral comparison of male and female adults with high functioning autism spectrum conditions. *PLoS One, 6*(6), e20835. doi:10.1371/journal.pone.0020835.

Lord, C., & Schopler, E. (1985). Differences in sex ratios in autism as a function of measured intelligence. *Journal of Autism & Developmental Disorders, 15*(2), 185–193.

Lord, C., Schopler, E., & Revicki, D. (1982). Sex differences in autism. *Journal of Autism & Developmental Disorders, 12*(4), 317–330.

Lord, C., Rutter, M., & Le Couteur, A. (1994). Autism diagnostic interview-revised: A revised version of a diagnostic interview for caregivers of individuals with possible pervasive developmental disorders. *Journal of Autism and Developmental Disorders, 24*(5), 659–685.

Lord, C., Petkova, E., Hus, V., Gan, W., Lu, F., Martin, D. M., Risi, S., et al. (2011). A multisite study of the clinical diagnosis of different autism spectrum disorders. *Archives of General Psychiatry.* doi:10.1001/archgenpsychiatry.2011.148.

Lord, C., Rutter, M., DiLavore, P. C., Risi, S., Gotham, K., & Bishop, S. (2012). *Autism diagnostic observation schedule* (2nd ed.). Torrance: Western Psychological Services.

Lotspeich, L. J., Kwon, H., Schumann, C. M., Fryer, S. L., Goodlin-Jones, B. L., Buonocore, M. H., Reiss, A. L., et al. (2004). Investigation of neuroanatomical differences between autism and Asperger syndrome. *Archives of General Psychiatry, 61*(3), 291–298.

Macintosh, K. E., & Dissanayake, C. (2004). Annotation: The similarities and differences between autistic disorder and Asperger's disorder: A review of the empirical evidence. *Journal of Child Psychology & Psychiatry, 45*(3), 421–434.

Mandy, W., Chilvers, R., Chowdhury, U., Salter, G., Seigal, A., & Skuse, D. (2012). Sex differences in autism spectrum disorder: Evidence from a large sample of children and adolescents. *Journal of Autism and Developmental Disorders, 42*(7), 1304–1313. doi:10.1007/s10803-011-1356-0.

Matson, J., Belva, B., Horovitz, M., Kozlowski, A., & Bamburg, J. (2012). Comparing symptoms of autism spectrum disorders in a developmentally disabled adult population using the current DSM-IV-TR diagnostic criteria and the proposed DSM-5 diagnostic criteria. *Journal of Developmental and Physical Disabilities.* doi:10.1007/s10882-012-9278-0.

Matson, J. L., Rieske, R. D., & Williams, L. W. (2013). The relationship between autism spectrum disorders and attention-deficit/hyperactivity disorder: An overview. *Research in Developmental Disabilities, 34*(9), 2475–2484. doi:10.1016/j.ridd.2013.05.021.

Mattila, M. L., Kielinen, M., Linna, S. L., Jussila, K., Ebeling, H., Bloigu, R., Moilanen, I., et al. (2011). Autism spectrum disorders according to DSM-IV-TR and comparison With DSM-5 draft criteria: An epidemiological study. *Journal of the American Academy of Child and Adolescent Psychiatry, 50*(6), 583–592e511. doi:10.1016/j.jaac.2011.04.001.

Mayes, S. D., Black, A., & Tierney, C. D., (2013). DSM-5 under-identifies PDDNOS: Diagnostic agreement between the DSM-5, DSM-IV, and checklist for autism spectrum disorder. *Research in Autism Spectrum Disorders, 7*(2), 298–306. doi:http://dx.doi.org/10.1016/j.rasd.2012.08.011.

Mazefsky, C. A., McPartland, J. C., Gastgeb, H. Z., & Minshew, N. J. (2013). Brief report: Comparability of DSM-IV and DSM-5 ASD research samples. *Journal of Autism and Developmental Disorders, 43*(5), 1236–1242. doi:10.1007/s10803-012-1665-y.

McKelvey, J. R., Lambert, R., Mottron, L., & Shevell, M. I. (1995). Right-hemisphere dysfunction in Asperger's syndrome. *Journal of Child Neurology, 10*(4), 310–314.

McLennan, J. D., Lord, C., & Schopler, E. (1993). Sex differences in higher functioning people with autism. *Journal of Autism & Developmental Disorders, 23*(2), 217–227.

McPartland, J. C., Reichow, B., & Volkmar, F. R. (2012). Sensitivity and specificity of proposed DSM-5 diagnostic criteria for autism spectrum disorder. *Journal of the American Academy of Child & Adolescent Psychiatry, 51*(4), 368–383. doi:10.1016/j.jaac.2012.01.007.

Mesibov, G. (1992). Treatment issues with high-functioning adolescents and adults with autism. In E. Schopler & G. Mesibov (Eds.), *High-functioning individuals with autism* (pp. 143–156). New York: Plenum.

Miller, J. N., & Ozonoff, S. (1997). Did Asperger's cases have Asperger disorder? A research note. *Journal of Child Psychology and Psychiatry, 38*(2), 247–251.

Mordre, M., Groholt, B., Knudsen, A. K., Sponheim, E., Mykletun, A., & Myhre, A. M. (2012). Is long-term prognosis for pervasive developmental disorder not otherwise specified different from prognosis for autistic disorder? Findings from a 30-year follow-up study. *J Autism Dev Disord, 42*(6), 920--928. doi: 10.1007/s10803-011-1319-5.

Ozonoff, S., South, M., & Miller, J. N. (2000). DSM-IV-defined Asperger syndrome: Cognitive, behavioral and early history differentiation from high-functioning autism. *Autism: the international journal of research and practice, 4*(1), 29–46.

Pina-Camacho, L., Villero, S., Fraguas, D., Boada, L., Janssen, J., Navas-Sanchez, F. J., Parellada, M., et al. (2012). Autism spectrum disorder: Does neuroimaging support the DSM-5 proposal for a symptom dyad? A systematic review of functional magnetic resonance imaging and diffusion tensor imaging studies. *Journal of Autism and Developmental Disorders, 42*(7), 1326–1341. doi:10.1007/s10803-011-1360-4.

Regier, D. A., Narrow, W. E., Clarke, D. E., Kraemer, H. C., Kuramoto, S. J., Kuhl, E. A., & Kupfer, D. J. (2013). DSM-5 field trials in the United States and Canada, Part II: Test-retest reliability of selected categorical diagnoses. *American Journal of Psychiatry, 170*(1), 59–70. doi:10.1176/appi.ajp.2012.12070999.

Ritvo, E., Freeman, B., Pingree, C., Mason-Brothers, A., Jorde, L., Jenson, W., Ritvo, A., et al. (1989). The UCLA-University of Utah epidemiologic survey of autism: Prevalence. *American Journal of Psychiatry, 146*(2), 194–199.

Rourke, B. P. (1989). *Nonverbal learning disabilities: The syndrome and the model.* New York: Guilford.

Saliba, J. R., & Griffiths, M. (1990). Brief report: Autism of the Asperger type associated with an autosomal fragile site. *Journal of Autism and Developmental Disorders, 20*(4), 569–575.

Scahill, L., & Martin, A. (2005). *Psychopharmocology.* In F. Volkmar, R. Paul, A. Klin, & D. Cohen (Eds.), *Handbook of autism and pervasive developmental disorders* (3rd ed., Vol. 2, pp. 1102–1117). Hoboken: Wiley.

Scott, F. J., Baron-Cohen, S., Bolton, P., & Brayne, C. (2002). Brief report: Prevalence of autism spectrum conditions in children aged 5–11 years in Cambridgeshire, UK. *Autism: the international journal of research and practice, 6*(3), 231–237.

Siegel, D. J., Minshew, N. J., & Goldstein, G. (1996). Wechsler IQ profiles in diagnosis of high-functioning autism. *Journal of Autism & Developmental Disorders, 26*(4), 389–406.

Skuse, D. H. (2012). DSM-5's conceptualization of autistic disorders. *Journal of the American Academy of Child & Adolescent Psychiatry, 51*(4), 344–346. doi:http://dx.doi.org/10.1016/j.jaac.2012.02.009.

Tager-Flusberg, H. (2013). Evidence weak for social communication disorder. http://sfari.org/news-and-opinion/specials/2013/dsm-5-special-report/evidence-weak-for-social-communication-disorder. Accessed 24 Sept 2013.

Tanguay, P. E. (2011). Autism in DSM-5. *American Journal of Psychiatry, 168*(11), 1142–1144. doi:10.1176/appi.ajp.2011.11071024.

Tentler, D., Johannesson, T., Johansson, M., Rastam, M., Gillberg, C., Orsmark, C., Dahl, N., et al. (2003). A candidate region for Asperger syndrome defined by two 17p breakpoints. *European Journal of Human Genetics, 11*(2), 189–195.

Tsai, L. Y., & Beisler, J. M. (1983). The development of sex differences in infantile autism. *The British Journal of Psychiatry, 142*(4), 373–378.

Vivanti, G., Hudry, K., Trembath, D., Barbaro, J., Richdale, A., & Dissanayake, C. (2013). Towards the DSM-5 criteria for autism: Clinical, cultural, and research implications. *Australian Psychologist, 48*(4), 258–261. doi:10.1111/ap.12008.

Volkmar, F., & Reichow, B. (2013). Autism in DSM-5: Progress and challenges. *Molecular Autism, 4*(1), 13.

Volkmar, F., Szatmari, P., & Sparrow, S. (1993). Sex differences in pervasive developmental disorders. *Journal of Autism & Developmental Disorders, 23*(4), 579–591.

Volkmar, F., Klin, A., Siegel, B., Szatmari, P., Lord, C., Campbell, M., Kline, W., et al. (1994). Field trial for autistic disorder in DSM-IV. *American Journal of Psychiatry., 151*(9), 1361–1367.

Volkmar, F., Klin, A., & Pauls, D. (1998). Nosological and genetic aspects of Asperger syndrome. *Journal of Autism & Developmental Disorders, 28*(5), 457–463.

Wing, L. (1981a). Asperger's syndrome: A clinical account. *Psychological Medicine, 11,* 115–129.

Wing, L. (1981b). Sex ratios in early childhood autism and related conditions. *Psychiatry Research, 5*(2), 129–137.

Wing, L., Gould, J., & Gillberg, C. (2011). Autism spectrum disorders in the DSM-V: Better or worse than the DSM-IV? *Research in Developmental Disabilities, 32*(2), 768–773. doi:10.1016/j.ridd.2010.11.003.

World Health Organization. (1993). *The ICD-10 classification of mental and behavioural disorders: Diagnostic criteria for research.* Geneva: World Health Organization.

Worley, J. A., & Matson, J. L. (2012). Comparing symptoms of autism spectrum disorders using the current DSM-IV-TR diagnostic criteria and the proposed DSM-V diagnostic criteria. *Research in Autism Spectrum Disorders, 6*(2), 965–970. doi:10.1016/j.rasd.2011.12.012.

Yeargin-Allsopp, M., Rice, C., Karapurkar, T., Doernberg, N., Boyle, C., & Murphy, C. (2003). Prevalence of autism in a US metropolitan area. *JAMA: Journal of the American Medical Association, 289*(1), 49–55.

Young, R. L., & Rodi, M. L. (2013). Redefining autism spectrum disorder using DSM-5: The implications of the proposed DSM-5 criteria for autism spectrum disorders. *Journal of Autism and Developmental disorders,* 1–8. doi:10.1007/s10803-013-1927-3.

Catherine Lord and Katherine Gotham

Collectively, we are part of exciting times in the history of psychiatry and psychology and the area of autism spectrum disorder (ASD) clinical practice and research. We write this just a few weeks after the release of the fifth edition of the *Diagnostic and Statistical Manual of Mental Disorders* (*DSM-5*; American Psychiatric Association 2013). This transition, like most, has evoked both excitement and trepidation within our field; in this chapter, we endeavor to consider the reasons for both. This commentary includes (1) a brief history of autism-related disorders in the DSM system, (2) specific changes in autism spectrum criteria from *DSM-IV* to *DSM-5,* (3) advantages of *DSM-5* classification of ASD, (4) common concerns about *DSM-5* changes to ASD criteria, with accompanying responses, and (5) questions that remain for future research.

Brief History of Autism-Related Disorders in the DSM System

The medical community began to take notice of autism and related disorders in the 1940s, based on the work of Leo Kanner and Hans Asperger. For the next several decades, these disorders generally were referred to as childhood schizophrenia ("schizophrenic reaction, childhood type" in the first edition of the *Diagnostic and Statistical Manual, DSM-I*; American Psychiatric Association 1952). In 1980, "infantile autism" was officially recognized as a category in the *DSM-III* (American Psychiatric Association 1980), marking the emergence of autism in the American Psychiatric Association's nosological system. At that time, individuals had to meet all specified diagnostic criteria in order to receive the diagnosis, which resulted in the classification primarily of more severely affected persons to whom we might refer today as having "classic autism." In *DSM-III,* "Child Onset Pervasive Developmental Disorder" was proposed as a distinct category characterized by social impairments and at least three of seven "mixed bag" symptoms that ranged from anxiety attacks to unusual use of speech to abnormal reactions to sensory stimuli. The *DSM-III-R* (American Psychiatric Association 1987) adopted this polythetic approach (i.e., individuals must meet a specific number of criteria within a provided range) for "Autistic Disorder," which broadened its developmental scope to include younger and/or more cognitively able individuals. *DSM-III-R* also

K. Gotham (✉)
Department of Psychiatry, Vanderbilt University Medical Center, Nashville, TN 37212, USA
e-mail: katherine.gotham@Vanderbilt.Edu

C. Lord
Center for Autism and the Developing Brain, Weill Cornell Medical College, New York-Presbyterian Hospital, New York, USA

marked the appearance of the residual category "Pervasive Developmental Disorder-Not Otherwise Specified" (PDD-NOS). In 2000, revisions in *DSM-IV* (American Psychiatric Association 2000) resulted in several categories under the pervasive development disorder umbrella, including Asperger's disorder, Rett's disorder, and Childhood Disintegrative Disorder.

DSM-5 workgroups were formed in 2007 to carry out revisions with a clear paradigm shift in mind: Across disorders, the *DSM-5* ideally would achieve dimensional diagnosis within a categorical system, for example, separating the constructs of impairment and disorder by adding continuous severity scales and reducing "-NOS" diagnoses in favor of broad categories with dimensional specifiers. These changes centered around a vision of incorporating neurobiological models into this manual and its subsequent versions (with nomenclature changed for ease of updates: *DSM-5.1*, *DSM-5.2*, etc.). Some of these objectives were achieved in large or small ways; for example, "NOS" (now "unspecified") categories are somewhat rarer in *DSM-5* (released May 2013; American Psychiatric Association 2013), and "Neurodevelopmental Disorders" replaces the major heading of "Disorders Usually First Diagnosed in Infancy, Childhood, or Adolescence" in order to emphasize the current understanding of brain development as the underpinning for child/adolescent disorders, as well as the continuance of many childhood-onset disorders into adulthood (Wakefield 2013). Other examples of the paradigm shift are detailed below as we discuss specific changes to autism-related classification. Later in this chapter, we comment on other forces, of equal or greater importance in *DSM-5* decision making around ASD, that tempered this shift to dimensional, neurobiologically indicated categories and criteria.

Specific Changes to Autism-Related Disorders from *DSM-IV* to *DSM-5*

Under *DSM-IV* (American Psychiatric Association 2000), the category of pervasive developmental disorders (PDDs) included five distinct disorders: autistic disorder, Asperger's disorder,

PDD-NOS, Rett's syndrome, and childhood disintegrative disorder (CDD). Diagnosis of Autistic disorder required a minimum of six behavioral criteria, at least two from the domain of social impairment and one each from communication and restricted, repetitive, stereotyped behavior domains. Asperger's disorder was identical to autistic disorder in terms of requiring two symptoms from the social domain and one from the stereotyped behavior domain, but its diagnosis could be made only in the absence of intellectual disability, language delay, or meeting any diagnostic criteria in the communication domain (because autistic disorder must have been ruled out before making an Asperger's disorder classification). PDD-NOS generally indicated a mild or subthreshold form of autism or a manifestation of PDD-like social impairment that was atypical in terms of onset or symptomatology such that the defining features of other PDDs were not met. Onset criteria in *DSM-IV* specified that some symptoms of the autistic disorder must have been manifest prior to age 3, though this was not necessary for a diagnosis of Asperger's disorder or PDD-NOS.

In *DSM-5*, the single broad category of "Autism Spectrum Disorder" has replaced the term PDD and subsumed all its subcategories into one (with the exception of Rett's syndrome, which, if associated with ASD, would be specified as a "known genetic condition"). The *DSM-IV* triad of symptom domains (i.e., social, communication, and stereotyped/repetitive behaviors) has been reduced to two domains: First, the social symptoms are combined with nonverbal and some language-related communication symptoms into a single area. Individuals must meet all of the three criteria in this domain, showing evidence of deficits in (1) social–emotional reciprocity, (2) nonverbal communicative behaviors used for social interaction, and (3) developing, maintaining, and understanding relationships and/or adjusting to social context. ASD diagnosis also requires the presence of two out of four criteria in a second symptom domain associated with restricted, repetitive behaviors (RRB). The RRB domain now includes sensory abnormalities and resistance to change as two of the four criteria; repetitive aspects of speech and play now are subsumed under the RRB criteria as well. ASD criteria may be met "currently or by history," and classification requires meeting the criterion that symptoms are/were present in the "early developmental period," though they "may not become fully manifest until social demands exceed limited capacities" and "may be masked by learned strategies later in life" (American Psychiatric Association 2013).

An attempt to dimensionalize ASD characteristics is evident in several ways within the new diagnostic rubric. Verbal skill, language delay, and cognitive ability are treated as dimensions outside of the diagnosis itself, rather than used to describe categories. Specifiers of intellectual impairment, language impairment (including description of current language functioning), known medical/genetic conditions and/or environmental factors, and other neurodevelopmental, mental, or behavioral disorders are all recognized now as necessary aspects of an ASD diagnosis under *DSM-5*. The supporting text includes a call for specific assessment of language skills (receptive and expressive separately) and cognitive ability (as verbal and nonverbal discretely). Further, the severity of social/communication and RRB symptom domains is specified by the "level of support" (requires support, substantial support, or very substantial support) that indicates the individual's level of clinical impairment by domain.

Of note, *DSM-5* text makes explicit that existing "well-established" *DSM-IV* ASD diagnoses should be grandfathered in. In other words, individuals with an existing ASD diagnosis under *DSM-IV* (including Asperger's disorder and PDD-NOS) should receive a *DSM-5* diagnosis of ASD without the need for reevaluation. (Concerns have been raised about individuals who would have met *DSM-IV* criteria but will receive a first diagnosis under *DSM-5*, making them ineligible for "grandfathering." See the several sections following for discussions of flexible, example-based criteria intended to increase the sensitivity of *DSM-5* diagnosis; the role of the new diagnostic category, Social (Pragmatic) Communication Disorder; as well as potential prevalence changes between *DSM-IV* and *DSM-5*, as these

topics directly address the issue of those who might be "left out" of *DSM-5*.)

A new, related diagnosis, social (pragmatic) communication disorder (SCD), is included in *DSM-5*. ASD must be ruled out before making a SCD diagnosis. SCD is defined by impairment in social use of verbal and nonverbal communication. These difficulties must be judged to impair social relationships and comprehension and must not be accounted for by problems with word structure, grammar, or general cognitive ability. To qualify for a SCD diagnosis, symptoms must be present in early childhood, though again they may not developmentally manifest until social expectations exceed limited capacities.

Advantages of and Theory Behind *DSM-5* ASD Criteria

Although *DSM-IV* criteria proved useful in diagnosing ASD in school-aged children, they performed less well when used to identify toddlers and preschoolers, adolescents, and young adults on the autism spectrum (Swedo et al. 2012). Further, deficits were noted in *DSM-IV* criteria in terms of sensitivity to ASD in girls and women, as well as in ethnic or racial minorities (Shattuck et al. 2009). *DSM-5* attempts to address these needs by providing criteria that are conceptual in nature about domains of deficit; each criterion includes developmentally specific examples of behaviors meeting the required domain. The goal is to provide clinicians with the flexibility to identify individual symptoms that relate to each particular domain, with guidelines provided for the changing manifestations of various autism symptoms across the life span, gender, ethnicity, or culture (Swedo et al. 2012). The new criteria also eliminate the confusion surrounding distinctions between *DSM-IV* subcategories of PDD in individuals without intellectual disability or language delay by subsuming all ASD within a broad category; individual difference in these other features (e.g., language delay, intelligence) are intended to be specified dimensionally in complement to the broad categorical diagnosis (Happe 2011; Lord and Jones 2012). This approach should clarify the unreliable, highly varied approaches that clinicians currently use to differentiate milder cases of autism from Asperger syndrome and PDD-NOS (Lord et al. 2012) and eliminate the common dilemma of the same individual receiving serial or concurrent diagnoses of PDD-NOS, autism, and Asperger syndrome from different diagnosticians depending on the clinician's own skill and/or biases (Klin et al. 2007; Lord et al. 2012; Miller and Ozonoff 2000; Sharma et al. 2012). In addition, individuals who meet criteria for ASD who have a known genetic condition, such as Fragile X or Rett Syndrome, receive a standard diagnosis of ASD to describe their behavior as well as a genetic specifier to describe these conditions. This strategy has the advantage of leaving room for new genetic and other biological findings that may shed light on etiology.

In addition to the potential for increased sensitivity among special populations and the practical benefits of streamlined diagnosis, *DSM-5* criteria for ASD have the advantage of being founded on more than a decade of research that did not exist at the conception of *DSM-IV* (but came to existence thanks in part to that document). We will enumerate several examples of increased validity in *DSM-5* criteria here, though this is not an exhaustive list:

- The *DSM-IV* criterion of a delay in or complete lack of development in expressive language has been eliminated in *DSM-5* due to findings that this characteristic is not specific to individuals with ASD (e.g., Hartley and Sikora 2010; Matson and Neal 2010; Solomon et al. 2011).
- The reduction of a three-domain model of symptoms (social, communication, and RRB) to a two-domain model (social–communication and RRB) is supported by factor analytic findings from many independent research teams analyzing several different measures of autism symptoms (Constantino et al. 2004; Frazier et al. 2008; Gotham et al. 2008; Lord et al. 2000; Robertson et al. 1999; Snow and Lecavalier 2008). Recent findings from large datasets have indicated that the *DSM-5* symptom dyad has greater validity than the *DSM-IV* triad, with the core impairments of ASD manifested as separable social–communication and RRB dimensions (Frazier et al. 2012; Mandy et al. 2012).

- Onset criteria have been "softened" to balance the need for ascertaining abnormal development in the early years with the acknowledgment that this is quite difficult in practice: The age at which caregivers recognize that something is not quite right and the age at which professionals diagnose autism or a related condition are not the same as the age of onset, and retrospective reports of dates are affected by the distance between the proposed event and the current date (i.e., "telescoping" effects; Hus et al. 2011).

- Childhood Disintegrative Disorder has been omitted as a distinct category in *DSM-5* based on the findings that later-occurring extensive regressions are extremely rare (Fombonne 2002) and are followed by a profile of behaviors that appears to be adequately described by an autism diagnosis (Volkmar and Rutter 1995). To retain a method of identifying these cases in *DSM-5*, there are specifier codings for age and type of onset, so this information is not lost.

- Sensory responses, including hyperreactivity and hyporeactivity to sensory input and unusual interest in sensory aspects of the environment, now are included in the RRB criteria domain to reflect research showing that these behaviors are prevalent in ASD, useful in distinguishing ASD from other disorders, and load on an RRB factor (Ben-Sasson et al. 2009; Billstedt et al. 2007; Leekham et al. 2007; Mandy et al. 2012; Tadevosyan-Leyfer et al. 2003; Wiggins et al. 2009).

Though the dimensional updates to the DSM have yet to be tested in the field, the call for a shift to more dimensional nosology was a result of research as well, and no doubt will come to represent a strong advantage of *DSM-5*. The field of neurobiology advanced the need for dimensions throughout psychiatry, with evidence that dimensional measurement provides both additional statistical power in quantitative analyses (beyond that which is offered by categories) and allows for the inclusion of more subjects in research samples, as milder cases or even noncases with some symptoms can be included (Ronald et al. 2011; see Lord and Jones 2012). Additionally, dimensions offer important theoretical underpinnings in the effort to link ASD-related behaviors and neurobiological mechanisms, such as those related to certain forms of anxiety (Juranek et al. 2006; Kleinhans et al. 2010) and to the social brain (Pelphrey et al. 2011). Again, the new diagnostic criteria in *DSM-5* (as well as the *International Classification of Diseases*, 11th revision, *ICD-11*; World Health Organization 2013) propose three principles in defining diagnostic features within the social dimension: social–emotional reciprocity; nonverbal communicative behaviors used for social communication; and deficits in developing and maintaining relationships and adjusting to social contexts. While these three subdomains are not empirically defined dimensions (but rather are descriptions of levels of social difficulties typically manifested in ASD), it is possible that some variation of these or related social factors (e.g., reciprocity/communication, social adaptation, withdrawal or motivation; Lord and Jones 2012) might provide a platform for neurobiological research into mechanisms associated with abnormal social development.

Because a formal system based on dimensions is relatively new to psychological and psychiatric research, we must also keep in mind some caveats in dimensional conceptualization. Existing research tells us that empirically validated dimensions within social communication vary greatly across developmental levels, and their specificity to ASD depends on the comparison population (Bishop et al. 2007). Many of the most theoretically important constructs proposed as core social deficits in ASD, such as theory of mind (Baron-Cohen et al. 1985), joint attention (Mundy et al. 1990), and social motivation (Dawson et al. 2005), are striking in their presence at some ages and in some individuals but are not necessarily observable in very young children, are no longer present in significant numbers of older children or adults, and/or are not specific to ASD (Bowler 1992; Gillespie-Lynch et al. 2012; Herold et al. 2002; Lord and Jones 2012). In addition to developmental effects, it could be that what we are describing as social deficits or RRBs in ASD are not truly valid dimensions of human behavior from the

"ground up" but represent theoretical "dimensions" based on our initial conceptualization of this categorical disorder (Lord and Jones 2012). Conversely, there could be an unknown dimensional mediator, such as a basic cognitive process, that has profound effects on social behavior and repetitive behaviors that would account for a more continuous distribution in symptoms across the ASD and typical populations (Dawson et al. 2005). On the other hand, dimensional social deficits and RRBs may have multiplicative effects on each other that set individuals with ASD apart as a group. Given these hypotheses, the *DSM-5* approach to ASD—as a category determined by dimensions but which, taken together, may result in more than the sum of its parts—makes sense within the limits of our current knowledge (Lord and Jones 2012; Pickles and Angold 2003).

Based on findings from both genetics and neuroscience, the assumption has been that when we have one or more strong biomarkers, the behaviors that comprise a diagnostic syndrome will be of less importance than measurable constructs (as a hypothetical example: recognition of biological motion) which link to these biomarkers. These constructs would link to biomarkers, biomarkers would link directly to neuropathophysiology, which in turn would link to medical treatment of a specific dimension, even if effective treatment for all core diagnostic features did not exist. In cancer research, for example, this approach has paid off with advances in personalizing treatments, albeit as much through knowing that a particular medication does *not* work as that it does with a specific genetic subgroup (McMahon and Insel 2012).

Nevertheless, there are many reasons to think that direct links between biology and mental health or cognitive and behavioral development will be less clear. Development and context within that development have extremely strong effects on behavior, and in general, approaches such as those mentioned above do not consider these effects. Ultimately, it is behavior—whether seen in a child's lack of response to other children, an adult's over-friendly approaches to strangers on the bus, or a toddler's distress when she cannot line up all the shoes in her mother's closet—that we are trying to shape or change in order to provide help to individuals and families.

Consequently, as basic researchers search for those links between biology and behavior, we need to be careful to avoid prioritizing neurobiological and genetics results over behavior; specifically, we must avoid the tautology of prioritizing behaviors that happen to fit well into these types of studies, as key concepts on which to build diagnostic models of ASD that then fit into the same neurobiological or genetic studies. This may promote research directions that are ultimately of limited value for understanding underlying core ASD pathophysiologies or etiologies of disorders of human behavior. A related risk is too much focus on one dimension, particularly one defined with minimal validity, which may move us away from underlying factors that may contribute to our understanding and treatment of the complex, multidimensional, developmental phenomenon of ASD. Similarly, we must be careful not to reify "dimensions" that in fact may not be truly continuous when considered carefully but are attractive to those interested in quantifying anything related to ASD that can be quickly measured in large samples (Hyman 2010). Finally, as a field, we should take care to avoid a "biology over all" approach that could lead us to neglect the aspects of development and behavior that limit the lives of children and adults with ASD right now and into the future.

On the opposite end of the spectrum from dimensions (although with complementary goals and combined utility), the ability to create meaningful subtypes within the autism spectrum may be another advantage to the new *DSM-5* criteria. Evidence suggests that cognitive deficits within ASD may be more common in females (Dworzynski et al. 2012; Nicholas et al. 2008; Szatmari et al. 1989; Wing 1981), in individuals with known genetic abnormalities (Herman et al. 2007; Muhle et al. 2004), and in those with dysmorphic physical characteristics (Miles et al. 2005), suggesting the possible existence of subgroups with unique etiologies or risk factors (Grzadzinski et al. 2013). Similarly, neurobiological evidence suggests that individuals with both ASD and language impairment show patterns of structural brain abnormalities in the core

language areas of the brain that are more similar to individuals with specific language impairment (SLI; without ASD) over those individuals with ASD who do not have language impairment (De Fossé et al. 2004), hinting at another potential etiological subtype of ASD. Research has demonstrated the utility of subgrouping within ASD based on specific social communication profiles (Ingram et al. 2008), though many subtyping efforts based on existing measures of ASD (notably, most of which are based on *DSM-IV* criteria) have failed to identify distinct subtypes. In an effort to increase the specificity of the diagnostic criteria, *DSM-5* identifies both core diagnostic symptoms and critical non-ASD-specific characteristics that vary within ASD populations. Taken together, the revisions encourage researchers to take a dimensional approach to "carving up" the heterogeneous autism phenotype, similar to approaches that have been used in population samples (Dworzynski et al. 2009; Grzadzinski et al. 2013). Perhaps with revisions to symptom measures based on *DSM-5* criteria, additional dimensions will emerge from which ASD subtypes for future study will be created.

Responses to Notable Concerns about *DSM-5* Changes

One of the earliest and enduring concerns about the changes associated with *DSM-5* has to do with the omission of the Asperger's disorder label. Many individuals with previous autism spectrum diagnoses, particularly cognitively able adolescents and adults, have used "Asperger's syndrome" (AS) as a rallying point both for self-exploration and identity and to find and forge relationships with others of similar interests, insights, and obstacles. These individuals and their families often view AS as less stigmatized and stigmatizing than labels that include the term "autism," while viewing AS as more circumscribed and politically or personally compelling than PDD-NOS. With the early drafts of the *DSM-5*, came a strong backlash against the loss of this label and the perceived dignity and identity that came with it. This was not the intention of the *DSM-5* workgroup. In addition to paving the way for a dimensional spectrum rather than a multicategorical model, the decision to omit Asperger's disorder from the *DSM-5* was based on more than a decade of research findings that failed to identify consistent behavioral or biological features that separated autism and AS. Further, and most importantly, the goal of the new criteria was to increase equity across the *DSM-IV* subcategories in terms of treatment coverage by third-party payers, most commonly, insurance companies and school districts, many of which covered services under diagnoses of autistic disorder but not AS and PDD-NOS. We hope, as does the *DSM-5* workgroup, that a single, broad ASD category in fact will open doors previously closed to certain individuals with ASD. Overall, it is important to bear in mind that the DSM is a manual for psychiatric and thus medical use; individuals and advocacy organizations alike can continue to use any term they see as beneficial or preferred for other purposes.

A second and more general concern about how to improve upon *DSM-IV* was the need for autism spectrum criteria to address a wide range of behaviors within the context of very different developmental levels. In response, *DSM-5* ASD criteria are designed to address the need for breadth by describing principles that define each subdomain (e.g., integration of verbal and nonverbal communication, social reciprocity, relationships, and adjusting to social contexts) and then providing examples that represent different ages and levels of development to represent these principles. This approach has created some confusion leading up to the *DSM-5* release: Data corresponding to the many possible examples often simply were not available within existing datasets, limiting attempts to match data from other frameworks onto the new criteria (Mattila et al. 2011; McPartland et al. 2012). This has been interpreted to mean that individuals would no longer receive diagnoses of ASD under *DSM-5*; however, this is not the intention and should not be the case, if clinicians use the new criteria appropriately. The expectation is that, when *DSM-5* criteria are used as intended, there would be no need for children and adults with existing ASD diagnoses to have to be re-diagnosed, given the

expected comparability of the inclusiveness of the former and new systems (Lord and Jones 2012). As an added safeguard, it is specifically stated in the manual that individuals with "well-established" *DSM-IV* ASD diagnoses qualify for a *DSM-5* ASD diagnosis by virtue of their previous diagnosis alone (American Psychiatric Association 2013).

An issue closely related to mapping previously collected data onto new diagnoses of ASD is the highly politicized question about whether *DSM-5* criteria will significantly alter ASD prevalence rates (Carey 2012; McPartland et al. 2012). A 2012 study by McPartland and colleagues used data archived from a field trial study for the *DSM-IV* to model sensitivity and specificity of *DSM-5* draft criteria, and thus estimated prevalence under the new set of criteria. Their findings, including sensitivity of 25 % in the subsample with Asperger's disorder, were met with professional and public outcry alike. A commentary by the *DSM-5* workgroup pointed out, however, that the purpose of the field trials (from which the McPartland et al. data arose) was to determine the comparability of *DSM-III-R* and *DSM-IV* criteria and not to assess the sensitivity of the (then) newly proposed *DSM-IV* criteria for identifying cases in the population. In fact, as the workgroup noted, "it was not possible to use the data to measure sensitivity when first collected two decades ago and it is not possible to do so now" (Swedo et al. 2012, p. 347). Further, because the original field trial was focused on comparing *DSM-III-R* and *DSM-IV* diagnostic criteria for PDD subcategories, it did not collect the information necessary to evaluate the specific criteria proposed for the *DSM-5* (Swedo et al. 2012). This points to the primary reason that archival datasets, particularly brief questionnaires or registries based on similar approaches, cannot adequately answer prevalence questions: A major strategy underpinning the *DSM-5* criteria, as noted above, is to expand both the possible examples with which to define each subdomain, as well as the range of nonoverlapping subdomains, beyond *DSM-IV* and *ICD-10* (Lord and Jones 2012). Therefore, existing datasets are very unlikely to contain these examples unless they include very comprehensive, systematic assessments (see Mandy et al. 2012; Huerta et al. 2012). In those groups that looked at more extensive, standardized types of data, the *DSM-5* has been found to exhibit increased validity over *DSM-IV* in representing the structure of ASD symptoms (Mandy et al. 2012), and to have increased specificity over *DSM-IV* with negligible loss of sensitivity (Huerta et al. 2012).

One specific concern related to prevalence rates is that *DSM-5* sensitivity would be lower as a result of requiring the presence of RRB symptoms for diagnosis (unlike PDD-NOS criteria in *DSM-IV*). In a 2012 study subsequent to McPartland's, Huerta and colleagues mapped symptoms from a comprehensive parent interview and a clinician observation onto *DSM-5* criteria and assessed the association between this proxy *DSM-5* diagnosis and best estimate clinical diagnoses made under *DSM-IV*. In post hoc examinations of why some children with PDDs did not meet *DSM-5* criteria in their combined dataset of 4,453 children aged 2–17 years, Huerta et al. reported that most children who did not meet the overall criteria for ASD in fact met the RRB criteria but showed subthreshold social and communication impairments. This may be because the third social criterion, involving relationships and adjusting to social contexts, requires broader information, particularly for more able adolescents and adults, than is available in most child-focused diagnostic screeners or interviews. This is also likely to be an issue for the next few years of Center for Disease Control (CDC) surveillance data, because their findings depend on extraction from records that are likely not to have this information available. With regard to the new RRB criteria, however, Huerta and colleagues interpreted their results to suggest that few children with ASD are likely to be misclassified as having social communication disorder by virtue of absent repetitive behaviors.

Overall, the *DSM-5* workgroup endeavored to be responsive to data analysis and theoretical commentary ongoing during *DSM-5* drafting, in terms of both number of specific criteria required (e.g., Frazier et al. 2012), content around criteria, and onset requirements (e.g., Huerta et al. 2012; Mattila et al. 2011), and additions to explanatory text (Wing et al. 2011). At this time, ASD

prevalence rates based on thorough clinical evaluations using *DSM-5* criteria are not yet known. However, in the *DSM-5* workgroup commentary on potentially altered prevalence under the new criteria, the authors emphasize that the *DSM-5* workgroup was charged with revising criteria to be more sensitive to ASD in younger and older individuals (whereas the *DSM-IV* showed good performance validity with school-aged children in particular), girls and women, and racial and ethnic minorities (Swedo et al. 2012). To treat prevalence rates based on *DSM-IV* criteria as a "gold standard" against which to judge *DSM-5*-associated prevalence rates represents a bias that should be recognized. Ultimately, prevalence rates of ASD have continued to increase under the *DSM-IV*; to understand these increases in prevalence, it is critical to know if they are due to recognition of more mild cases or to increased numbers of all types of cases. Given the confusion among *DSM-IV* subcategories (autistic disorder, Asperger's disorder, PDD-NOS), such patterns are difficult to discern (Bertrand et al. 2001; Lord and Jones 2012). It is our expectation that *DSM-5* will lead to negligible changes in prevalence estimates, with improved validity where prevalence does differ from *DSM-IV*.

We discussed the advantages of a dimensional approach in *DSM-5* criteria previously. Another controversy around the *DSM-5* stemmed from suggestions that neurobiology and dimensions of behavior should be emphasized over DSM criteria and categories altogether. One proposed method for doing so is the Research Domains Criteria initiative (RDoC; National Institute of Mental Health 2013a), which enumerates several dimensional constructs for study, and methods by which these dimensions must be explicated (for example, from genes, through circuits, physiology, behavior to "paradigms"; see National Institute of Mental Health 2013a for more information). RDoC has been referred to as a "taxonomy for mental health disorders" in publications from the National Institute of Health (National Institute of Mental Health 2013b), leading some to view this system as an alternative to *DSM-5*. This is not the case. In short, neurobiological disorders do not match up with behavior adequately at this point to involve them directly in nosology. Approaches such as RDoC may yield valuable information in the long run about links between biology and behaviors that cross diagnoses. However, particularly for ASD, where the reliability and prognostic validity of standardized diagnoses are well established, RDoC dimensions will not provide the same practical or even empirical information as an ASD diagnosis accompanied by information about other key factors (e.g., language level, intelligence, comorbid features; Haslam et al. 2012). At this stage in history, we must continue to document behavior, look for patterns that group behaviors into syndromes, and then document genetic and neurobiological conditions that are associated with these syndromes.

Biological research consistently yields examples of multifinality (one "cause" leading to multiple outcomes) and equifinality (multiple "causes" leading to the same outcome). Not only are many different genetic patterns associated with autism (Veenstra-VanderWeele et al. 2004), but many of these same patterns are also associated with numerous other psychological and psychiatric disorders (Guilmatre et al. 2009; Lord and Jones 2012). Similarly, imaging and other neurobiological approaches seldom provide data on an individual level, do not yet have well-accepted standards for replicability across time or site (Lotspeich et al. 2004), and have rarely addressed questions of the specificity of findings to ASD as opposed to other psychiatric or developmental disorders (Lord and Jones 2012). Thus, genetic and other biological descriptions are an important basis for future research but are in no way a replacement for a behavioral diagnosis, as their links to autism are not unique or universal (Walsh and Bracken 2011). To access the information typically associated with a diagnosis (e.g., course, response to treatment, risk factors, associated conditions), we must return to behavior (Charman et al. 2011; Shattuck et al. 2009).

As an additional caveat, by breaking behavior apart into too finely descriptive dimensions, it is easy to lose *patterns*. In other words, a child who presents with several descriptive qualifiers (e.g., sensory avoidance, receptive language delay, unusual gait, poor social skills) but no primary diagnosis (when ASD would explain many of those

qualifiers) loses a crucial chance at informed treatment and prognosis. The child's family also loses an orienting foundation for understanding the needs of the child and other relevant data, such as genetic risk to future children. At this point in history, RDoC or similar dimension-only rubrics can function as a useful research framework and a strategic plan (National Institute of Mental Health 2013a); however, we must continue to link (i.e., lump) behaviors in addition to pulling things apart (i.e., splitting) for practical reasons that impact research as well as clinical considerations.

SCD, the new category marked by social deficits not associated with a more well-established categorical disorder, is likely the current aspect of *DSM-5* ASD-related classification that is most similar to the RDoC approach (and as such, may prove to be representative of its strengths and weaknesses; H. Tager-Flusberg, personal communication, May 29, 2013). At this point in time, minimal evidence exists for SCD as a valid, stand-alone syndrome. This category is intended to describe individuals who have significant social and communication difficulties similar to those in ASD but without repetitive or restricted behaviors. Language impairments overlap with ASD behaviorally and by neural circuitry and genetics (Bishop 2010; De Fossé et al. 2004; Pickles et al. 2013). It is possible that individuals diagnosed with SCD under *DSM-5* will have a history of either or both SLI or repetitive behaviors that are no longer in evidence at the time of assessment (and about which the clinician does not inquire sufficiently). A particular concern is the use of SCD as a tentative diagnosis in situations when no one wants to bring up ASD or when a speech and language pathologist or educational practitioner is uncomfortable making a "psychiatric" diagnosis. The potential exists for this category to become the confusing and potentially over-diagnosed successor of PDD-NOS.

Collectively, these are valid concerns, and they reflect the phenomenon we have seen under the *DSM-IV*, in which lack of psychometrically valid categories leads to the same individual getting two distinct diagnoses from separate assessments by two different clinicians with discrepant skills and biases (Lord et al. 2012). In truth, the number of individuals who will fall into the SCD category is not clear. SCD is similar to what Dorothy Bishop described many years ago as semantic–pragmatic disorder (Bishop 1989), with more explicit ruling out of children who meet the new ASD criteria (Lord and Jones 2012). No data are yet available about its reliability or prevalence, though some initial reports have supported its validity with limited data (Gibson et al. 2013; Greaves-Lord et al. 2013). This is the aspect of *DSM-5* ASD-related classification around which there is the most disagreement and the least amount of useful data from standardized measures. However, as important as psychometrically valid categories are, the process of drafting *DSM-5* criteria involved a give-and-take between empirical evidence (e.g., such as that which led to the removal of Asperger's disorder and PDD-NOS) and public health ramifications (e.g., striving to avoid leaving a subset of people, who would have qualified for *DSM-IV* PDD-NOS without a diagnosis under *DSM-5*).

Overall, *DSM-5* revisions do not reflect a strictly scientific process, but rather the intersection between empiricism and scientific decision making (e.g., do we have valid dimensions?) and political and practical decision making (e.g., who will get left out and how can we circumvent that?). In terms of avoiding the recreation of ambiguous PDD-NOS diagnoses, *DSM-5* text emphasizes the need to rule out ASD first. Unfortunately, some diagnosticians may see this new, unknown disorder as less stigmatizing and prefer it, thus failing to adequately ask about or observe potential RRBs and/or other features of ASD, either by history or by current presentation. If this diagnosis remains in the DSM system, we will need instruments that differentiate it from ASD, Attention deficit hyperactivity disorder (ADHD), and related disorders in order to establish reliability of SCD diagnosis across practitioners.

Future Directions for ASD Research Under *DSM-5*

We are in an exciting period of ASD research, standing as we are at the precipice of a new, more dimensional nosology. The future directions are

myriad not only for ongoing research into the neurobiological and genetic makeup of ASD and effective treatments across ages and symptom profiles but also for research more directly applicable to the reliability, validity, and prevalence estimates associated with the *DSM-5* conceptualization of ASD. At this point, one of the most crucial future directions bridging these research areas is the need for quantitative measures that accurately map *DSM-5* and other ASD-related dimensions, independent of developmental factors such as age, language level, and IQ. Such new or revised measures may have particular value in increasing cohesion of global autism research under *DSM-5* and *ICD-11* (scheduled for 2015 release); though revisions to both classification systems are intended to complement the other, the *ICD-11* is guided by somewhat different priorities, concerns, and questions (World Health Organization 2013).

Clearly, prevalence estimates of the *DSM-5* are an important proximal research question. As discussed above, leading up to the release of the *DSM-5* in May 2013, prevalence estimates of the new criteria were based on *DSM-IV* questions used to classify via *DSM-5* criteria, which consequently gave a skewed view of sensitivity under the new criteria. Soon we will begin to hear reports on the sensitivity and specificity associated with the developmentally flexible, example-based *DSM-5* criteria as it is applied to new data. We emphasize that using *DSM-IV* as if it were a true gold standard comparison with regard to prevalence estimates is not appropriate given evidence that specificity of *DSM-IV* (especially for PDD-NOS) was not good. The *DSM-5* appears to have improved but still with moderate specificity (Huerta et al. 2012), in which case borderline cases may continue to receive ASD classification. In other words, in terms of balancing over- and under-identification, *DSM-5* criteria seem more likely to classify children without ASD as having ASD rather than excluding children who truly have ASD. In addition, because both symptom domains are codable based on history in *DSM-5,* specificity is not likely to improve vastly from *DSM-IV*. However, for the same reason, sensitivity of the *DSM-5* should be very high when there is adequate current and historical information (this is another example of information that was not available in *DSM-IV* datasets based on review of medical and educational records). There is clearly much room for improvement with respect to specificity, which likely will be a goal of *DSM-5.1* and beyond. In the meantime, there is a great deal to learn about the field performance of the *DSM-5,* and a National Institute of Health interagency workgroup will be among the first reporting on this as early as July 2013.

We hope that dimensions will be useful for future research, particularly with regard to understanding the pathways to social deficits. Social behavior, typical or impaired, is so complex that it likely needs to be represented as more fine-grained dimensions before it can be linked successfully to neurobiological mechanisms. RDoC and similar dimensional research endeavors share a hope of someday being able to identify risk factors (likely in the form of biomarkers) so that we can essentially "diagnose" future autism before behavioral symptoms become manifest, and thus intervene before the syndrome goes on to develop. At this time, however, our multidisciplinary field understands relatively little about the pathophysiology underlying the autism spectrum. It is clearly a neurodevelopmental disorder, but it is not clear exactly what is developing abnormally in the brain on a molecular, cellular, or systems level. Thus, while it holds great promise, neurobiological research has had little direct bearing on our understanding of what ASD is or how to treat it. Examples of gains in neurobiological understanding within other research fields, and the outcome of those gains to this point, give us both reasons for optimism (e.g., cancer) as well as skepticism (Huntington's disease, Down syndrome, steps to get from MECP2 to treatment). An immediate approach would be to attempt to better delineate meaningful behavioral dimensions that can serve as indicators of the need for different services and of response to treatments, as well as risk for associated problems. Behavioral dimensions may also become the indicators of how neurobiological changes occur, how they are intermeshed, and how developmental pathways might be modified or built upon (Cicchetti

et al. 2011; Rutter and Sroufe 2000). This approach would involve reconsidering the meaning of the complex findings from genetics and to some degree, from neuroscience, based on categorical conceptions of ASD and very broad dimensions. Over time, hopefully, we can enrich future versions of the DSM with more subgroup specifiers pertaining to biology and genetics. SCD may come to be seen as a dimension that cuts across, for example, autism, schizophrenic and depressive spectra, rather than a stand-alone category. These goals require more attention to the specificity of behaviors associated with ASD, and when nonspecific dimensions are of interest, their interactions with core features (Lord and Jones 2012). This calls for continued research that, as proposed for RDoC, includes several categorical disorders (e.g., ASD, ADHD, anxiety) within a single study to identify both commonalities and differences.

Again, subtyping from dimensions is another important future direction in ASD research. The medical community is turning to "precision medicine" by asking, for example, what distinguishes cancer patients from each other, and studying those factors as keys to successful intervention within subgroups. In the *DSM-5*, the core diagnosis of ASD can be accompanied by specifiers (in essence, lumping and splitting at the same time), including additional diagnoses such as ADHD. Ideally, these new diagnoses will reflect individual patterns that clinicians previously noted but which were not explicitly documented in the past. This may provide a more successful way to characterize individuals that group together in meaningful ways. ADHD, as well as anxiety and several other associated diagnoses/specifiers, receive specific acknowledgment in the *DSM-5* text for their dual-diagnosis prevalence with ASD. This fits into the dimensional view of comorbidities emphasized in the *DSM-5* and may be helpful in reorienting collection of research samples for study of shared mechanisms.

Quite obviously, there is room for all comers: categories, subtypes within categories, and dimensions within ASD research, and in fact, the artful combination of all three may be the key to groundbreaking discoveries in etiology and intervention. As discussed by Lord and Jones (2012), arguing for the exclusive use of either categories or dimensions creates a false dichotomy: Rather than contrasting categories versus dimensions, we might more usefully ask, for what purposes do we define and measure dimensions: To more accurately describe, predict, and be able to change behavior? Or, to link with neurobiological findings? And what are the relationships among diagnostic descriptions (often reflecting different behaviors or behavioral categories), dimensions, and categories such as disorders? Without a doubt, there is much to be gained from fine-grained analyses of behavior patterns that are reliably manifest across time in at least some subsets of individuals with ASD and are either independent or that interact in a predictable fashion with intelligence and language level. At the same time, more efficient clinical measures of severity, ideally within dimensions, are also needed, particularly for studying the boundaries of ASD.

In summary, the *DSM-5* attempts to improve description of the core features of ASD and other dimensions that interact with them, and to provide more valid and reliable ways to quantify these features both for research and clinical purposes. Additional research with these goals in mind, as well as field testing of *DSM-5* and *ICD-11* and the development of finer measures of ASD dimensions, will advance both practice and science with regard to the autism spectrum.

References

American Psychiatric Association. (1952). *Diagnostic and statistical manual of mental disorders* (1st ed.). Washington, DC: American Psychiatric Association.

American Psychiatric Association. (1980). *Diagnostic and statistical manual of mental disorders* (3rd ed.). Washington, DC: American Psychiatric Association.

American Psychiatric Association. (1987). *Diagnostic and statistical manual of mental disorders* (3rd ed., rev.). Washington, DC: American Psychiatric Association.

American Psychiatric Association. (2000). *Diagnostic and statistical manual of mental disorders* (4th ed., text rev.). Washington, DC: American Psychiatric Association.

American Psychiatric Association. (2013). *Diagnostic and statistical manual of mental disorders* (5th ed.). Washington, DC: American Psychiatric Association.

Baron-Cohen, S., Leslie, A. M., & Frith, U. (1985). Does the autistic child have a "theory of mind"? *Cognition, 21*(1), 37–46.

Ben-Sasson, A., Hen, L., Fluss, R., Cermak, S., Engle-Yeger, B., & Gal, E. (2009). A meta-analysis of sensory modulation symptoms in individuals with autism spectrum disorders. *Journal of Autism and Developmental Disorders, 39*(1), 1–11.

Bertrand, J., Mars, A., Boyle, C., Bove, F., Yeargin-Allsopp, M., & Decoufle, P. (2001). Prevalence of autism in a United States population: The Brick Township, New Jersey, investigation. *Pediatrics, 108*(5), 1155–1161.

Billstedt, E., Gillberg, I. C., & Gillberg, C. (2007). Autism in adults: Symptom patterns and early childhood predictors. Use of the DISCO in a community sample followed from childhood. *Journal of Child Psychology and Psychiatry, 48*(11), 1102–1110.

Bishop, D. V. (1989). Autism, Asperger's syndrome and sematic-pragmatic disorder: Where are the boundaries? *The British International Journal of Language and Disorders of Communication Disorders, 24*(2), 107–121.

Bishop, D. V. M. (2010). Overlaps between autism and language impairment: Phenomimicry or shared etiology? *Behavioral Genetics, 40*, 618–629.

Bishop, S., Gahagan, S., & Lord, C. (2007). Re-examining the core features of autism: A comparison of autism spectrum disorder and fetal alcohol spectrum disorder. *Journal of Child Psychology and Psychiatry, 48*(11), 1111–1121.

Bowler, D. M. (1992). "Theory of mind" in Asperger's Syndrome. *Journal of Child Psychology and Psychiatry, 33*(5), 877–893.

Carey, B. (2012). New definition of autism may exclude many, study suggests. *The New York Times*, A1.

Charman, T., Jones, C. R. G., Pickles, A., Simonoff, E., Baird, G., & Happe, F. (2011). Defining the cognitive phenotype of autism. *Brain Research, 1380*, 10–21.

Cicchetti, D. V., Koenig, K., Klin, A., Volkmar, F. R., Paul, R., & Sparrow, S. (2011). From Bayes through marginal utility to effect sizes: A guide to understanding the clinical and statistical significance of the results of autism research findings. *Journal of Autism and Developmental Disorders, 41*(2), 168–174.

Constantino, J. N., Gruber, C. P., Davis, S., Hayes, S., Passanante, N., & Przybeck, T. (2004). The factor structure of autistic traits. *Journal of Child Psychology and Psychiatry, 45*(4), 719–726.

Dawson, G., Webb, S. J., & McPartland, J. (2005). Understanding the nature of the face processing impairment in autism: Insights from behavioral and electrophysiological studies. *Developmental Neuropsychology, 27*(3), 403–424.

De Fossé, L., Hodge, S. M., Makris, N., Kennedy, D. N., Caviness, V. S., McGrath, L., et al. (2004). Language-association cortex asymmetry in autism and specific language impairment. *Annals of Neurology, 56*(6), 757–766.

Dworzynski, K., Happé, F., Bolton, P., & Ronald, A. (2009). Relationship between symptom domains in autism spectrum disorders: A population based twin study. *Journal of Autism and Developmental Disorders, 39,* 1197–1210.

Dworzynski, K., Ronald, A., Bolton, P., & Happé, F. (2012). How different are girls and boys above and below the diagnostic threshold for autism spectrum disorders? *Journal of the American Academy of Child and Adolescent Psychiatry, 51,* 788–797.

Fombonne, E. (2002). Prevalence of childhood disintegrative disorder. *Autism: The International Journal of Research and Practice, 6*(2), 149–157.

Frazier, T. W., Youngstrom, E. A., Kubu, C. S., Sinclaire, L., & Rezai, A. (2008). Exploratory and confirmatory factor analysis of the autism diagnostic interview-revised. *Journal of Autism and Developmental Disorders, 38*(3), 474–480.

Frazier, T. W., Youngstrom, E. A., Speer, L., Embacher, R., Law, P., Constantino, J., et al. (2012). Validation of proposed *DSM-5* criteria for autism spectrum disorder. *Journal of the American Academy of Child & Adolescent Psychiatry, 51*(1), 28–40.

Gibson, K., Adams, C., Lockton, E., & Green, J. (2013). Social communication disorder outside autism? A diagnostic classification approach to delineating pragmatic language impairment, high functioning autism and specific language impairment. *Journal of Child Psychology and Psychiatry, 54*(11), 1186–1197. (Electronic publication ahead of print).

Gillespie-Lynch, K., Sepeta, L., Wang, Y., Marshall, S., Gomez, L., Sigman, M., & Hutman, T. (2012). Early childhood predictors of the social competence of adults with autism. *Journal of Autism and Developmental Disorders, 42*(2), 161–174.

Gotham, K., Risi, S., Dawson, G., Tager-Flusberg, H., Joseph, R., Carter, A., et al. (2008). A replication of the autism diagnostic observation schedule (ADOS) revised algorithms. *Journal of the American Academy of Child and Adolescent Psychiatry, 47*(6), 642–651.

Greaves-Lord, K., Eussen, M. L., Verhulst, F., Minderaa, R., Mandy, W., Hudziak, J., et al. (2013). Empirically based phenotypic profiles of children with pervasive developmental disorders: Interpretation in the light of the *DSM-5*. *Journal of Autism and Developmental Disorders, 43*(8), 1784–1797.

Grzadzinski, R., Huerta, M., & Lord, C. (2013). *DSM-5* and autism spectrum disorders (ASD): An opportunity for identifying ASD subtypes. *Molecular Autism, 4*(1), 1–6. doi:10.1186/2040-2392-4-12.

Guilmatre, A., Dubourg, C., Mosca, A. L., Legallic, S., Goldenberg, A., Drouin-Garraud, V., & Campion, D. (2009). Recurrent rearrangements in synaptic and neurodevelopmental genes and shared biologic pathways in schizophrenia, autism, and mental retardation. *Archives of General Psychiatry, 66*(9), 947–956.

Happe, F. (2011). Why fold Asperger syndrome into autism spectrum disorder in the DSM-5? Simons Foundation Autism Research Initiative News and Opinion. http://sfari.org/news-and-opinion/viewpoint/2011/why-fold-asperger-syndrome-into-autism-spectrum-disorder-in-the-dsm-5. Accessed 29 June 2013.

Hartley, S. L., & Sikora, D. M. (2010). Detecting autism spectrum disorder in children with intellectual disability: Which *DSM-IV-TR* criteria are most useful? *Focus on Autism and Other Developmental Disabilities, 25*(2), 85–97.

Haslam, N., Holland, E., & Kuppens, P. (2012). Categories versus dimensions in personality and psychopathology: A quantitative review of taxometric research. *Psychological Medicine, 42*(5), 903.

Herman, G. E., Butter, E., Enrile, B., Pastore, M., Prior, T. W., & Sommer, A. (2007). Increasing knowledge of PTEN germline mutations: Two additional patients with autism and macrocephaly. *American Journal of Medical Genetics Part A, 143A*(6), 589–593.

Herold, R., Tenyi, T., Lenard, K., & Trixler, M. (2002). Theory of mind deficit in people with schizophrenia during remission. *Psychological Medicine, 32*(06), 1125–1129.

Huerta, M., Bishop, S. L., Duncan, A., Hus, V., & Lord, C. (2012). Application of *DSM-5* criteria for autism spectrum disorder to three samples of children with *DSM-IV* diagnoses of pervasive developmental disorders. *American Journal of Psychiatry, 169*(10), 1056–1064.

Hus, V., Taylor, A., & Lord, C. (2011). Telescoping of caregiver report on the autism diagnostic interview-revised. *Journal of Child Psychology and Psychiatry, 52*(7), 753–760.

Hyman, S. E. (2010). The diagnosis of mental disorders: The problem of reification. *Annual Review of Clinical Psychology, 6,* 155–179.

Ingram, D., Takahashi, T. N., & Miles, J. (2008). Defining autism subgroups: A taxometric solution. *Journal of Autism and Developmental Disorders, 38*(5), 950–960.

Juranek, J., Filipek, P. A., Berenji, G. R., Modahl, C., Osann, K., & Spence, M. A. (2006). Association between amygdala volume and anxiety level: Magnetic resonance imaging (MRI) study in autistic children. *Journal of Child Neurology, 21*(12), 1051–1058.

Kleinhans, N. M., Richards, T., Weaver, K., Johnson, L. C., Greenson, J., Dawson, G., & Aylward, E. (2010). Association between amygdala response to emotional faces and social anxiety in autism spectrum disorders. *Neuropsychologia, 48*(12), 3665–3670.

Klin, A., Saulnier, C. A., Sparrow, S. S., Cicchetti, D. V., Volkmar, F. R., & Lord, C. (2007). Social and communication abilities and disabilities in higher functioning individuals with autism spectrum disorders: The Vineland and the ADOS. *Journal of Autism and Developmental Disorders, 37*(4), 748–759.

Leekham, S. R., Nieto, C., Libby, S. J., Wing, L., & Gould, J. (2007). Describing the sensory abnormalities of children and adults with autism. *Journal of Autism and Developmental Disorders, 37*(5), 894–910.

Lord, C., & Jones, R. M. (2012). Annual research review: Re-thinking the classification of autism spectrum disorders. *Journal of the American Academy of Child and Adolescent Psychiatry, 53*(5), 490–509.

Lord, C., Risi, S., Lambrecht, L., Cook Jr, E. H., Leventhal, B. L., DiLavore, P. C., & Rutter, M. (2000). The Autism Diagnostic Observation Schedule—Generic: A standard measure of social and communication deficits associated with the spectrum of autism. *Journal of autism and developmental disorders, 30*(3), 205–223.

Lord, C., Petkova, E., Hus, V., Gan, W., Lu, F., Martin, D. M., et al. (2012). A multisite study of the clinical diagnosis of different autism spectrum disorders. *Archives of General Psychology, 69*(3), 306–313.

Lotspeich, L. J., Kwon, H., Schumann, C. M., Fryer, S. L., Goodlin-Jones, B. L., Buonocore, M. H., et al. (2004). Investigation of neuroanatomical differences between autism and Asperger syndrome. *Archives of General Psychiatry, 61*(3), 291–298.

Mandy, W. P., Charman, T., & Skuse, D. H. (2012). Testing the construct validity of proposed for *DSM-5* autism spectrum disorder. *Journal of the American Academy of Child and Adolescent Psychiatry, 51*(1), 41–50.

Matson, J., & Neale, D. (2010). Differentiating communication disorders and autism in children. *Research in Autism Spectrum Disorders, 4*(4), 626–632.

Mattila, M. L., Kielinen, M., Linna, S. L., Jussila, K., Ebeling, H., Bloigu, R., et al. (2011). Autism spectrum disorders according to *DSM-IV-TR* and comparison with *DSM-5* draft criteria: An epidemiological study. *Journal of the American Academy of Child and Adolescent Psychiatry, 50*(6), 583–592.

McMahon, F. J., & Insel, T. R. (2012). Pharmacogenomics and personalized medicine in neuropsychiatry. *Neuron, 74*(5), 773–776.

McPartland, J. C., Reichow, B., & Volkmar, F. R. (2012). Sensitivity and specificity of proposed *DSM-5* diagnostic criteria for autism spectrum disorder. *Journal of the American Academy of Child and Adolescent Psychiatry, 51*(4), 368–383.

Miles, J. H., Takahashi, T. N., Bagby, S., Sahota, P. K., Vaslow, D. F., Wang, C. H., et al. (2005). Essential versus complex autism: Definition of fundamental prognostic subtypes. *American Journal of Medical Genetics, Part A, 135*(2), 171–180.

Miller, J. N., & Ozonoff, S. (2000). The external validity of Asperger disorder: Lack of evidence from the domain of neuropsychology. *Journal of Abnormal Psychology, 109*(2), 227–238.

Muhle, R., Trentacoste, S. V., & Rapin, I. (2004). The genetics of autism. *Pediatrics, 113*(5), e472–e486.

Mundy, P., Sigman, M., & Kasari, C. (1990). A longitudinal study of the joint attention and language development in autistic children. *Journal of Autism and Developmental Disorders, 20*(1), 115–128.

National Institute of Mental Health. (2013a). NIMH research domain criteria (RDoC), Draft 3.1, June 2011. http://www.nimh.nih.gov/research-priorities/rdoc/nimh-research-domain-criteria-rdoc.shtml. Accessed 25 June 2013.

National Institute of Mental Health. (2013b). *DSM-5* and RDoC: Shared interests, a press release. http://www.nimh.nih.gov/news/science-news/2013/dsm-5-and-rdoc-shared-interests.shtml. Accessed 25 June 2013.

Nicholas, J. S., Charles, J. M., Carpenter, L. A., King, L. B., Jenner, W., & Spratt, E. G. (2008). Prevalence and characteristics of children with autism-spectrum disorders. *Annals of Epidemiology, 18*(20), 130–136.

Pelphrey, K. A., Shultz, S., Hudac, C. M., & Vander Wyk, B. C. (2011). Research review: Constraining heterogeneity: The social brain and its development in autism spectrum disorder. *Journal of the American Academy of Child and Adolescent Psychiatry, 52*(6), 631–644.

Pickles, A., & Angold, A. (2003). Natural categories or fundamental dimensions: On carving nature at the joints and the rearticulation of psychopathology. *Development and Psychopathology, 15*(3), 529–551.

Pickles, A., St. Clair, M., & Conti-Ramsden, G. (2013). Communication and social deficits in relatives of individuals with SLI and relatives of individuals with ASD. *Journal of Autism and Developmental Disorders, 43*(1), 156–167.

Robertson, T. J. M., Tanguay, P. E., L'Ecuyer, S., Sims, A., & Waltrip, C. (1999). Domains of social communication handicap in autism spectrum disorder. *Journal of the American Academy of Child and Adolescent Psychiatry, 38*(6), 738–745.

Ronald, A., Larsson, H., Anckarsater, H., & Lichtenstein, P. (2011). A twin study of autism symptoms in Sweden. *Molecular Psychiatry, 16*(10), 1039–1047.

Rutter, M., & Sroufe, L. A. (2000). Developmental psychopathology: Concepts and challenges. *Developmental Psychopathology, 12*(3), 264–296.

Sharma, S., Woolfson, L. M., & Hunter, S. C. (2012). Confusion and inconsistency in diagnosis of Asperger syndrome: A review of studies from 1981 to 2010. *Autism: The International Journal of Research and Practice, 16*(5), 465–486.

Shattuck, P. T., Durkin, M., Maenner, M., Newschaffer, C., Mandell, D. S., Wiggins, L., et al. (2009). Timing of identification among children with an autism spectrum disorder: Findings from a population-based surveillance study. *Journal of the American Academy of Child & Adolescent Psychiatry, 48*(5), 474–483.

Snow, A. V., & Lecavalier, L. (2008). Sensitivity and specificity of the modified checklist for autism in toddlers and the social communication questionnaire in preschoolers suspected of having pervasive developmental disorders. *Autism: The International Journal of Research and Practice, 12*(6), 627–644.

Solomon, M., Olsen, E., Niendam, T., Ragland, J. D., Yoon, J., Minzenberg, M., & Carter, C. S. (2011). From lumping to splitting and back again: Atypical social and language development in individuals with clinical-high-risk for psychosis, first episode schizophrenia, and autism spectrum disorders. *Schizophrenia Research, 131*(1), 146–151.

Swedo, S. E., Baird, G., Cook, E. H. Jr., Happé, F. G., Harris, J. C., Kaufmann, W. E., et al. (2012). Commentary from the *DSM-5* workgroup on neurodevelopmental disorders. *Journal of the American Academy of Child & Adolescent Psychiatry, 51*(4), 347–349.

Szatmari, P., Bartolucci, G., & Bremner, R. (1989). Asperger's syndrome and autism: Comparison of early history and outcome. *Developmental Medicine and Child Neurology, 31*(6), 709–720.

Tadevosyan-Leyfer, O., Dowd, M., Mankoski, R., Winklosky, B. R. I. A. N., Putnam, S. A. R. A., McGrath, L., et al. (2003). A principal components analysis of the autism diagnostic interview-revised. *Journal of the American Academy of Child & Adolescent Psychiatry, 42*(7), 864–872.

Tager-Flusberg, H. (29 May 2013). Live *DSM-5* discussion: A virtual roundtable featuring Thomas Insel, Catherine Lord, and Helen Tager-Flusberg. Hosted by the Simons Foundation Autism Research Initiative (SFARI). https://sfari.org/sfari-community/community-blog/2013/live-dsm-5-discussion. Accessed 16 July 2013.

Veenstra-Vander Weele, J., Christian, S. L., & Cook, E. H. Jr. (2004). Autism as a paradigmatic complex genetic disorder. *Annual Review of Genomics and Human Genetics, 5*, 379–405.

Volkmar, F. R., & Rutter, M. (1995). Childhood disintegrative disorder: Results of the *DSM-IV* autism field trial. *Journal of the American Academy of Child and Adolescent Psychiatry, 34*(8), 1092–1095.

Wakefield, J. C. (2013). *DSM-5*: An overview of changes and controversies. *Clinical Social Work Journal, 41*,1–16.

Walsh, K. M., & Bracken, M. B. (2011). Copy number variation in the dosage-sensitive 16p11.2 interval accounts for only a small proportion of autism incidence: A systematic review and meta-analysis. *Genetics in Medicine, 13*(5), 377–384.

Wiggins, L. D., Robins, D. L., Bakeman, R., & Adamson, L. B. (2009). Brief report: Sensory abnormalities as distinguishing symptoms of autism spectrum disorders in young children. *Journal of Autism and Developmental Disorders, 39*(7), 1087–1091.

Wing, L. (1981). Sex ratios in early childhood autism and related conditions. *Psychiatry Research, 5*(2), 129–137.

Wing, L., Gould, J., & Gillberg, C. (2011). Autism spectrum disorders in the *DSM-V*: Better or worse than the *DSM-IV*? *Research in Developmental Disabilities, 32*(2), 768–773.

World Health Organization. (2013). The international classification of diseases, 11th revision. ICD-11 announcement. http://www.who.int/classifications/icd/revision/en/. Accessed 25 June 2013.

Index

A
Anxiety 4, 11, 21–24, 32, 38, 47, 48, 54, 114, 139
  assessment 63–65
  disorders 31, 32, 34–37, 41, 42, 49, 61–63
  provoking situations 66
  sensitivity 37
  symptoms 38–41, 63, 64
Applied behavior analysis 8
Assessment 51, 55, 61, 62, 69, 77
  clinical 6
  diagnostic 7
  recommendations 110–112
  tools 110
Attention-Deficit/Hyperactivity Disorder
    (ADHD) 21, 25, 47, 49, 50, 51, 191, 235
  diagnosis of 235
Autism 3–5, 8–10, 81, 113, 132, 143, 161, 166,
    172
  spectrum 6, 10, 16, 17, 36, 42, 48, 52, 75, 125,
    171

B
Behavior 56, 66–68, 76, 123, 124, 127, 129, 175,
    203, 206
  adaptive 15, 20, 24
  and psychiatric problems 20–22
  direct observation of 160, 161
  interviews 157, 158
  negative 123
  positive 123
  repetitive 19, 81, 82, 92, 108, 109, 111, 114,
    131, 155, 205, 207
  ritualistic 76
  transdiagnostic 93
  treatment 162
Behavioral assessment 146, 156, 157, 166, 208
Behavior therapy *See* Cognitive behavior therapy
    (CBT) 24

C
Children 3, 4, 6, 9, 11, 16, 20, 24, 31, 32, 35, 39,
    53, 62
  anixiety-prone 38
  school-aged 18, 55, 83
Cognition 139, 206
  catastrophic 139
  negative 34
Cognitive-behavioral therapy (CBT) 24, 39, 40,
    41, 65–69, 112, 113, 131, 147, 162, 165,
    171–173, 180, 185, 192
  intervention 41, 42, 69, 180, 191, 195
Comorbidity 31, 35, 51, 76, 110, 114, 124, 141,
    142, 144, 148, 204, 235
  differential diagnosis and 123, 124
  rates 48, 55, 62, 68
Compulsions 32, 80, 82, 107–109, 111, 112, 114,
    115
Controversies 8, 9
Course 5, 18, 23, 31, 35, 37, 67, 110, 124, 219,
    237

D
Depressive disorders 47, 54, 55
Developmental levels 15
Developmental psychopathology 125
Diagnosis 3, 7, 15, 18, 23, 31, 63–65, 108,
    121–123, 237, 242
  comorbid 49
  dimensional approaches to 223, 224
  primary 41
  psychiatric 6, 218
Diagnostic and statistical manual (DSM) 20, 21,
    32, 63, 78, 80, 122, 139
Diagnostic and statistical manual (DSM)-5 32,
    36, 48, 50, 52–54, 56, 80, 84, 114, 115,
    132, 139, 142, 148, 149, 224–226, 231–
    233, 239
  strengths of 233–235

CPSIA information can be obtained at www.ICGtesting.com
Printed in the USA
LVOW03*0910021114

411655LV00003B/19/P